ERIN
Moore
626 441 -2007

Birth in the Age of AIDS

Birth in the Age of AIDS

Women, Reproduction, and HIV/AIDS in India

Cecilia Van Hollen

Stanford University Press
Stanford, California

For Lila and Jasper

Stanford University Press
Stanford, California

Printed in the United States of America on acid-free, archival-quality paper

Library of Congress Cataloging-in-Publication Data

Van Hollen, Cecilia Coale, author.
  Birth in the age of AIDS : women, reproduction, and HIV/AIDS in India / Cecilia Van Hollen.
    pages cm
  Includes bibliographical references and index.
  ISBN 978-0-8047-8422-1 (cloth : alk. paper) — ISBN 978-0-8047-8423-8 (pbk. : alk. paper)
  1. AIDS (Disease) in pregnancy—India. 2. Pregnant women—Services for—India. 3. HIV-positive women—Services for—India. 4. HIV infections—Transmission—India—Prevention.
5. AIDS (Disease)—Social aspects—India. 6. Childbirth—Social aspects—India. 7. Medical anthropology—India. I. Title.
  RG580.A44V36 2013
  362.19697'9200954—dc23
                                   2012040243

Typeset by Bruce Lundquist in 10/14 Minion

Contents

Acknowledgments

This book has been a project long in the making, and countless individuals and institutions have helped to make it possible. First and foremost, I would like to extend my heartfelt thanks to all the women living with HIV/AIDS and the pregnant women I met in maternity hospitals who agreed to participate in my research. I hope that this book accurately reflects their experiences, perspectives, and opinions and that the publication of this book will lead to improvements in policies and programs for the prevention and treatment of HIV/AIDS and the care of people living with HIV/AIDS in India and around the globe.

I am extremely grateful to the networks of people living with HIV/AIDS who let me participate in their activities. I have mentioned these organizations in the book, but I want, in particular, to thank the Positive Women's Network (PWN+), the Society for Positive Mothers Development (SPMD), and the HIV Ullor Nala Sangam (HUNS) network for their support and, above all, P. Kousalya, of PWN+, for allowing me to have a six-month affiliation with that network. Thanks also to R. Meenakski, of SPMD; Jeypaul of both the Indian Network for Positive People (INP+) and HUNS; Rama Pandian of the Tamil Nadu Network for Positive People (TNP+); and K. K. Abraham of INP+. I am also greatly indebted to Dr. P. Kuganantham, coordinator of the joint Tamil Nadu State AIDS Control Society (TNSACS)and the UNICEF Prevention of Parent to Child Transmission (PPTCT) program, for facilitating my research in government maternity hospitals in Chennai; Dr. Suniti Solomon and A. K. Srikrishnan, who made arrangements for my research at YRG Care; and Janaki Krishnan, who organized my research with the Zonta Resource Centre. Thanks also to all the counselors, lab technicians, doctors, and nurses in numerous hospitals throughout Tamil Nadu who participated in this research and allowed me to observe them at work with their patients. I would also like to thank the following individuals in India and the United States for giving me the time to interview them and for their valuable information and advice based on their expertise in the field of HIV/AIDS prevention and care in India: Bill Pick (United States Agency for International Development [USAID]); Christopher Castle and Ellen Weiss (Population Council); Dr. P. L. Joshi (National AIDS Control Organization [NACO]); Dr. Bitra George and Laura Kayser (Family Health International [FHI]); Drs. Bimal Charles and Devashish Dutta (AIDS Prevention and Control Project [APAC]); Supriya Sahu (Tamil Nadu Department of Health and Family Welfare); Mr. Dheenabandhu and Mr. Muruganandh (TNSACS); Dr. Srilata, Dr. Bir Singh, Tim Schaffter, Vidhya Ganesh, and Aruna Rathnam (UNICEF); Drs. P. Paramesh, S. Rajasekaran, and O. R. Krishnarajasekhar (Tambaram Hospital); Drs. R. Shoba and A. Sundaravalli (Institute for Obstetrics and Gynecology [IOG]); Jacob Varghese (Centers for Disease Control and Prevention [CDC]); Shyamala Natarajan (South Indian AIDS Action Programme [SIAAP]); Geeta Ramaseshan (Chennai High Court); T. A. Majeed (Fair Pharma); Vandhana Mahajan (United Nations Development Fund for Women [UNIFEM]); Dr. P. Manorama (Community Health Education Society [CHES]); and Magdalene Jeyarathnam (Health First).

This research would not have been possible without the hard work of S. Padmavathy, Beulah Rajakumari, Ms. Punitha, Jasmine Obeyesekere, and Sharon Watson, who have worked as research assistants on this project both in India and the United States, and Rajeswari Prabhakaran, Dr. Dasaratan, Sheela Chavan, and members of the YRG Care research team, who helped with the transcription and translation of recorded interviews. Thanks also to Haripriya Narasimhan for guidance on the English transliteration of Tamil words.

Many colleagues and graduate students have provided fruitful feedback on the book manuscript and on presentations of my research at numerous conferences. For this I would like to thank, in particular, Susan Wadley, Ann Gold, Maureen Schwarz, Patricia Whelehan, Lawrence Cohen, Stacy Pigg, Marcia Inhorn, Carolyn Sargent, Carole Browner, Aditya Bharadwaj, Jeremy Shiffman, Susan Erikson, Margaret Lock, Martha Selby, Melissa Pashigian, Barbara Koenig, Crista Craven, Lalit Narayan, Jocelyn Killmer, and Chen-I Kuan. I would also like to thank my editors at Stanford University Press, Stacy Wagner and Michelle Lipinski, as well as the anonymous reviewers of my manuscript for their constructive comments.

This research was made possible by the generous financial support from the following institutions: the Fulbright Foundation, the American Institute for Indian Studies, the University of Notre Dame, and Syracuse University.

Note on Statistics
and Transliteration

This book was written while I was on leave from teaching in 2009–2010. The statistics, therefore, reflect updated statistics at that time. Epidemiological statistics and statistics on public health programs are constantly changing, but I believe that the statistics included in this book from 2009–2010 accurately depict the current trends as of 2012, when the book manuscript went in to press.

I have chosen not to use diacritical marks for transliteration of non-English words to facilitate reading.

Abbreviations

AFASS	Affordability, Feasibility, Acceptability, Sustainability, Safety
APAC	AIDS Prevention and Control
ART	Antiretroviral therapy
CAPACS	Corporation AIDS Prevention and Control Society
CBO	Community-based organization
CDC	Centers for Disease Control and Prevention
CEDAW	Convention on the Elimination of All Forms of Discrimination Against Women
CHES	Community Health Education Society
CPK+	Council of People Living with HIV/AIDS in Kerala
GIPA	Greater Involvement of People Living with or Affected by HIV/AIDS
HAART	Highly active antiretroviral therapy
HUNS	HIV Ullor Nala Sangam
ICTC	Integrated Counselling and Testing Centre
IEC	Information, Education, Communication
INP+	Indian Network for Positive People
IOG	Institute for Obstetrics and Gynecology
MCH	Maternal-child health
MSM	Men who have sex with men

MTP   Medical termination of pregnancy

NACO   National AIDS Control Organization

NAPCP   National AIDS Prevention and Control Program

NGO   Nongovernmental organization

NIH   National Institutes of Health

PLHA   People Living with HIV/AIDS

PMTCT   Prevention of mother to child transmission

PPTCT   Prevention of parent to child transmission

PWN+   Positive Women's Network

SACS   State AIDS Control Society

SIAAP   South Indian AIDS Action Programme

SIP+   South India Positive Network

SPMD   Society for Positive Mothers Development

STD   Sexually transmitted disease

TNP+   Tamil Nadu Network for Positive People

TNSACS   Tamil Nadu State AIDS Control Society

TRIPS   Trade-Related Aspects of Intellectual Property Rights

UNAIDS   United Nations Programme on HIV/AIDS

UNICEF   United Nations Children's Fund

UNIFEM   United Nations Development Fund for Women

USAID   United States Agency for International Development

VCTC   Voluntary Counselling and Testing Centre

WHO   World Health Organization

WLHA   Women Living with HIV/AIDS

WTO   World Trade Organization

Birth in the Age of AIDS

Prologue

Into the Well and Out Again

SARASWATI[1] WAS 24 YEARS OLD AND LIVING WITH HIV/AIDS when I met her in 2004 in Namakkal, a nondescript town nestled below the Kolli Hills in the state of Tamil Nadu and the hub of the South Indian trucking industry. She told me the story of her HIV diagnosis, her pregnancy, child's birth, and early motherhood experiences.

Saraswati hailed from a nearby village, and her father, like many of the men in her village, worked as a lorry driver when she was growing up. At the age of 17, after she had completed the tenth standard of school, her marriage was arranged to her mother's brother's son—a common practice in Tamil Nadu. Her husband was 22 years old at the time of their wedding, and he too was a lorry driver who spent much of his time on the road away from home. Saraswati moved in with her husband's family after their marriage, and, to everyone's delight, within a year and a half she was pregnant and would soon give birth to her first child: a son. By the time this son was 18 months old, Saraswati was a widow.

Saraswati discovered her HIV-positive status when she went to the hospital for her first prenatal visit in the fifth month of her pregnancy and was tested for HIV, although she was not informed that the test was being done until after the fact. The medical personnel urged her husband to also be tested, but he refused. Soon afterward, Saraswati discovered that even before their marriage, her husband had been taking medicines from Majeed's Fair Pharma clinic in Kerala—medicines that Majeed claimed would cure AIDS. Armed with that knowledge, Saraswati and her parents conspired to get her husband tested on some other pretense, and it was revealed that he too was HIV-positive. Despite all this, her husband and in-laws accused her of having infected her husband.

They harassed her so vehemently that one day she climbed down the rusty steps of the ladder into the village well with the intent of drowning herself, but when she reached the bottom rung of the ladder, thoughts of the child in her womb made her reconsider and she climbed back out. Saraswati's own parents were the only others who knew of her HIV status at that time. They were supportive and wanted to rescue her from the abuse of her in-laws (even though Saraswati's father-in-law was also her mother's brother). Saraswati refused their offer, fearing that, because of her HIV status, her presence in their home would jeopardize her younger sister's marriage prospects.

Contending with the mistreatment of her in-laws was not Saraswati's only challenge. She also faced many obstacles as she sought medical care for her pregnancy and childbirth. Several doctors told her openly that they would not care for her because of her HIV status, and in other cases she found herself being referred from doctor to doctor for no apparent reason. The doctor who finally agreed to oversee her delivery only did so for an exorbitant fee, and even in that clinic the nursing staff refused to touch her or change her glucose drips for fear of being infected. The only medical practitioners who did not hesitate to treat both Saraswati and her husband were unlicensed biomedical and Ayurvedic "doctors"; they claimed that they could cure AIDS and charged high fees for their miracles.

After the birth of her son, Saraswati's doctor advised her to avoid breastfeeding because HIV can be transmitted through breast milk. Despite the financial difficulty of this and despite the shame of going against a deep-seated cultural prerogative to breast-feed, Saraswati was able to follow this advice. But Saraswati's grandmother could not bear the nagging criticism of the neighbors about Saraswati's choice to bottle-feed her baby, and the grandmother finally spilled the beans about Saraswati's HIV status to the community to justify her granddaughter's decision not to breast-feed. This only added fuel to the fire of the cruel treatment of her in-laws. When Saraswati's husband died as a result of AIDS shortly thereafter, her in-laws publicly blamed Saraswati for his death, threw her and her young son out of the house, and denied her rights to inherit her husband's property. In the end, Saraswati reluctantly moved back in with her parents, even though her sister's marriage had not yet been arranged.

When I met her, Saraswati was living with her parents and she was still battling her in-laws for her rights to a share of her husband's property in the form of cash compensation and the return of some of her jewels, which were part of her dowry. She sought help through the local *panchayat*,[2] the police, a "self-help" organization for women, and the courts, but all these attempts were in vain.

She was on the verge of giving up hope when a local network for people living with HIV/AIDS and a larger national network for women living with HIV/AIDS stepped in to help. A lawyer on the High Court in Chennai was offering legal services pro bono to these networks to help women living with HIV/AIDS fight against AIDS-related forms of discrimination and to gain access to what should legally be theirs. That lawyer worked with Saraswati on her inheritance claim. Furthermore, Saraswati had recently been employed as an outreach worker for one of the local HIV/AIDS support group networks. With her modest but respectable monthly salary of 4,000 rupees (US$91),[3] she became the primary breadwinner in her household, supporting her child, her mother, and her father, who was no longer working as a truck driver. When I asked her about meeting with the lawyer, she said that it was the first time in years that she had some hope, albeit guarded, for her future and for the future well-being of her son, who was now 4 years old and HIV-negative. When I asked her about her new job, she said, "I don't try to hide my status anymore. I am able to talk freely and am free of fear. I like meeting others, and I am able to encourage others to get rid of fear and shame."

Over the course of my research on HIV/AIDS and childbirth in Tamil Nadu from 2003 to 2008, I interviewed seventy low-income women living with HIV/AIDS. Although each woman's story is unique, Saraswati's experiences of her HIV diagnosis during pregnancy and the ripple effects are in many ways iconic of the experiences of most of the women I met. Throughout this book I flesh out the details of Saraswati's narrative and of the narratives of many other women, some of whom faced far fewer challenges than Saraswati and some far greater. But this story serves as a good vantage point from which to begin to examine the social impact of HIV/AIDS and of HIV prevention and care programs on the lives of young mothers in India at the turn of the twenty-first century.

1 Birth in the Age of AIDS

THIS IS A BOOK ABOUT HIV/AIDS AND CHILDBIRTH—two phenomena that may seem incongruous. One conjures up illness and loss; the other life and hope. Yet of the 2 million children living with HIV worldwide, 90% have acquired the virus from an HIV-positive mother during pregnancy, birth, or breastfeeding (UNAIDS 2008: 33–37). We often read about such demographic statistics generated by organizations such as the Joint United Nations Programme on HIV/AIDS (UNAIDS), the World Health Organization (WHO), or the Centers for Disease Control and Prevention (CDC). But what do we know about the experiences of these women? What is it like to go through pregnancy knowing that you are an HIV-positive woman? How do you decide whether to give birth to a baby if you are HIV-positive? Is the birth event itself different for an HIV-positive woman? And how does being HIV-positive affect the experience of feeding your newborn? In short, does being HIV-positive transform the experience of becoming a mother? If so, how? The answers to these questions are as numerous and varied as the number of women involved and are influenced by the contexts of their lives, such as their nationality, class, ethnicity, race, religion, sexual orientation, kinship arrangements, and the year in which they are pregnant.

In this book I explore the lived experiences of pregnancy, childbirth, and motherhood in the age of AIDS among low-income and lower caste women living in the South Indian state of Tamil Nadu in the early twenty-first century (see Map 1). My focus is on the impact of the Prevention of Parent to Child Transmission (PPTCT) of HIV program on women's lives in India. This program, jointly organized by UNICEF and the Government of India, provides free HIV counseling and testing to pregnant women in government mater-

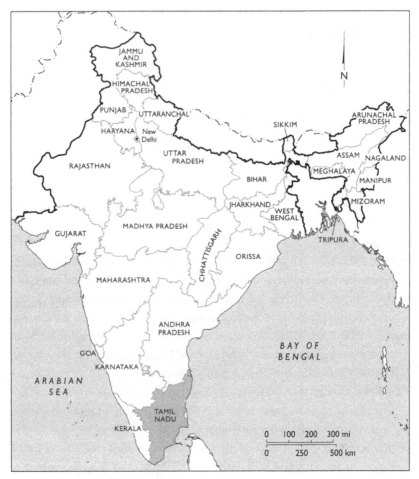

Map 1 India, with the state of Tamil Nadu shaded.

nity hospitals and provides free single-dose antiretroviral therapy to pregnant mothers who test HIV-positive and their newborns. The program was piloted in 2000 and formally inaugurated in Tamil Nadu in September 2002. Women may come to learn of their HIV-positive status before, during, or after their pregnancy (or not at all). Because I am particularly interested in the impact of this PPTCT program, in this book I foreground the experiences of those women who learned of their HIV-positive status during pregnancy.

The adult HIV prevalence rate in India is low—currently reported to be 0.34% (UNAIDS 2009)[1]—but because of India's large population (more than 1 billion people),[2] the country ranks third worldwide in actual number of people living with HIV/AIDS—2.4 million—behind South Africa and Nigeria (UNAIDS 2008). Of those 2.4 million people, only 50% were thought to be aware of their HIV status in 2008–2009, thus making the population vulnerable to a potentially dramatic spike in the number of HIV-positive people (NACO 2009: 15). However, reported HIV prevalence rates for India have fluctuated wildly[3] and have been hotly contested. Regardless of statistical disputes or irregularities, as the country with the highest number of HIV-positive people in all of Asia, India is clearly confronting a daunting epidemic, and global health organizations and governments around the world are responding.

The HIV/AIDS epidemic is more challenging to manage for cultural and political reasons than for biology reasons alone. As a medical anthropologist, I draw my attention to these sociocultural dynamics of HIV/AIDS. As an anthropologist interested in the impact of global and national policies and programs on local communities and individual lives, I recognize that although a program such at the PPTCT program makes good public health sense, its social effect transcends the health arena. In this particular case, in which low-income mothers are the targets of this health policy, structures of gender, socioeconomic class and caste, and global economic and political inequalities among nations influence both how the program is implemented and the repercussions that it has on women's bodies and lives—within their families, in interactions with medical practitioners, and with organizations providing care and support for people living with HIV/AIDS. As Didier Fassin has so aptly stated in his poignant ethnography of HIV/AIDS in South Africa, the experiences of people living with HIV/AIDS in places around the globe that may seem remote from any given standpoint should not be viewed as foreign but rather as part of a shared humanity that we must think about "less in terms of difference than inequality, less a matter of culture than history" (Fassin 2007: xv). Describing the experiences of those women in India whose lives have been touched by HIV/AIDS and by this global health program to prevent the transmission of HIV from mother to child is thus also a way to portray the local embodiment of world history.

To foreground inequality is not, however, to deny the significance of cultural variation. Medical anthropologists view illness and disease as a window into understanding social life and cultural forms. We can learn much about societies' belief systems, including our own, by observing responses to disease. Likewise, a deep look into what causes illness, why certain people get sick, why certain people die, and how diseases travel reveals a great deal about human social organization and value systems. HIV/AIDS is arguably one of the most salient diseases to think about anthropologically precisely because it evokes intense moral responses that both reinforce and challenge cultural norms and because it reveals so blatantly the gross inequalities of our world. As Arthur Kleinman and Paul Farmer wrote in the early years of the HIV/AIDS pandemic, "All illnesses are metaphors. They absorb and radiate the personalities and social conditions of those who experience symptoms and treatments. . . . The way in which a person, family, or a community responds to AIDS may reveal a great deal about core cultural values" (Farmer and Kleinman 2001: 353–56).

Anthropologists and other social scientists have found that in India AIDS is interpreted predominantly through the lens of the morality of sex. The prevailing view is that HIV/AIDS comes about as a result of premarital and extramarital sexual relationships, both of which fall outside the prescribed norm in India. Recent studies have revealed that sexual practice does not always conform to the stated ideals (Puri 1999; Verma et al. 2004). Nevertheless, the norms prevail. Thus, to be HIV-positive is to be marked with a grave social transgression, and the disease is intensely stigmatized. Media reports of HIV-positive people being ostracized in all arenas of social life in India—the family, the workplace, medical settings, and the community—are commonplace. Such discrimination fosters a culture of secrecy in which HIV-positive people avoid disclosing their status as a coping strategy. It also can lead to high rates of depression and even suicide among this population (Chandra et al. 1998; Steward et al. 2008). As a result, the government, nongovernmental organizations (NGOs), and community-based organizations (CBOs), which are known as networks run by and for people living with HIV/AIDS in India, are not only engaged in HIV prevention and treatment but also waging a campaign to prevent the stigma and discrimination that plagues those affected by the disease. In this book I draw from Erving Goffman's seminal theoretical discussion on stigma (Goffman 1963), but I do so in the same vein as Richard Parker and Peter Aggleton, who argue that stigma must be viewed not simply as an individual psychological process but as a key component of social power and as "central to the constitution of the social order" (Parker and Aggleton 2003: 17).

Anthropologists who study reproductive health similarly argue that the management of and beliefs about the processes of reproduction both reflect and transform sociocultural systems and get to the heart of ideas about the body, life, gender, family, and, increasingly, technology. As Faye Ginsburg and Rayna Rapp wrote in the introduction to their edited volume, *Conceiving the New World Order: The Politics of Reproduction,* "Regardless of its popular associations with notions of continuity, reproduction also provides a terrain for imagining new cultural futures and transformations" (Ginsburg and Rapp 1995: 2). In this book I thus explore how responses to HIV/AIDS in the context of birth and motherhood both reflect and transform social relations and cultural value systems. For example, although the stigma experienced by HIV-positive people, particularly women living with HIV/AIDS, serves to reproduce and enforce Indian and Tamil cultural norms of sexual morality, the presence of HIV/AIDS and its spread to rural areas and to individuals who are not associated with high-risk groups, as has become increasingly evident through widespread prenatal testing, also reveals the cracks between imagined cultural ideals and actual practice, leading to increased self-reflection about the unstable and changing nature of cultural identity. Furthermore, although HIV-related stigma may serve to bolster preexisting forms of gender-based discrimination, such as taboos against widow remarriage and denial of inheritance rights of women, HIV-positive women who become affiliated with feminist, human rights–based organizations to combat discrimination against HIV-positive women are publicly pushing back against both of these social conventions; in doing so, they may help to open up the social space to combat these forms of gender discrimination not only for HIV-positive women but also for women in Tamil Nadu or in India more broadly.

Focusing on HIV/AIDS and birth compels me to draw from the anthropology of reproduction and the anthropology of AIDS, both robust subfields within medical anthropology. This project is the first of its kind to deeply explore the intersections of reproduction and HIV/AIDS from an ethnographic perspective, bringing forth the voices of women from one part of the world as they struggle and strive to make sense of the effect that HIV/AIDS and programs that have emerged in response to this disease have had on their reproductive lives.

Global Health Policy: Local Reality

Both reproductive health and HIV/AIDS have been major foci of global health organizations involved in what has broadly been called international development. The international development agencies, which first emerged in the post–World War II era, were and continue to be an important factor in the processes of globalization, with new international organizations, such as UNAIDS and the Global Fund to Fight AIDS, Tuberculosis, and Malaria, coming into play and new foundations, such as the U.S.-based Bill and Melinda Gates Foundation, the Clinton Foundation, and the Gere Foundation, supplementing earlier household names, such as the Ford Foundation and the MacArthur Foundation. Programs designed within the arenas of such international development organizations to combat HIV/AIDS and maternal and infant mortality and morbidity are implemented globally and attempt to both work within and transform local practices and systems of knowledge to improve health outcomes. The proliferation of such organizations working in health-related fields in India along with the rise in local NGOs has been a direct result of the neoliberal turn in India and the government's retrenchment from the provision of health services (Finn and Sarangi 2008). Anthropologists have been keenly interested in examining the relationships between such global initiatives and discourses and their local manifestations. In the introduction to their 2000 edited volume *Global Health Policy, Local Realities: The Fallacy of the Level Playing Field*, Linda Whiteford and Lenore Manderson argue that "too often international health planners design programs based on the assumption that 'all else is equal' and that each recipient nation shares the same 'level playing field.' The assumption of uniformity may be necessary to the process of planning global health programs but also may create needless barriers to their effective execution" (Whiteford and Manderson 2000: 1–2). These writers call for more studies of the localization of international health policies and programs, and my work is a contribution to that end. Understanding how global health policies and discourses about HIV/AIDS and reproduction intersect with local realities and inform everyday practices for poor women in Tamil Nadu is a primary goal of this book.

Global health policies are, of course, not developed in a vacuum. Typically these policies are rooted in local U.S.-based or European contexts or they emerge out of globalizing processes themselves, such as colonialism, postcolonial development projects, and currently the global spread of neoliberalism. In this sense these global health policies carry with them core cultural and political values and interests of those contexts. This book is a historically specific ethnographic study of the intersection of such global health policies, state policies, and local practices on the reproductive lives of HIV-positive women in Tamil Nadu, South India, at the beginning of the new millennium.

What I found is that there are unintended consequences of the PPTCT program. My research suggests that low-income pregnant women who are the targets of this program are given little choice over whether or not to get tested for HIV and how to proceed with the pregnancy once they receive an HIV-positive diagnosis. My research also demonstrates that as a result of this program, women are being diagnosed as HIV-positive before their husbands, and this can have negative repercussions on the status of women within the extended patrilocal, patrilineal family structure, because women are accused of being promiscuous and are blamed for bringing HIV/AIDS into the family, thereby exacerbating preexisting gender inequalities. As a result of their HIV-positive status, these women, like Saraswati, may be ostracized from their husband's family. Many become AIDS widows at a young age, and their HIV status becomes a justification for their husbands' families to force them out of the home. With little or no education, they face grave difficulties supporting themselves and their children. Even though women are tested for HIV in the interest of improving public health, their HIV-positive status often leads to stigma and discrimination within the medical arena itself, even when seeking basic obstetric care.

To make matters worse, during the first half of 2004, when I conducted most of my ethnographic interviews, although the government was providing antiretroviral medicine to prevent HIV transmission from mother to child, it was not providing antiretroviral treatments for the mothers themselves. Thus an HIV-positive diagnosis during pregnancy was sometimes experienced as both a social and a physical death sentence for these women. Since that time the government has established an antiretroviral therapy (ART) program for such women, and networks and governmental bodies have worked hard to overcome the public stigma associated with HIV/AIDS in India. This has led to some improvement in the quality of life of women who test positive through the PPTCT program, although at the tail end of my research in 2008 ART was still difficult for some to access and the stigma associated with HIV/AIDS was far from eradicated.

The choices of lower class and lower caste women are limited within the context of decisions about HIV testing during pregnancy and in relation to the experience of birth and infant feeding for HIV-positive women. These choices are highly influenced by structures of global health policies and by national and state public health policies and services, international and national policies concerning the manufacture and sales of pharmaceuticals, transnational human rights and feminist organizations and discourses, gender and kinship structures, and social class and caste. Nevertheless, although my work makes these structures apparent, I also highlight the ways in which women use their agency to navigate these structures in pragmatic and creative ways.

Structure, Agency, and Gender

It is assumed in the United States (and elsewhere) that women in India are subjugated and have little or no control over their reproductive lives, the implication being that North American and European women have substantially more decision-making power and act as free individuals. Much has been written about the ways in which such "othering" discourses on "non-Western" or "third world women" primarily serve to create a sense of superiority in the "West" (Mohanty 1991; Abu-Lughod 1993). I recognize that the reproductive decisions of the women I met were constrained by social and cultural structures, including gender inequality. This is true of women everywhere. But, using Laura Ahearn's definition of agency as "the culturally constrained capacity to act" (Ahearn 2001: 54), I draw attention to women's agency as they frame their decisions in response to the previously mentioned set of factors.

Ever since Anthony Giddens's theory of "structuration," which in one social theory accounts for both the "strategic conduct" of agents that results in potentially transformative action and institutional structures that reproduce social systems (Giddens 1979: 95), anthropologists have sought to achieve this balance in their ethnographic analyses. Feminist anthropology since the 1990s has highlighted the ways in which women around the world exert their agency in the face of local and global structures of patriarchy in ways that can sometimes be described as "accommodating protest" (MacLeod 1991), because "resistance and compliance are not mutually exclusive" (Mankekar 1999: 29). Although agency may be expressed as resistance or may demonstrate the necessary foundations for resistance (Raheja and Gold 1996), it "may also involve complicity with, accommodation to, or reinforcement of the status quo" (Ahearn 2001: 55). Furthermore, "all too often, compliance is the most effective way to resist an oppressive power" (Seizer 2005: 325). My work contributes to these poststructural feminist understandings of agency and structure insofar as I examine many structures and agentive engagements with these structures that HIV-positive women demonstrate as they navigate the terrains of pregnancy, birth, and motherhood, sometimes reinforcing sociocultural norms but sometimes opening up spaces for the possibility of social change.

Feminist medical anthropologists and historians engaged in the study of reproduction, particularly the medicalization of reproduction, have similarly shifted their theoretical attention away from earlier feminist approaches, which foregrounded the links between medicalization, biopower, and the control of women's bodies (Martin 1987; Jordan 1993), toward an increasing emphasis on explaining and documenting how women actively engage with new forms of medical science and technology in complex, context-specific, and sometimes contradictory ways (Rapp 2000; Inhorn and Van Balen 2002; Van Hollen 2003a). As Margaret Lock and Patricia Kaufert wrote in the introduction to their 1998 edited volume, *Pragmatic Women and Body Politics*, women's responses to medicalization "may range from selective resistance to selective compliance, although women may also be indifferent" (Lock and Kaufert 1998: 2). Ultimately, they suggest that "ambivalence coupled with pragmatism may be the dominant mode of response to medicalization by women" (2). Given that the women in my research were engaging with the medicalization of their reproductive processes within the unique context of HIV testing and HIV-positive diagnoses, indifference was never a response that I encountered. However, ambivalence coupled with pragmatism perfectly characterizes the nature of these women's responses and decision-making processes. It is precisely this kind of ambivalence coupled with pragmatism that I hope to convey through this ethnography.

Women and HIV/AIDS

Social scientific studies on women and HIV/AIDS globally focus primarily on women's vulnerability and risk of contracting HIV, resulting in the feminization of the HIV/AIDS epidemic such that the number of HIV-positive women has now exceeded the number of HIV-positive men globally. Women now make up 52% of the infected population (UNAIDS 2010: 23). Scholars have shown how "structural violence" associated with gender discrimination increases women's vulnerability, with particular attention to commercial sex work, domestic and sexual violence, and women's lack of power to negotiate safe sex (Schoepf 1992; Farmer 1999; Epele 2002; Mill and Anarfi 2002). Studies on HIV/AIDS and women in India also emphasize women's vulnerability to HIV in a patriarchal social context (Ashraf and Godwin 1998; Majumdar 2004; Shanti 2004; Ghosh et al. 2009). These studies point out that lack of education, lack of decision-making power related to health care, and lack of access to information and health care services, combined with a taboo against speaking about sex or AIDS, make women more vulnerable to contracting HIV than men.

Conversely, some have pointed to the ways in which increased autonomy for women in India helps reduce their vulnerability to HIV (Bloom and Griffiths 2007). Many of those scholars conducting ethnographic research in India with the aim of improving HIV prevention efforts have sought to better understand sexual practices and awareness of sex and HIV/AIDS among various groups within the population, including women (Nag 1996; Verma et al. 2004) and adolescent girls (Bhan et al. 2004; Mahajan and Sharma 2005). Special attention has been given to the study of female commercial sex workers (Asthana and Oostvogels 1996; Guntupalli 2008), especially in relation to the empowerment of sex workers in the Sonagachi project in Kolkata (Pardasani 2005; Ghose et al. 2008; Swendenman et al. 2009) and also in relation to *devadasis*[4] (Orchard 2007) and the often hostile interaction between sex workers and the police (Biradavolu et al. 2009).

Another key topic of research on women and HIV/AIDS globally is the relationships between gender, stigma, and HIV/AIDS; studies suggest that HIV-positive women throughout the world face greater stigma and discrimination than do HIV-positive men (Bond et al. 2003; Ogden and Nyblade 2005). Research from India corroborates these more global findings, with reports of in-laws (with whom many women live) accusing women of infecting their sons. Women in India who become AIDS widows at a young age face added discrimination in a society in which not only AIDS but also widowhood itself is stigmatized (Bourdier 1997, 1998; CFAR and PWN+ 2003; Van Hollen 2010).

A third area of research on women and HIV/AIDS that is relevant to my own study addresses the issue of reproductive health. Social scientists exploring this topic have examined such things as HIV-positive women's experiences with sterilization to prevent pregnancy (Hopkins et al. 2005), how HIV contributes to infertility (Inhorn and Van Balen 2002), morbidity and mortality associated with pregnancy among women living with HIV/AIDS (Berer 1999), debates about infant feeding for low-income HIV-positive mothers (Blystad and Moland 2009; Desclaux and Alfieri 2009; Traoré et al. 2009), and ethical and political issues of providing ART to prevent mother-to-child transmission in the global south (Hankins 2000; Richey 2011).

Maria de Bruyn provided an important report on women's decision-making processes and difficulties in preventing pregnancy or dealing with wanted or unwanted pregnancies based on a broad review of the literature on HIV/AIDS and a comparison of interviews with women in four different countries (de Bruyn 2002). Others have addressed the same topic by focusing on one country (Kirshenbaum et al. 2004). To date, the most comprehensive study of women, reproductive health, and HIV/AIDS in India is Patrice Cohen and Suniti Solomon's *AIDS and Maternity in India: From Public Health to Social Science Perspectives—Emerging Themes and Debates* (2004); this edited volume aims to bridge perspectives of the social and medical sciences on the topic of mother-to-child transmission of HIV in India. The book's contributors first contextualize women's reproductive concerns within broader sociocultural factors concerning gender inequality in India; these factors make women vulnerable to HIV infection and make HIV-infected women vulnerable to discrimination and to economic and social suffering (Geetha 2004; Shanti 2004). The contributors then move on to consider what work has been done on women's perspectives about HIV transmission during pregnancy, birth, and infant feeding. Finally, in the last chapters the contributors point to the need for more detailed studies examining the lived experiences of HIV-positive women during birth and for more studies to examine how measures to prevent HIV transmission from mother to child are in fact being carried out on the ground (Hancart Petitet 2004; Lingam and Mankad 2004).

In this book I provide precisely the kind of ethnographically grounded study that the contributors to Cohen and Solomon's book say is needed. This kind of richly textured ethnographic analysis is critical so that policy makers, health care providers, and social workers engaged in designing HIV/AIDS prevention and care programs can provide women with the information and options necessary to make informed reproductive choices.

From There to Here

My interest in studying the intersections of HIV/AIDS and reproduction emerged in the mid- to late 1990s when I was engaged in my dissertation research on the medicalization of childbirth in Tamil Nadu, a study that resulted in the publication of my book *Birth on the Threshold: Childbirth and Modernity in South India* (Van Hollen 2003a). Talk of AIDS was beginning to percolate into conversations with doctors, community health workers, and friends during my dissertation research. I recall two conversations in particular.

> A friend asks in hushed tone: "What does AIDS look like? You must see it in America, no?" I reply: "There is a virus called HIV and you can have that for a long time without having it affect your health. But after some time, you develop AIDS and then your immune system begins to break down and you can get other diseases that your body cannot fight against." He persists: "But what does it *look* like? How can I know if someone has AIDS?" I say, "You may

be able to see that people have some disease that their immune system cannot fight, but you cannot know that they have AIDS just by looking at them." He seems frustrated by my answer. I tell him that I really don't know much about it myself. (Chennai, February 1995)

I am interviewing an obstetrician in one of the Corporation hospitals in Chennai (which was then still called Madras). At the end of the interview, she says: "Now, if you don't mind, may I please ask you a question?" "Yes, of course" I say. And she asks me: "What are people in America doing to prevent the spread of HIV/AIDS? What are people doing in the hospitals there?" "Well," I say, "there are lots of advertisements about the importance of using condoms. You see them in public places, like the metro stops and in magazines." I am thinking about a particular advertisement I remember seeing in a San Francisco magazine which says "Sex is Good"[5] and which has a picture of a heterosexual couple and a gay couple, each naked in an erotic embrace. The advertisement was encouraging responsible, safe sex and health awareness. I find I am too uncomfortable to describe this ad to this Indian doctor, thinking it might seem improper to her. Later I realize I am the one being prudish. She presses me again with her question: "What are people doing about this in the hospitals there?" I sheepishly tell her that I don't really know about that. (Chennai, July 1995)

With each of these encounters the presumption was that I, as an American, would have a wealth of information about HIV/AIDS that could be helpful to share in India for either personal or professional reasons. Although the first case of AIDS in India was detected in 1986 in a sex worker in Chennai (the capital of Tamil Nadu), the initial response among government officials and the general public was one of denial that this disease could become a problem in India. It was assumed that because Indians had a highly traditional sense of morality when it came to sexual practice, they would not be affected by this disease in the way that seemingly promiscuous societies, such as the United States and countries in sub-Saharan Africa, would be (Dube 2000; K. Jain 2002: 156). It was not until the mid-1990s that policy makers in India began to wake up to reality and had to step away from their moral superiority complex in the face of a mounting epidemic. As it turned out, Chennai was then emerging as a hub of civic activism to tackle this disease and provide care and dignity to those suffering from it, and the Tamil Nadu state government was demonstrating a unique political commitment to addressing the problem of HIV/AIDS. I was not aware of all these developments in Chennai when people were turning to me for advice. These queries made me more aware of how little I myself knew about social responses to HIV/AIDS around the world, other than what I had seen of gay activism in the United States, especially in the San Francisco Bay Area, where I had been living.

Anthropologists argue that blame is the primary universal response to the HIV/AIDS crisis and that imagined national and ethnic identities are forged in the construction of the dangerous "other" responsible for AIDS lurking "out there" and threatening "our" borders and bodies (Farmer 1992; Hyde 2007). As Paul Farmer writes, "Of all the responses registered, accusation—the assertion that human agency had a role in the etiology of AIDS—is the dominant leitmotiv" (Farmer 1992: 192). Indeed this was a widespread response when AIDS was first detected in India. Yet, in those few moments when HIV/AIDS snuck into conversations during my research in 1995, it was not in the spirit of blame but in the form of a sincere interest in cooperation.

In this book I present the voices and opinions of many players involved at the intersection of HIV/AIDS and reproduction, most notably the voices of those who often go unheard: lower class women living with HIV/AIDS, women attending public maternity hospitals, and counselors working in these hospitals. The discourse of blame runs throughout these ethnographic accounts, whether the object of blame is a husband, a nurse, a doctor, a hospital, an NGO, or the government. I relay these critiques not in the interest of exacerbating the cycles of blame but in the spirit of cooperation, with the belief that how people interpret and respond to this disease—and the concerns they have about how the disease and the social responses to the disease affect their lives—needs to be heard so that the international community, national and local governments, and NGOs can continue to strive not only to stem the tide of HIV/AIDS but to provide care and treatment to people affected by this disease in the most humane way possible. Lamenting the inadequacies of the global response to HIV/AIDS in the world at the beginning of the twenty-first century, former secretary-general of the United Nations Kofi Annan once said, "What sort of people are we? Can we use the words compassion, humanity, dignity of our fellow man and woman? They all become hollow."[6] Countless people have, of course, responded with compassion, humanity, and dignity worldwide, but there is always room for more, and I hope this book is a further contribution to that end.

In the spring of 2000 I learned that the government of India was piloting the new PPTCT program in select Government Hospitals around the country. Three of the eleven hospitals selected to pilot this program were in the state of Tamil Nadu, all in Chennai (Kuganantham 2004: 117). Given that Tamil Nadu was considered one of five high-prevalence states for HIV and given the long history of Tamil Nadu's (particularly Chennai's) prominence in hospitalized births in India (Van Hollen 2003a), it was not surprising that this state would play a leading role in this new program. My interest was piqued. I wanted to know more about what pregnant women attending these hospitals would think about such a program. How would this fit into their broader experiences of childbirth, medical institutions, and the state about which I had already been writing?

After meeting in Washington, D.C., in the fall of 2002 with several people who were affiliated with governmental and nongovernmental organizations engaged in HIV/AIDS prevention projects in India, in December 2002 I stepped off a plane at the Chennai International Airport with my family and Sharon Watson, one of my undergraduate students from the University of Notre Dame (where I was then on the faculty) who had come along to work as my research assistant. I had received support from the University of Notre Dame to explore the possibility of doing research on HIV/AIDS and reproduction in the context of the government's goal to formally integrate its PPTCT program into its maternity hospitals.

During this one-month exploratory study in India, I traveled to Chennai, Delhi, and Kochi to meet with members of governmental and nongovernmental organizations and with medical practitioners involved in HIV/AIDS prevention and care projects whose work in one way or another related to maternity health care and the PPTCT program. This brief visit provided me with an overview of the landscape of organizations working on HIV/AIDS prevention and care in India generally and in Tamil Nadu in particular. I was encouraged by all to return for further ethnographic study.

But my lasting impression from that trip was this: Over the course of my trips to India in 1991, 1993, 1995, and 1997 for dissertation research, I saw many changes. After all, 1991 was the year that India liberalized its economy, and the shift to a consumer-oriented culture, driven by the rising income of the middle class, was palpable in Chennai: Foreign cars and the new compact Indian Marutis were quickly filling the streets and replacing the rounded white Indian Ambassador cars, and new, gleaming buildings, including high-rise Internet technology offices and grandiose shopping arcades, were sprouting up in the center of the city and in the newly emerging suburbs. Despite all this change, though, one thing remained constant: the ubiquitous inverted red triangle, a symbol of the Family Planning program in India since the 1960s. Often accompanied by the phrase "We Two, Ours One" (thus the two top points of the triangle leading down to the one), the red triangle could be seen on posters in hospitals, outside shops, at bus stands, and always on the back of the three-wheeled auto-rickshaws that plied the busy streets. By the end of 2002, however, the red triangle was scarcely visible, except in faded form on the rickshaws and on the walls of some hospitals for obstetrics and gynecology. Something else had taken its place, something that would have seemed unimaginable only a few years ago. In the place of prominence that had once been occupied by the red triangle throughout the bustling streets of Chennai, there now sat—or rather danced—a cartoon of a smiling condom guy. On one sign the condom guy stands with a shield in one hand and a spear in another, saying (in Tamil), "To prevent AIDS, I alone can help. Wear a condom. Prevent AIDS." In another ad the condom guy stands with his arms held high, his hands creating a cover over his head. The caption reads (in Tamil), "For a house, a thatch roof is important. For safe sex, a condom is important. There is no medicine for AIDS. There is no treatment. One can avoid AIDS. There is no cure." And on a huge 6 by 3 foot banner I saw a comic strip (also in Tamil) with several scenes in which the condom guy is having a conversation. The conversation begins with a woman named Rani; she is complaining to the condom guy that she cannot suggest to her husband that he use a condom without raising his suspicions. Next the condom guy has a longer conversation with the husband, Ravi, in which he tries to convince Ravi of the birth control and preventive health benefits of using a condom, dispel Ravi's concerns that sex with a condom is less pleasurable (the pleasure lasts longer!), and reassure Ravi that condoms made in India are of high quality (they are even exported to other countries!). In the end, Ravi accepts the condom, and for this newlywed couple "happiness bloomed in their family life."

The condom guy and the international symbol of the HIV/AIDS red ribbon were two of the new icons of the Information, Education, Communication (IEC) materials being produced with the help of the USAID-funded AIDS Prevention and Control (APAC) Project (an NGO) and the Tamil Nadu State AIDS Control Society (TNSACS). When I visited the APAC office, I came away with a stack of these IEC materials, including five different illustrated pamphlets of "side-splittingly hilarious condom jokes" (in English) and a Snakes and Ladders board game in Tamil (known as Chutes and Ladders in the United States). Snakes and Ladders is an ancient Indian game originally created to teach children lessons about Hindu morality, karma and moksha. Here too it was being used to teach morality to prevent the spread of HIV and AIDS: Have a monogamous married relationship or wear a condom, and you climb the ladders to become a winner; have sex with a sex worker, and you slide down a snake to end up in a hospital bed with an IV drip. HIV/AIDS was no longer something hidden and only to be discussed in hushed tones. It was becoming part of the fabric of mainstream public culture.

By 2004, when I returned to Chennai, the PPTCT program had been officially inaugurated with technical support and training from UNICEF. This time I had received funding from the Fulbright Foundation to spend six months conducting ethnographic research (the project title was "AIDS, Medicine, and Gender in India: How Pregnant Women Negotiate Options to Prevent Mother-To-Child Transmission of HIV in Tamil Nadu, India"). I made one more return visit to Chennai in 2008 for one month of research on the same project with funding from the American Institute for Indian Studies. The material presented in this book comes from all three trips to India (2002–2003, 2004, and 2008). The bulk of the ethnographic data come from the 2004 and 2008 research trips.

One of my anthropology professors at Berkeley, where I did my doctoral work, once told me that the primary methodology of anthropology was serendipity and that we must remain open-minded and flexible to allow for that serendipity. Of course we must have well-developed methods, but flexibility is a premium in cultural anthropology because we never know precisely what we will be able to do or what will be most important to do methodologically until we are in fact making our way through the social landscapes we planned to investigate.

I faced my share of the mundane and predictable frustrations of waiting long hours to meet with government officials or medical personnel, who may not have even showed up for the appointment, and of needing to be flexible and change course to focus more on the networks when government permissions to carry out research in certain hospitals were not granted as quickly as I had hoped. Indeed, the shift in focus proved to be rewarding. Throughout, I knew that what mattered most about my research method and what makes the anthropological method unique was the quality of the interactions I had (the interviews, observations, and participatory research)—the attention to understanding individuals within the context of their life histories and within the context of the local, national, and global contours of the historical moment in which they live. One of the strengths of anthropology is to be witness to people's lives and to present the voices of people and to situate those voices within their broader social and cultural contexts. I sometimes am envious of those researchers working with large teams who can access enormous amounts of data—both qualitative and quantitative—to generate generalizations about patterns of behavior and thought. The smaller scale, more localized research of solo anthropologists working in concert with a small group of research assistants may in some respects be less generalizable. Yet there is something profound about the kind of embodied knowledge that can be gained by individual anthropologists that is simultaneously analytical and emotional, allowing for empathy. In the realm of ethnographic research on a topic such as childbirth and HIV/AIDS, this kind of embodied knowledge is crucial to understanding women's lived experiences. My hope is that this ethnography provides the analytical rigor necessary to understand the complexity of context while simultaneously conveying empathy.

Given the inherent flexible nature and contingencies of the ethnographic method and its attention to long-term qualitative research, it is impossible to fully describe everything that goes into the research process itself. Nevertheless, what follows is a snapshot of how I went about gathering the information on which this book is based.

A central component of this research involved ethnographic interviews with seventy women living with HIV/AIDS.[7] The interviews, which I conducted in 2004 and 2008, focused on how these women came to know about their HIV status, how they and others responded to their HIV-positive diagnosis, what role they think gender plays in social responses to people living with HIV/AIDS, and their recommendations for improving HIV/AIDS prevention and care. Thirty-two of these women knew their HIV status before giving birth to all of their children. Interviews with these thirty-two women included discussions about how they made decisions to continue (or not) with their pregnancy and delivery after receiving an HIV-positive diagnosis, what their experiences were like during birth, how they made decisions about infant feeding, and what they thought about the decisions they had made.

I met thirty-seven HIV-positive women through networks of HIV-positive people in Chennai, Namakkal District (a largely rural district and home to one of India's trucking centers), and Coimbatore (a major industrial city) (see Map 2). Twenty of the women I met were recruited through the Y. R. Gaitonde Centre for AIDS Research and Education (YRG Care), where they were receiving maternity health care.[8] I met three women living with HIV/AIDS in government maternity hospitals, where they had recently delivered babies through a PPTCT program. I met eight women who were living in a home on the outskirts of Chennai and were receiving care and support through an NGO called Zonta Resources. Finally, I met two HIV-positive women through a PPTCT counselors' evaluation meeting because they had been hired as counselors in the government PPTCT program.

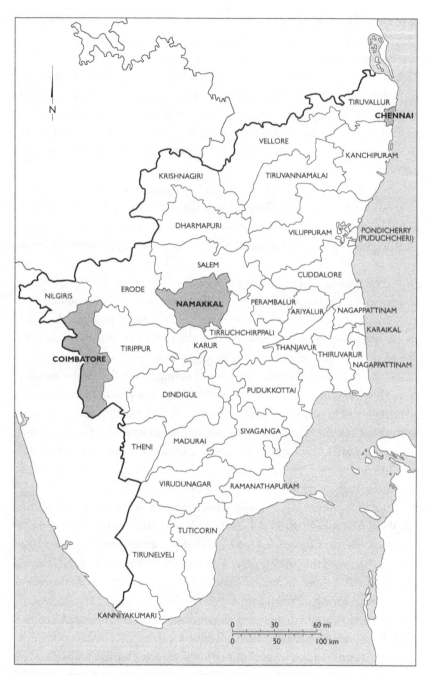

Map 2 Tamil Nadu and its districts, with Chennai, Namakkal, and Coimbatore shaded.

Several of the networks for positive people—including the Positive Women's Network (PWN+), HIV Ullor Nala Sangam (HUNS), the Society for Positive Mothers Development (SPMD), the Indian Network for Positive People (INP+), the Tamil Nadu Network for Positive People (TNP+), the South India Positive Network (SIP+), and the Council of People Living with HIV/AIDS in Kerala (CPK+)—allowed me to take part in their support group meetings.[9] PWN+, which was the network with which I was most closely affiliated, also invited me to participate in their public meetings to educate the media about concerns of people living with HIV/AIDS and in public meetings to educate HIV-positive people about their legal rights; at these meetings I served as a note taker and helped to compile follow-up reports for the organization.

In addition to interviews and participant observation with HIV-positive women, during my research in 2004 I also conducted sixty-five interviews with pregnant women who were receiving prenatal care in Government Hospitals with PPTCT projects, and I observed patient-counselor interactions in those hospitals.[10] None of those sixty-five pregnant women were known to be HIV-positive. The hospitals where this portion of the research was conducted were the Institute for Obstetrics and Gynecology (IOG) at the Government Hospital for Women and Children in Egmore and three Corporation hospitals: the Saidapet Health Post, the Vadapalani Health Post, and the Pulianthope Health Post. All were public maternity hospitals in Chennai where I received government permission to conduct the research. These interviews focused on women's experiences with and opinions about HIV testing for themselves and their partners during pregnancy and explored their opinions about the risks of HIV in India and recommendations for prevention.[11]

In addition to the interviews with HIV-positive women and with other pregnant women attending public maternity hospitals, I also met with policy makers and others working for international and local governmental and nongovernmental organizations involved in HIV/AIDS prevention and treatment programs in Chennai, Delhi, and Washington, D.C., including the National AIDS Control Organization (NACO), TNSACS, the Tamil Nadu Health and Family Welfare Department, UNICEF, the United Nations Development Fund for Women (UNIFEM), WHO, the United States Agency for International Development (USAID), the CDC, Family Health International, APAC, the South Indian AIDS Action Programme (SIAAP), Zonta Resources, the Community Health Education Society (CHES), and Health First. I also interviewed a lawyer with the High Court in Chennai who was providing legal aid to people living with HIV/AIDS.

Finally, I met doctors and counselors at the Government Hospital for Thoracic Medicine in Tambaram (near Chennai), IOG–Egmore, the Corporation
hospitals in Saidapet, Vadapalani, and Pulianthope mentioned earlier, the private
YRG Care hospital in Chennai, and the Taluk District Hospital in Rasipuram
(Namakkal District). I also interviewed two practitioners of Ayurveda and a
practitioner of Siddha who were treating HIV/AIDS patients. Ayurveda and
Siddha are both indigenous Indian systems of medicine. Interviews with policy
planners, members of NGOs, and medical personnel explored their assessment
of the successes and future needs of HIV/AIDS prevention and care programs,
with particular emphasis on mother-to-child transmission.

Profile of the HIV-Positive Women Interviewed

The ethnographic data presented in Chapters 5–9 make up the heart of this
book and are drawn primarily from interviews with the seventy HIV-positive
women I met. These women came primarily from the lower socioeconomic
segment of society. This is due in part to the method that I used to make contact with them; few middle- or upper-class women participated as members
of the networks or attended Government Hospitals or YRG Care for their
maternity health care needs. However, as far as income levels are concerned,
my sample is reflective of overall global trends, because HIV is now known
to disproportionately affect people living in poverty. Poverty curtails access
to health care, nutrition, and education and may contribute to high rates of
migration and drive people into sex work for pay or into substance abuse, all
factors that place people at risk for HIV (Singer 1994a, 1994b; Farmer 1999).
Fourteen of the women I met were living in institutional centers, such as the
Zonta Resource Center, or at a hostel set up by World Vision (an international
charitable organization) or were unemployed but temporarily supported by
World Vision and therefore did not have any household income. Two other
women were homeless, engaged in sporadic commercial sex work, and had no
steady household income. Of the remaining women the average total household income, as reported by the interviewees, was 3,726 rupees per month. This
was the equivalent of US$85 per month, or US$1,020 per year.[12] Twenty-six of
the seventy women interviewed had some kind of employment that substantially supplemented the household income. This is in part due to my research
method rather than a reflection of the actual income levels of HIV-positive
women's households in general because several of the women were working
for the networks and two worked as counselors in the government's PPTCT
program in maternity hospitals, reflecting the government's attempt to practice

a GIPA (Greater Involvement of People Living with or Affected by HIV/AIDS) policy. Others had low-paying daily wage jobs in factories or on farms. The remaining forty-four women either identified themselves as housewives or were unemployed because they were being supported by institutions.

Education levels of most of these women were low. This is not surprising given that many were born into families living in poverty. Sixteen (23%) of the interviewed women reported that they had never received any formal education at all. The average level of education of all seventy was between the seventh and eighth standard (seventh and eighth grade).[13] Most of the women came from lower caste *dalit* communities (also known as the Scheduled Castes). Fifty-one of the women were Hindus. Seventeen were Christian, sixteen of whom had recently converted from Hinduism. (The reasons for this large number of recent Christian converts is discussed in Chapter 6). Two women were Muslim. The average age of these women was 28.[14] Most had been married at some point (most of the first marriages were arranged, but a sizable minority had entered into love marriages). Thirty-three (47%) had already become widows; their husbands had died as a result of HIV/AIDS. Despite cultural taboos against widow remarriage and, in some cases, even despite acknowledgment of their HIV-positive status, some women were in their second marriages when I met them (as is discussed further in Chapter 9). Twelve of the women had a history of commercial sex work (including some who were married at the time of the interviews). Fifty-seven (81%) of the women either had children or were pregnant with children; thirteen were childless and not pregnant, representing a high rate of childlessness given the sociocultural context that places a premium on motherhood and given the expectation that a woman should bear a child as soon after marriage as possible, usually within the first year of marriage.

My focus in this book is on heterosexual HIV-positive women's commentary and perspectives. This obviously results in biased opinions. Interviews among HIV-positive heterosexual men or among men and women with non-heterosexual sexual identities, including "third gender" groups (such as *hijras*, who are discussed in Chapter 2), would undoubtedly reveal different viewpoints. Furthermore, studies based on observations of social interactions of HIV-positive men and women within households and in public contexts would further yield a more nuanced perspective than a study, such as this one, based primarily on interviews. Finally, as a result of my recruiting method, a disproportionate number of the interviewed women were in one way or another associated with networks or with NGOs and therefore had been influenced by a transnational discourse on rights of HIV-positive people and, more specifically, a transnational feminist discourse critiquing the discrimination against women living with HIV/AIDS. This too no doubt results in a bias in the comments of my consultants. Research with a larger pool of HIV-positive women who were not affiliated with networks or NGOs might bear different ethnographic data. These methodological limitations do not, however, invalidate the importance of understanding the perspective of the seventy HIV-positive women in Tamil Nadu who participated in my study.

Navigating the Minefields of Stigma

I cannot say that all of my research went off without a hitch. My previous major research project on childbirth had been demanding. I had worked mostly in poor urban and semi-urban neighborhoods with squalid living conditions, and it had been difficult to decipher tape-recorded interviews because there was always a cacophony of sounds of children, chickens, and scolding grandmothers in the background. I had slogged through Chennai's traffic to get to hospitals, to NGOs, to archives, returning home exhausted to a hungry baby of my own. To a large extent the pattern of my days was much the same with my new research project as it had been before: searching for addresses in crowded public housing projects all around Chennai and visiting government maternity hospitals where nurses wore starched white dresses and caps and the scent of Dettol antiseptic was omnipresent. With my previous research on childbirth, however, I had the satisfaction of feeling as though the women I met enjoyed telling me their birth stories. In fact, oftentimes, when I was trying to interview one woman, her neighbors would catch wind of the conversation and want to come in and regale me with their birth stories as well. Before I knew it, the room would fill with a group of several women, all sharing their lives, laughing, and creating a deep sense of community among themselves and between me and them as I shared my own birth experiences. Nothing could have been further from this in my experiences interviewing HIV-positive women about their birth experiences. Fears of stigma and discrimination coupled with experiences of sorrow, suffering, and anger framed the contours and filled the content of these interviews. The joys of childbirth were not absent, but they seemed to take a back seat in these women's narratives.

To begin with, there was the difficult question of where to conduct the interviews. I left this choice up to the women themselves, giving them the options of meeting in my own apartment, in their homes, or in another place—a park or the gardens outside a restaurant where we could sit and have a picnic. I was aware that many had not disclosed their HIV status to all of their family members or to neighbors and that my presence in their homes (especially as a white foreigner) could evoke curiosity and could lead to them being "outed." I explained that I did not want to cause such problems. I was also aware that meeting outside the home could be difficult for women who had a heavy work-load at home—taking care of young children and sometimes in-laws, cooking, cleaning, getting water from the water tanks—and that their husbands might not allow them to leave all this behind or might not approve of them going out to a public park on their own to meet me. I was equally aware that women from poor backgrounds might feel extremely uncomfortable coming to my simple but distinctly middle-class apartment, the kind of space where people typically sit on chairs rather than on the floor and where people from the lower class usually enter as servants, not as guests.

In some cases I interviewed women who worked for the networks, and in those cases I could simply interview them in a private room at their office, where everyone knew of their status. In other cases, such as in Namakkal, I met women in my room at the Golden Palace Hotel (a fine hotel but one far less grandiose than its name might suggest), since they had come to the same hotel for a network meeting earlier that same day. In Coimbatore I was able to inter-view women in the SPMD building, where I was invited to help cut the ribbon at the opening ceremony to inaugurate their new building. I met five women in hospitals where they had recently delivered their babies; they were either al-ready alone in a postpartum room, or we were given a private room to conduct the interviews. The twenty interviews with HIV-positive women coming for prenatal or postnatal care at YRG Care were all interviewed in a doctors' room that was made available to me when the doctors did not need them. The inter-views conducted through Zonta Resources were all conducted under the shade of a tree on the organization's private compound beyond earshot of others.

But for other women none of the options were ideal. I tried to impress upon them that doing the interview was voluntary, so if it was too risky or too time-consuming to meet, I would understand. Only one woman asked to be inter-viewed in my home, and she was the most educated and financially well-off woman I interviewed; that was the one interview conducted in English by her choice. A few women chose to be interviewed in the park at the Gandhi Manda-pam, and one woman opted to meet in the shade of some neem trees on the grounds of the Hotel Woodlands drive-in restaurant. Several women gave me their addresses and asked me to come to their homes for the interviews.

For the most part these home visits went smoothly, with two exceptions. Unfortunately it is often the exceptions that haunt you. The first exception was when Padma (my primary research assistant) and I arrived at a woman's apartment complex in a new government housing project on the far outskirts of Chennai at our appointed time, but nobody was home. As a white woman in Chennai, I rarely go anywhere unnoticed, but when I pull up to a housing project in a rented car, it is bound to cause a stir. It wasn't long before first the children in the neighborhood and then adult neighbors came up to me to ask who I was looking for and why. I explained that I was looking for Muthamma and that we had arranged a meeting. That did not prove to be a satisfactory answer, and the questions kept coming. Padma and I agreed to say that we were part of a women's "self-help scheme" and that we were meeting Muthamma in conjunction with the self-help group. Because self-help groups for women's empowerment—mostly involving various microfinancing schemes—have mushroomed in India as part of the neoliberal trend, this seemed like a plausible explanation and also seemed to calm the curiosity of the growing crowd. Another woman then came down the lane and said that Muthamma had just asked her to tell us that she would be here soon and to please wait just a little longer. As it turned out, Muthamma was involved with a self-help scheme through World Vision and she had been on her rounds selling oil for that scheme when we arrived. We were lucky that our pretense turned out to be so close to the truth, but I always wondered whether, after our departure later that afternoon, Muthamma had had to fend off a barrage of questions from all those people who had gathered in her absence and whether my presence had made life difficult for her in her neighborhood.

The second uncomfortable incident concerning the location of interviews once again involved World Vision. In this case I had made arrangements with four women at a PWN+ support group meeting to interview them. They told me that they all lived together in a house, and they gave me their address and asked me to come there for the interview. It was an attractive house near a church at the end of a road, a quiet spot in an otherwise crowded section of Chennai. When I arrived, I learned that the building was owned and run by World Vision as a hostel for HIV-positive women and their children. World Vision was providing room and board for these women for up to six months, and the organization helped them learn some skills to become economically self-sufficient so that they would be able to live on their own after the six-month period. Upon entering the house, I met the "warden" who lived with and supervised the women in the hostel. She said that it was fine for me to conduct interviews there. I also met the cook who lived nearby and came to the hostel to prepare meals for the women staying there. Amudha, one of the women staying at the hostel at that time, also had a son living with her. Her son was 8 years old, but he looked closer to 6 because of his height and he walked with a slight limp. Amudha recounted how he had not walked for several years until she converted to Christianity and her prayers were heard and he began to walk. The son was also HIV-positive. His CD4 count[15] had dipped to a dangerous low of 85, and he was receiving ART from World Vision. Shakila, who was also staying at the hostel, had a 5-year-old daughter, and the two children played together.

I sat down on the floor with the warden and the four women—all young widows—and once again explained my project to them and received informed consent to interview each of them individually. I came to the house on three occasions to complete these interviews. It was a spacious, clean house, and we would sit on the hard, cool floor of the main room until the sun went down and the heat subsided enough that we could move to sit on the floor of the veranda to enjoy a slight breeze. Shakila's daughter tried to fiddle with my tape recorder during my interviews, and I was constantly fending her off with an ample supply of Marie biscuits. In between interviews I shared tea with the women and let Amudha's son and Shakila's daughter play with my minidisc recorder, singing songs into it and playing them back. I admired the embroidered cards that these women had learned to make as a self-help scheme with World Vision. I bought several of these cards: one of a blue elephant and others of brightly colored birds. They were selling them for 50 rupees each and, although beautifully crafted, in my head I questioned the ability of these women to support themselves on the sales of these cards once their time at the hostel and their free supply of antiretroviral drugs ran out.

On the day of my third visit I was sitting on the veranda, conducting my final interview there with Kumutha. She was telling me about her marriage at the age of 12 to a 30-year-old man who had died four years earlier, leaving her alone with five children who were staying in her village near Salem. I was in the middle of a conversation with her, asking her to explain what exactly she meant when she said that the doctors had told her that she "only had seventy percent HIV," when all of a sudden three middle-class women, wearing brightly colored saris, came striding onto the veranda. I turned off my tape recorder and stood up to meet them, and Kumutha also rose to her feet.

These three women were alarmed to find me there. They were supervisors, working with World Vision, and they were on a periodic visit to inspect how things were going at the hostel. They spoke to me in English so that the other women could not understand what they were saying. After inquiring about what I was doing, one woman said that I should have gotten permission from the World Vision director to come to the hostel, and another woman accused me of "barging into someone else's house uninvited" and wanted to know how I had gotten the address. I explained that I had gotten the address from someone at a PWN+ meeting who had agreed to participate in the research and had given me permission to come to the house. Upon hearing this, they became angry that someone at PWN+ had given me the address, and I had to clarify that it was not a PWN+ employee but someone from the hostel who had come to a PWN+ support group meeting. They then wanted me to tell them exactly who had given me the address. Afraid of implicating the woman who had given me the address, I mumbled that I couldn't really remember exactly who it was but that because the women lived in the hostel, I thought they were entitled to provide me with their address, and they had invited me to meet them there as opposed to meeting elsewhere. I explained that the warden had also agreed to my interviewing in the hostel. But I also apologized for not getting permission from the World Vision director, and I assured them that I would contact the director to get permission before conducting further interviews at the hostel. I wrote down the phone number for the director and gathered up my things to go.

As I was leaving, I could hear the supervisors interrogating the women to find out who had given me the address and telling them that no one should be permitted to visit without permission from the director. I cringed at the thought that I could have jeopardized these women's ability to receive care and support from this organization. I wondered if it had been irresponsible of me not to think that I should have contacted the director before carrying on with the research on that first day when I had arrived and realized what kind of a home it was. Or, was this a manifestation of a common complaint I had heard from people at both PWN+ and TNP+ about the tendency for NGOs to become territorial about "our HIV-positive people" in the battle over funds in the global AIDS industry.

Some HIV-positive people I met were strategic about enticements that organizations used to get them to participate in that particular organization's activities. For example, people living with HIV/AIDS were often provided with 50 rupees and a free lunch to attend monthly support group meetings at the networks. Although the organizations framed this in terms of covering transportation expenses and time away from paid labor, some people living with HIV/AIDS viewed this as a way for CBOs and NGOs to increase their membership base so that they could report high attendance rates to their funders. Those same people who were cynical about such handouts, however, also took pride in their ability to take full advantage of the situation. For example, one homeless sex worker I met calculated that she received 200 rupees monthly and four free lunches for attending support group meetings of four different such networks in Chennai.

The anthropologist Vinh-Kim Nguyen (2010) argues that in Côte d'Ivoire the incipient "moral economy" that emerged initially in response to the AIDS epidemic quickly transformed into triage and a competition for resources as NGOs scrambled for "body counts" of HIV-positive people to justify their need for international funds; Côte d'Ivoirian citizens were driven to get tested for HIV and to come forward with public testimonials about their HIV-positive status to access not only treatment for HIV/AIDS but also basic resources to survive to which the average citizen was not otherwise entitled. This led to what Nguyen describes as a form of "therapeutic citizenship," "as people living with HIV developed a powerful sense of rights and responsibilities inherent to their medical predicament" (Nguyen 2010: 9). João Biehl's ethnographic account of the political and social effects of the Brazilian government's much touted universal antiretroviral rollout, which was implemented in 1996 and was the first of its kind in a developing country, similarly demonstrates how certain categories of people who can conform to a particular set of moral codes come to be deemed worthy of this kind of therapeutic citizenship while the most economically and socially marginalized members of society become further marginalized through their exclusion from the rights to such therapeutic citizenship and thus to AIDS therapies and other forms of social services (Biehl 2007). The women I met who made the rounds of multiple networks and gave their testimonials in support group meetings to access much needed cash and food can also be seen as desperately attempting to lay claim to a limited kind of therapeutic citizenship.

I called the World Vision office the next morning and left a message for the director with the receptionist. I called again toward the end of that week and left another message. I called a third time the following week. I never heard back from World Vision. However, when I went to interview two other women, they had just been notified by World Vision that they should not speak to me. It turned out that, although they did not live in the hostel, they were receiving ART from World Vision. The interviews were canceled. The next time I visited the PWN+ office, I received a distinctly cold shoulder from the women working there, unlike my previous visits to the office over the past four months. It turned out that World Vision had also contacted PWN+ and complained about this incident.

That week I traveled to Namakkal with a PWN+ group to attend a workshop on sex and gender education and legal literacy that was being organized by PWN+ and HUNS. A PWN+ employee had recommended that I attend this meeting and had helped make my travel arrangements. When I arrived at the hotel where the workshop was to take place, however, a group of PWN+ employees told me that they were not sure that I would, in fact, be permitted to attend the workshop. Although they would not say exactly why they had the sudden change of heart, I thought that it must have something to do with the sudden chill in my relations with PWN+ as a result of the World Vision incident. The workshop was about to begin, and I had to wait in the lobby while they discussed my case in a hotel room. When they finally emerged, they said that they had decided that I could attend the workshop, and we all went together to the meeting room. It seemed to take a few weeks, though, before the tension fully melted away. The moment of reprieve came when PWN+ asked me to attend a press event they were holding and asked if I would be a note taker at the event. I gladly accepted the invitation.

This series of events was a reminder of how crucial and yet delicate the process of trust building and reciprocity is to ethnographic research. Any introductory anthropology textbook will tell you so. But in conducting research on something as intensely stigmatized as AIDS within a highly contentious field of governmental and nongovernmental organizations who are competing for funds earmarked specifically for HIV/AIDS that were flowing into the country from abroad, the development of trust went beyond the personal to the political.

Building trust, negotiating the politics of access, and navigating the minefields of stigma were big issues, to be sure. Coping with the emotional challenges of bearing witness to stories of HIV-positive women's social, psychological, and physical suffering was even more challenging. During my six months of research in 2004, my two children (Lila and Jasper) attended the American International School in Chennai (with a few other American students and many from Korea and several other countries) in the beautifully landscaped spacious new campus in Tharamani. Their teachers—Ms. Nanda and Ms. Padma—were welcoming and provided them with a great educational experience. Their futures seemed bright, and the reassurance that came from that allowed me to pursue my own work. Yet so many of the women I met through my research lived with a constant, deep sense of anxiety about the future of their children as a result of their economic status, and that anxiety was severely compounded by the uncertainty of their own futures that had been handed to them with an HIV-positive diagnosis. Sometimes tacking back and forth between these two worlds was jarring. In the daytime I would receive stories of women whose children had died from AIDS or whose husbands had committed suicide following an HIV-positive diagnosis, leaving their wives and young children alone with no source of income; I would hear of parents who had placed their children in an orphanage because they could no longer work as a result of AIDS-related illnesses and they did not expect to live long enough to raise their children. In the evenings I would celebrate the birthday of Jasper's favorite stuffed animal puppy (Sammy) with candles stuck into little cakes or celebrate Lila's own birthday with henna designs applied to the hands of all her friends who came for a sleepover.

There is a powerful romance to the image of the cultural anthropologist being fully integrated into the daily lives of the people she is studying. This image has been challenged by critical inquiries into ethnographic fieldwork (A. Gupta and Ferguson 1997) and seems rather quaint and outdated to some, and yet it remains in some sense paradigmatic of the ethnographic method. But it does not represent my own experience with my research on low-income women and HIV/AIDS. In some sense it could not, given, first, the politics of stigma and my concerns about outing HIV-positive women just by virtue of my presence in their homes, and second, the fact that HIV-positive women in Tamil Nadu do not constitute a geographically bounded community. Their community manifests when some of them come together (often secretly) in meetings organized by networks. Most do not even risk participating in such gatherings for fear of exposing their status. They remain otherwise an imagined community. This romance of integration also does not represent my experience by my own choice because, while living in Chennai with my family, I chose to live in a middle-class residence and chose to place my children in an elite educational institution that was well suited to accepting international students for short-term arrangements.

I usually needed a moment to myself to pause as I shifted between the worlds of my home and my work. At times I recognized that the differences were not always as great as they appeared. For example, when I was in Chennai, I received news that a family friend had committed suicide, and my conversations about suicide with women in my research somehow helped me to come to terms with this death. Another example was when my children accompanied me to a support group meeting and played chess with the HIV-positive children of the women who had come for the meeting. I understand the dangers of essentializing or universalizing motherhood, and yet in my view the shared experience of motherhood can indeed sometimes be a powerful avenue for transcending differences. If nothing else, for me it helped to appreciate what is at stake in the differences between rights and privileges—to understand that my ability to live with my children, to provide them with a solid education, and to feel relatively secure that I will see them thrive and grow to adulthood is a privilege and not a fundamental right. It is a privilege that comes with the social structural hand I was dealt, and that is vastly different from what most of the women I met experienced; their position of class, caste, gender, and global political geography made them vulnerable to contracting HIV and less able to live a long life and to have confidence that their children would survive. It is a privilege that arguably should be a right.

Medical anthropologists have provided clear examples of the ways in which socioeconomic status affects rates of HIV transmission and rates of morbidity and mortality resulting from HIV in various communities (Farmer 1999; Farmer and Kleinman 2001; Lane et al. 2004). Appreciating the impact of these structural factors firsthand through my meetings with the women whose stories are presented here helps me to recognize the dire need for social change. For this reason, throughout this book I try to illuminate lessons learned from my research and point to steps that can be taken to mollify the vulnerabilities that low-income women living with HIV/AIDS in India face. These suggestions emerge partly through my broad analysis of the structures and impact of the PPTCT program, from the point at which women are presented with the option of HIV testing through to the stage in which new HIV-positive mothers must figure out how to feed their babies. My recommendations are also revealed through the insights and concerns of the many people who I met and who participated in this research, including not only the HIV-positive women but also women receiving prenatal care in the PPTCT center, the counselors and doctors involved in this program, and policy makers and members of international and local governmental and nongovernmental organizations.

One of the things that struck me most during this research was the resilience of those women who had suffered the most as a result of the social responses to HIV/AIDS. Despite their stories of social and physical suffering and despite a sense of despair that they felt when contemplating their futures and the futures of their children, many also learned how to combat that despair with a kind of optimism that came from their participation in the activist-oriented networks promoting a transnational discourse of positive living. Along with demonstrating the structures that constrain their lives, in this book I also seek to demonstrate how the women I met were reshaping their lives in the face of HIV/AIDS and gender- and class-related discrimination through their participation in forms of collective activism. This activism not only helped them to cope but also gave them hope and in some cases enabled them to take control of their lives (e.g., in the realm of employment, marriage and kinship, or demands for improved medical care) in a way that they said had not been possible before their participation in such organizations.

Mark Finn and Srikant Sarangi argue that the discourse of positive living is part and parcel of broader global discourses on quality of life and empowerment that promote a neoliberal form of governmentality. They argue that proponents of these concepts (of positive living, quality of life, and empowerment) advocate for self-management and individual entrepreneurship, thereby abdicating the government from responsibility for providing social services, such as health care, to the population (Finn and Sarangi 2008). This critique has merit and has links to the notion of therapeutic citizenship (Nguyen 2010) or "patient citizenship" (Biehl 2007: 97) that I have found fruitful in my own analysis. At the same time, however, I argue that the networks promoting positive living in India were also at the forefront of making demands on the government to improve access to medical and legal care and to enforce antidiscrimination laws. And those networks that catered specifically to women living with HIV/AIDS also collectively fought for legal rights for women and created a space for women to challenge broader patriarchal gender norms.

2 India Responds to the Epidemic

BEFORE TURNING TO MY OWN ETHNOGRAPHIC RESEARCH ON HIV/AIDS AND BIRTH, it is important to sketch a picture of governmental and civil society responses to HIV/ AIDS in India. It is not my intention to write the social history of this epidemic in India. Many such rich accounts have already been written by scholars and journalists (e.g., Godwin 1998; Dube 2000; K. Jain 2002; Panda et al. 2002; Bourdier 2004; R. N. Gupta 2004; Narain 2004; Chandrasekaran et al. 2006). Rather, I hope to point to some general trends in India as a whole and to demonstrate the crucial role that Tamil Nadu has played in formulating responses to HIV/AIDS and in developing the PPTCT program.

Responses to HIV/AIDS in India

When the first case of HIV in India was detected in 1986 in a sex worker in Chennai, many Indians speculated that because of the cultural fabric of Indian society, HIV/AIDS would never surface as a major threat to India as a nation and would remain not only a low-prevalence disease but also one sequestered to the margins of society, among commercial sex workers in major urban ports. By 2003, however, India's then prime minister Atal Bihari Vajpayee stated that "HIV/AIDS is not only a grave global challenge. . . . It is equally a national concern."[1] The first international trip that Sonia Gandhi (the wife of former prime minister Rajiv Gandhi and current president of the Indian National Congress Party) took after her Congress-led United Progressive Alliance Coalition came to power in May 2004 was to the Fifteenth International Conference on AIDS, held in Bangkok. There she gave a keynote address that publicly acknowledged to the world the severity of the AIDS epidemic in India while simultaneously vowing that the Indian government was committed to combating AIDS and

AIDS-related stigma as a global problem. Since that time, Manmohan Singh, the prime minister of India, has continued to make statements about the need for ongoing vigilance on the part of the government and civil society to control the spread of HIV and to provide care and support for people living with HIV/AIDS in India.

After the announcement of the first case of HIV in 1986, the national government responded by putting together a comprehensive surveillance plan to monitor the prevalence and risk of HIV in India and a preventive plan to increase awareness of risk reduction through, for example, condom promotion, regulation of blood supplies, and control of sexually transmitted diseases (STDs) closely associated with increased HIV risk. With funding from WHO and other multilateral agencies (K. Jain 2002: 156), India's Ministry of Health and Family Welfare launched the National AIDS Control Programme in 1987, and beginning in 1992 this effort was formalized through the establishment of the National AIDS Control Organization (NACO) and the National AIDS Prevention and Control Program (NAPCP), two umbrella organizations designed to coordinate all HIV/AIDS policies and programs, including NGO programs (Sethi 2002).

The period 1987–1992 was marred by state and city governmental blunders, which have been likened to the draconian sterilization campaigns under India's Emergency in 1975 (K. Jain 2002: 156). As Siddharth Dube explains, during this period the government treated HIV/AIDS as a law and order problem, and "police and health officials forcibly tested thousands of sex workers and drug users" and "those found to be HIV-positive or with AIDS were quarantined or jailed" (Dube 2000: 25–27). Indian Railways banned HIV-positive people from traveling on trains. In 1988, "Dr. A. S. Paintal, the then head of the Indian Council of Medical Research, the government's top advisory body on health, proposed that sex with foreigners be banned" (Dube 2000: 26). Mandatory HIV testing of foreigners, especially Africans, traveling to India was implemented; infected foreigners were to be deported (Dube 2000: 26). It was also during this time, in 1990, that the now infamous raid of brothels in Mumbai took place in which the Tamil Nadu and Maharashtra police "rescued" 824 Tamil sex workers in Mumbai and herded them onto a train euphemistically called the Mukti (liberation) Express, only to have them returned to Chennai, where they were met by hordes of media and thus openly labeled as sex workers. After being forcibly tested for HIV, those who tested positive—of which there were many—faced the double stigma of being a sex worker and HIV-positive. Several of these women promptly committed suicide. Fourteen years later, in 2004, while I was conducting my research, I would meet two of the survivors. They were being cared for by Zonta Resources International with Government of India funding and were living on the margins of society on scrubland owned by the army in something reminiscent of, but not as sinister as, what Biehl described as "zones of abandonment" for HIV-positive people in Brazil (Biehl 2005). For the two women I met, memories of this past episode had been willfully obliterated.

NACO Phase I: 1992–1999

Such tactics could not last long in a vibrant democracy like India. Human rights groups protested vociferously. Thus in Phase I of NACO's planning (1992–1997, extended to 1999) the more coercive approaches to the policy were abandoned, and the emphasis shifted to addressing HIV/AIDS as a health problem.[2] Nevertheless, Geeta Sethi (2002) argues that in Phase I the government was unsuccessful in operationalizing its plans because of the resistance of some people within and outside the government who denied that HIV was or would become a problem meriting substantial governmental resources. Bureaucratic red tape also proved to be an obstacle to implementing plans because the increasingly large sums of money coming from international sources and from the government were not distributed efficiently. Sethi and others (K. Jain 2002: 159) have also critiqued some of the early approaches of the NACO plan and a sensationalist media for focusing too exclusively on high-risk groups, such as commercial sex workers, truck drivers, recipients of blood transfusions, and intravenous drug users, with the result that members of these groups suffered extreme forms of stigma and discrimination. For example, I met families involved in the trucking business in Namakkal District of Tamil Nadu who told me of the enormous difficulties they faced in arranging marriages for their sons just because of all the intervention projects and media attention focused on truck drivers, especially truck drivers from Namakkal. Equally problematic with this approach was the fact that people who were not identified with these groups were led to believe that they were not at risk and therefore that they need not engage in preventive behavior. In reality, everyone is at risk. It has been argued that, in a cultural context where women have little bargaining power to insist that their husbands use condoms and where failing to produce children can be grounds for a husband to divorce his wife, for many women in India marriage itself can be considered a risk factor for HIV (CFAR and PWN+ 2003).

Perhaps the strongest critique of the approach taken in Phase I was that the policy was based on the assumption that awareness programs themselves could transform behavior. Insufficient attention was given to the complex social fac-

tors, such as poverty and gender inequality, that shape the construction of behaviors that put people at risk for HIV—factors that may leave individuals with
little control over their sexual or drug use practices. Anthropologists often refer
to this set of factors as forms of structural violence. Structural violence has
been defined as "preventable harm or damage . . . where there is no actor committing the violence or where it is not meaningful to search for the actor(s);
such violence emerges from the unequal distribution of power and resources
or, in other words, is said to be built into the structure(s)" (Weigert, quoted in
Lane et al. 2004: 320). Medical anthropologists working around the world have
provided compelling ethnographic examples of the ways in which structural
violence makes certain groups of people vulnerable to HIV (e.g., Farmer 1992,
1999; Schoepf 1992).

Furthermore, an overemphasis on education as a solution ignored the fact
that severe inadequacies in India's health care delivery system (e.g., the unsuccessful control of STDs, the lack of access to HIV testing and counseling, and
human rights abuses faced by HIV-positive people in hospitals) proved to be
major obstacles to individual attempts to engage in preventive behaviors. So
long as NACO approached HIV/AIDS as a health problem rather than as a social, economic, or political issue, it could not garner the political attention and
resources it needed because, as Kalpana Jain pointed out in 2002, "Health issues
are low among national priorities" (K. Jain 2002: 159). When Jain interviewed
Sushma Swaraj, an influential member of the then ruling Bharatiya Janata Party,
she was told: "Health and such issues may be the concern of rich nations like
the U.S.; for us it's providing basic bread and butter that are more important"
(K. Jain 2002: 160). Before this, in her position as Minister of Information and
Broadcasting in the late 1990s, Swaraj had banned sex education broadcasts
on the radio, believing them to encourage adultery (Gosh 2005: 494). Furthermore, in 2003 she was appointed the Minster of Health and Family Welfare,
during which time she began a campaign against condom promotion, which
she argued promoted promiscuity (Joshi 2003).

NACO Phase II: 1999–2007

As a result of some of the concerns just mentioned, Phase II of the NACO
plan (1999–2004, extended to 2007) was developed to try to provide a more
"enabling environment" for individuals to be able to engage in lower risk behaviors in the first place. This second phase acknowledged that in order to better comprehend what was required to create such an enabling environment in
diverse communities throughout India, a more decentralized and multisectoral

planning approach would be of paramount importance, including a move to include HIV-positive people as active collaborators in the planning process. Decentralization under Phase II also meant giving states more control over programs.

The mobilization of and by commercial sex workers in Kolkata's Sonagachi red light district, a movement that has attracted international media attention, has been viewed as a positive model for decentralized, community-generated efforts. These efforts are not just limited to HIV/AIDS awareness and prevention; they also emphasize the importance of economic, political, and social empowerment as a prerequisite for creating an enabling environment that will facilitate a reduction in the spread of HIV, in this case by enabling sex workers to insist on condom use (Jana et al. 2002; Pardasani 2005). Despite the touted successes of this one project, however, many thought that the government was still too focused on condom distribution among high-risk populations and that the central government was ineffective in changing health policy at the state level, because most health issues remained under the control of the states (K. Jain 2002: 161–76). NGOs working on HIV prevention were proliferating, and funds were pouring into what is referred to as behavioral change communication. However, the primary way that the government could evaluate the success of these NGOs was through numbers, such as the number of condoms distributed, the number of "peer educator" contacts with sex workers, and so on—none of which can be a barometer for real change (K. Jain 2002: 169–73).

Noteworthy among various programs initiated under Phase II was the launching of the government's ART program in the second half of 2004 to provide free antiretroviral medicines through select Government Hospitals. Activists involved in the networks for people living with HIV/AIDS were instrumental in advocating for this program, arguing that the government (and international aid organizations) had been overly focused on prevention efforts while neglecting the needs of people afflicted with this disease.

The issue of ART production, pricing, and distribution has been mired in the global controversy over the role of the World Trade Organization (WTO) in establishing and enforcing international patent laws. In 1996 the development of HAART (highly active antiretroviral therapy)—a combination therapy that delays the onset of AIDS—led to a dramatic reduction in the death rates in developed countries. Because of the exorbitant costs of HAART, however, these medicines remained out of reach of most people living with HIV/AIDS in the rest of the world until the beginning of the new millennium, when the Indian pharmaceutical company Cipla created a generic version at substantially reduced prices. This competition led to a price war that forced prices for brand name drugs to drop as well. Whereas in 1996 the cost of HAART was US$10,000–$15,000 per person per year, between 2004 and 2008 the most widely used first-line ART combination cost as little as US$88 per person per year in some countries, including India (Avert.org 2010). Largely because of these price reductions, the Indian government was able to roll out its free ART program in 2004. The Indian pharmaceutical industry has become a major exporter of these drugs throughout the world, particularly to sub-Saharan African countries hit hardest by the HIV/AIDS pandemic.

The future of this government-subsidized ART program, however, hangs in the balance because of WTO laws. In 1995 the Agreement on Trade-Related Aspects of Intellectual Property Rights (TRIPS) "introduced intellectual property law into the international trading system for the first time and applies to all members of the World Trade Organization" (Avert.org 2010). At that time developing countries, including India, were given a ten-year deadline—until 2005—by which time they would be required to fully comply with the TRIPS agreement. It was within that timeframe that the Indian pharmaceutical industry was able to develop generic ARTs, and these make up the bulk of the ARTs that are used by HIV/AIDS patients in India today. Increasingly, however, biological resistance to these first-line drugs is emerging, and newer, second-line drugs are being developed in response. Studies suggest that "10–15% of people taking antiretrovirals will develop resistance to the combination of drugs they are taking within 4–5 years" (Avert.org 2010). Furthermore, newer drug combinations are less toxic and easier to take than the first-line drugs. The manufacture of these new drugs, developed after 2005, must now abide by the TRIPS agreement, and, as a result, prices have once again begun to rise dramatically, making these drugs too expensive for most people in India (and other parts of the world) and threatening the viability of the government's ART program.

Organizations such as the Clinton Foundation, Médecins Sans Frontiers, and UNITAID have come on board to negotiate price deals with drug manufacturers to keep prices down. These negotiations have led to a system of tiered pricing, which means that "the price at which the big pharmaceutical companies sell their drugs is calculated using formulas based on average income per head, leading to lower prices in poor countries" (Avert.org 2010). The concern is that this system is "over-dependent on the goodwill of Big Pharma" (Avert.org 2010) and that should such voluntary agreements falter, WTO member countries would be forced to comply with the TRIPS agreement or risk being penalized by the WTO and prices would once again skyrocket as a result. Proponents of the TRIPS agreement argue that without such laws there is a disincentive for pharmaceutical companies to invest heavily in the research and development required to develop and patent new drugs if other companies have the right to make generic copies of the final product at reduced prices. Critics argue that there is a moral prerogative to make lifesaving drugs affordable to all people, regardless of their income level in the face of a pandemic such as HIV/AIDS. The numbers of people developing resistance to first-line drugs is steadily increasing. Because it is unlikely that the TRIPS agreement will be abolished in the near future, new solutions will need to be found to guarantee that ART prices will not once again become prohibitive to people in need of these drugs, most of whom live in the global south.

NACO Phase III: 2007–2012

Phase III of NACO, running from June 2007 until 2012, moved toward further decentralization to implement programs at the district level, and they have used a new cadre of rural community level "link workers" to spread awareness about culturally taboo subjects related to HIV prevention (such as sex and sexuality), with the assumption that local members of rural communities will be better positioned to broach such topics with other villagers. These measures were taken to spread HIV/AIDS awareness among young people in rural areas throughout India, following the trajectory of the disease. To that end, NACO and other partner organizations, such as UNICEF, sponsored the world's largest mass mobilization campaign on HIV/AIDS with the Red Ribbon Express. This train crisscrossed the nation for a year, reaching more than 50,000 villages; it carried HIV/AIDS educational information, including admonitions against stigmatizing people with HIV/AIDS. Sonia Gandhi gave a speech at Delhi's Safdarjung Railway Station as the train set off on its journey on December 1 (World AIDS Day), 2007. She said, "Many men and women in the prime of their youth have been lost to the disease. Sadly, through no fault of theirs, children have become victims. I do hope the Red Ribbon Express will succeed in educating young people and thereby carry forward the battle against this disease. It is a battle which can and must be won."[3] The contrast between this and the Mukti Express seventeen years earlier could not be more apparent.

Although Phase III set out to increase care for HIV-positive people—especially through ratcheting up its ART distribution program—its primary focus continued to be on prevention among high-risk groups, because HIV/AIDS continues to be categorized as a "concentrated epidemic" in India; that is, the HIV prevalence rate among high-risk groups is much higher than that among the general population. NACO now encourages members of these risk groups to organize themselves into CBOs to reduce dependence on NGOs and foreign funding and to ensure sustainability. Some people have criticized the disproportionate amount of foreign aid flowing into India in the wake of the HIV/AIDS epidemic. Critics argue that in India and other developing countries far more deaths are caused by such conditions as diarrhea, malnutrition, and anemia than by AIDS, and yet the amount of foreign aid flooding into these countries to combat HIV/AIDS far exceeds the amount given for what they see as more pressing public health needs (Shiffman 2006, 2008). They have also voiced concerns that the sudden availability of AIDS money has led to the proliferation of ersatz NGOs, which use funds for personal profit.

Under Phase III the targeted high-risk groups included commercial sex workers, intravenous drug users, truck drivers, migrant workers, and "men who have sex with men" (MSM). In India this MSM category covers a wide range of gender identities and is not exclusive to the gay community. *Hijras*, who have been described by some as "neither man nor woman" (Nanda 1990), are one of many other distinctive Indian gender categories that would be subsumed within the public health category of MSM. As Gayatri Reddy reports, the *hijras*—a community of people who are born either with ambiguously sexed genitalia and consider themselves female or with male genitalia but undergo ritualized castration and consider themselves female—have been hit hard by the HIV/AIDS epidemic, in part because they have lost their ability to earn money through their more traditional occupation of singing and dancing at births and weddings (Reddy 2005). Because they are marginalized and stigmatized in India, they have difficulty getting other jobs and have had to resort to sex work to make a living. At the same time, members of this community are considered to have special ritual powers, and the society does sometimes respect their desire to be identified as female. For example, in Tamil Nadu the state government allows *hijras* to stay in the women's ward of the Government Hospital of Thoracic Medicine in Tambaram on the outskirts of Chennai. This hospital has the largest number of AIDS patients in India, and the presence of *hijras* in its women's ward was noticeable on my visits there. To a certain extent, the fact that this community has been hard hit by HIV/AIDS has resulted in their political mobilization for human rights and recognition. On November 12, 2009, the Indian election authorities granted an independent identity to intersex and transsexual individuals on the country's voter lists. They now have the option of checking "O" for Other when indicating their sex or gender identity on voter forms.[4]

Indeed, somewhat like the gay rights movement in the United States, the devastating impact of HIV/AIDS on so-called MSM groups in India more broadly has helped to galvanize rights-based advocacy movements around sexual orientation (Humsafar Trust 1995; Bhaskaran 2004: 72–73; Joseph 2005: 86–87; Kavi 2007: 395). This advocacy led to a landmark ruling on July 2, 2009, by the Delhi High Court that overturned Section 377 of the Indian Penal Code and thereby abolished the criminalization of consensual homosexual sex between adults. This ruling should help ease the tension between those working in the field of HIV/AIDS prevention and care and the police. Such tensions remain, however, in the area of prostitution. The presence of HIV/AIDS has similarly led to growing movements in India (like that of the Sonagachi project and the Karnataka Sex Workers Union) to decriminalize activities associated with sex work and to recognize the rights of sex workers as part of the greater HIV prevention effort. In India as a whole, however, the views of detractors of these movements, who argue that sex work is inherently degrading (especially to women), still prevail.

Tamil Nadu: The Pioneer State

The Sonagachi project was touted as one successful intervention project, but the activities in the state of Tamil Nadu have also been celebrated for their proactive, progressive response to the AIDS epidemic. Tamil Nadu—Chennai in particular—emerged as a hub for the development of both governmental and civil society responses to HIV/AIDS, not only in terms of prevention but also in terms of advocacy for care and treatment of people living with HIV/AIDS. The care and treatment issue gained traction in mid-2004 with the new government ART program, after having been largely neglected by governmental and nongovernmental programs funded by international donors such as USAID and the Gates Foundation that had focused on prevention. In many respects Tamil Nadu has been the pivotal state in India in terms of both epidemiology and social and political responses to HIV/AIDS.

First, with regard to the epidemiology of HIV in India as a whole, it is important to note that HIV prevalence rates in India vary across regions. Currently Andhra Pradesh is the only state reported to have HIV prevalence rates greater than or equal to 1% (based on prenatal care attendees). However, six other states also have had a history of higher HIV prevalence rates than other parts of India: Karnataka, Maharashtra, Manipur, Mizoram, Nagaland, and Tamil Nadu (NACO 2008: 21). Geographically, these states are clustered in the south and northeast regions of India. Higher rates in the northeastern states have been attributed to high intravenous drug use. Because this region borders the Golden Triangle, it is a transit point for the heroin trade and is also known to have opium poppy cultivation.

The other higher prevalence states are all located in South and Central India. Andhra Pradesh and Maharashtra have the highest numbers of HIV cases, with nearly 500,000 each (NACO 2008: 23). The four South Indian states (Andhra Pradesh, Karnataka, Kerala, and Tamil Nadu) contribute 60% of all HIV cases in the country (NACO 2008: 23). In my discussions with members of governmental and nongovernmental HIV/AIDS organizations three explanations for this pattern emerged. Some point to the fact that HIV/AIDS entered India through the major port cities of Chennai and Mumbai, where commercial sex workers were the first reported victims of the disease. The higher rates in Tamil Nadu and Maharashtra and in the adjacent states of Andhra Pradesh and Karnataka could therefore be attributed to the fact that the virus had a longer period of time to spread in the region. Others suggest that the south and central regions have been hit hard by this disease because of the industrial and Internet technology growth in the south following the liberalization of India's economy in 1991. This has resulted in high levels of migration in the region as people move for new employment opportunities, not only in the high-tech sector but also in construction and other service sectors that support the emerging Internet technology industry. Migration is known to be a contributing factor to the spread of HIV throughout the world, particularly when men migrate as temporary wage laborers. It is well documented that when men leave wives and children behind in search of work, they often engage in sexual relationships with sex workers (Herdt 1997; Campbell 2004). Thus the category "Migrant Workers" is considered a high-risk category in NACO programs.

The third explanation given for higher prevalence rates in South and Central India is that the rates are simply a reflection of better epidemiological surveillance in this region and that rates may be much higher than reported in other states but are not accounted for because of a less developed HIV surveillance infrastructure. Indeed, although declines in HIV prevalence rates are evident in these higher prevalence states, several states that were previously considered to have lower prevalence rates (such as Gujarat, West Bengal, Orissa, and Rajasthan) are witnessing an increase in HIV prevalence rates (NACO 2008: 18). This increase could be an indication that interventions, which were put into place in higher prevalence states but not in the lower prevalence states, do work. On the other hand, increases in the previously low prevalence states could also be attributed to improvement in HIV surveillance in these states. Whereas none of the "newly identified districts with >1% HIV prevalence among ANC Clinic attendees" are in the states previously recognized as higher prevalence states, four of the nine districts mentioned are in Bihar and Orissa, states that are known to have had underdeveloped public health service infrastructure (NACO 2008: 18).

Tamil Nadu has been a central focus for HIV/AIDS in India for two reasons. On the one hand, it is known as the state in which the first case of AIDS in India was ever detected.[5] Earlier in the epidemic Tamil Nadu was also reported to have had prevalence rates as high as 1.1% (this was the official rate at the time of my research in 2004) (TNSACS 2003).[6] These statistics were subsequently recalibrated downward, suggesting a prevalence rate of 0.67% for Tamil Nadu in 2004 (NACO 2008: 20). Nevertheless, Tamil Nadu is still viewed as one of the higher prevalence states, and it has several very high prevalence districts within its borders. In 2008 NACO reported that there were ten districts in India that had "very high" prevalence rates of greater than or equal to 3%. Four of these ten districts were located in Tamil Nadu, more than in any other state: Coimbatore, Namakkal, Salem, and Viluppuram Districts (NACO 2008: 18).

On the other hand, Tamil Nadu is also recognized as the state that has been the most proactive in developing programs for HIV/AIDS prevention and care, both at the governmental and the nongovernmental level (Parameswaran 2004). Programs developed in Tamil Nadu have been used as models for other states. Under Phase II of the NACO plan, in the interest of decentralization, State AIDS Control Societies (SACSs) were established with the intent of improving the implementation of NACO's broader goals in local states (K. Jain 2002: 183). To this end, the central government used the model of TNSACS, which had been established in 1994 and was the first of its kind. TNSACS is only one of a long list of other groundbreaking organizations born in Tamil Nadu that have since become models for the country.

The networks in India—support and advocacy organizations run by and for people living with HIV/AIDS that are modeled after other international HIV-positive rights-based organizations—first took hold in Tamil Nadu. These networks formed as HIV-positive people organized to combat the extreme forms of stigma and discrimination that they faced at home, in the workplace, and in medical institutions.[7] Several of the individuals who formed these networks had been working at NGOs involved in HIV prevention, but even in those organizations they felt marginalized because of stigma. Rama Pandian formed TNP+ in 1994 (registered in 1995). Since then, virtually every state has developed its own state-level network. INP+, with a national agenda, was established in Chennai soon thereafter in 1997 as a central organizing body for the newly emerging state-based networks. INP+, which had twelve founding members, including the charismatic Ashok Pillai (now deceased) and K. K. Abraham, the past president of INP+, is still headquartered in Chennai today. PWN+, with four founders, including the current president P. Kousalya, was founded in 1998 and is also headquartered in Chennai. PWN+ was the first women-specific network of its kind in India and now has branches in Delhi and six states across the country. The common goals of all these networks are to promote social acceptance of people living with HIV/AIDS and overcome stigma and discrimination, to protect the human rights of HIV-positive people (e.g., by providing legal aid), to provide HIV-positive people with access to information and medical treatment, to promote the employment of people living with HIV/AIDS, and to provide a forum for networking and counseling. Funding for these organizations has come through a variety of sources, including Family Health International, USAID, UNIFEM, the Gates Foundation's Avahan AIDS Initiative, and governmental bodies such as NACO and the various SACSs.

YRG Care is a nonprofit organization founded by Dr. Suniti Solomon, one of the leading experts in the treatment and care of HIV/AIDS patients and the first scientist to discover HIV in India. This organization, established in 1993 in Chennai, is involved in education, care and support, and research and training in the field of HIV and AIDS and is one of the preeminent organizations of its kind in India.

International donors also focused their attention early on in the state of Tamil Nadu. The USAID-funded APAC Project was first established in India in 1995 through an affiliation with Voluntary Health Services, a nonprofit community health organization located on the outskirts of Chennai that also houses the YRG Care clinic. Not far down the road, in Tambaram, lies the Government Hospital of Thoracic Medicine (formerly, and still colloquially, known as the Tambaram Sanatorium for tuberculosis). Because tuberculosis is one of the most common opportunistic infections associated with HIV/AIDS in India, the hospital began to see HIV-positive patients in 1993. Both TNSACS and NACO provided support to this hospital for the treatment of AIDS patients. It has since become the largest AIDS care center in all of India, and physicians from around the country go there for training in treatment and care of HIV/AIDS patients. The CDC has provided substantial technical support to this hospital. The Tambaram hospital, along with the Christian Medical College hospital in Vellore, which is also in Tamil Nadu, were identified as two of only four centers in India to initiate the government's ART program in 2004,[8] underscoring once again the vital role of Tamil Nadu in HIV/AIDS care and prevention efforts in India.

And the list goes on. It is these interventions in Tamil Nadu that have been credited with reducing the prevalence rate by 50% in the state from 2003 to 2007, bringing it down to 0.25% (NACO 2008: 20).

When I first met Rama Pandian in December 2002, I asked him why Tamil Nadu had been such a pioneer state in its response to the HIV/AIDS epidemic in India. He smiled and jokingly said (in English), "We Tamilians are just superior." He then went on to say that NGOs were strong in Tamil Nadu, that the general public in Tamil Nadu was more open to discussing HIV/AIDS than elsewhere, and that, although the Tamil Nadu government had done a good job in the area of prevention, it was failing in the area of care and treatment.[9] I asked a number of people this question and never got a clear answer. Indeed a similar question arose when I was conducting my earlier research on reproductive health care in India, because Chennai (then Madras) had emerged as the center for the provision of biomedical maternal and child health care as early as the nineteenth century. In the twentieth and twenty-first centuries Tamil Nadu has been considered a model state in terms of rates of institutional deliveries, low maternal and infant mortality rates, and low fertility rates. Several explanations emerge that might explain why Tamil Nadu has been so pivotal both in reproductive health care and in HIV/AIDS prevention and care over time.

The explanation, as I see it, has four components: historical, cultural, economic, and political. These are not mutually exclusive categories. I suspect that the answer lies at the intersection of all four. Put simply, the historical argument would have us believe that because the city of Madras (built by the British) and the Madras Presidency were so crucial to the British colonizers and because the British and American missionaries were particularly active in southern India during the colonial era, allopathic health care institutions proliferated and flourished in the region early on; the colonizers took an interest in keeping their labor pool healthy, and the missionaries made the development of health and educational institutions a central part of their religious calling, which also proved to be instrumental to their interests in conversion (R. Jeffery 1988; Arnold 1993; Van Hollen 2003a). This legacy could have contributed to the active role of the state and NGOs in public health services in the postcolonial era.

The cultural argument—also highly simplified—suggests that gender equity is greater in South India than in North India (Wadley 1980; Miller 1981; Dyson and Moore 1983; Agarwal 1994). Greater gender equity relates to higher levels of education and literacy for girls and women. And education—although not a panacea—is, of course, key for both HIV/AIDS prevention and care efforts. It is also possible that greater gender equity might translate into women having more leverage over their own sexuality both within and outside marriage. Greater gender equity could also contribute to a cultural climate that is more comfortable with and receptive to media and educational programs for HIV/AIDS (and reproductive health) that address sensitive topics of sexuality.

The economic argument for relatively better responses to both reproductive health issues and HIV/AIDS in Tamil Nadu in the late twentieth and early twenty-first centuries—the time period coinciding with the history of HIV/AIDS in India—is that both economic liberalization since 1991 and the high-tech boom centered in South India (with Chennai as one of the hubs) has led to the creation of a larger middle class with greater access to education and increased resources to spend on health care. However, the flip side of the economic argument is that liberalization and the high-tech boom have compounded the health problems in the region, particularly HIV/AIDS, because new jobs in urban centers have led to increased migration, which is correlated with increased HIV transmission. Liberalization has also led to increasing privatization of health care, which has arguably further disenfranchised the impoverished members of society (Banerjee 2004).

The fourth argument is the political argument, which maintains that it is the unique populist nature of Tamil Nadu state politics that accounts for greater attention to health care within the population, particularly among the poor. In her dissertation, "Public Policy and Maternal Mortality in India" (Smith 2009), Stephanie Smith asks why maternal mortality rates in Karnataka far exceed those in Tamil Nadu even though the two states have similar sociocultural contexts. Her analysis suggests that the health policy making and implementation processes in these two states diverged significantly because of differences in political will. Smith notes that differences in health policy can diverge significantly in India.

> Constitutionally, health policy is on India's concurrent list—a responsibility shared by the national and state governments. The federal government has some influence as it sets national health policy goals, develops programs and funds a portion of states' health activities. In practice, India's states are largely responsible for health policy and implementation, including a significant role in service delivery. States fund the greater proportion of public health services and activities. (Smith 2009: 33)

Echoing the comments of Sushma Swaraj from North India, Smith found that politicians in Karnataka simply did not view health as a political priority and that civil society organizations were not mobilizing around health as a rights issue. As Smith writes, "There is little evidence that health has [cachet] as a political issue amongst parties at the state-level, or is of any particular historically or socially based political value for health policy" (Smith 2009: 98). The contrast with Tamil Nadu was unmistakable.

> Tamil Nadu's long record of initiative for health is grounded in a social movement that fostered a long-term pattern of political commitment between two major parties to values for social equity and politicization of health in the state. These created conditions in the health bureaucracy that promoted interest and investment in health system development and programs of action that showed priority for social welfare and public health. As a result, Tamil Nadu has been at the fore for promoting nutrition, family planning, and safe motherhood, in addition to such health system-strengthening measures as reliable and affordable drug supply. Ongoing political attention to these issues is facilitated by shared priority and intense competition in state level politics. (Smith 2009: 117)

Indeed, Tamil Nadu has a long and illustrious history of populist politics and egalitarian movements aimed at battling caste and gender-based forms of discrimination. Some note continuous threads of such movements dating as far back as the South Indian Hindu devotional bhakti movements of medieval India. Certainly there is continuity dating back to the early-twentieth-century Dravidian movements, such as Periyar E. V. Ramasamy Naicker's Self Respect Movement, founded in 1925 (Irschick 1969; Ramaswamy 1997).

Although no one of these theories alone can explain why Tamil Nadu has held such an important position in HIV/AIDS prevention and care and reproductive health care efforts within India, I contend that together they illuminate a great deal and provide a satisfactory (if incomplete) answer to this vexing question. In this light, it is also not surprising that Tamil Nadu has played a key role in India's PPTCT program.

The Emergence of the PPTCT Program

Given the place of prominence that Tamil Nadu has occupied in the arenas of both reproductive health and HIV/AIDS, it is no surprise that three of the eleven hospitals in India selected by NACO to pilot the PPTCT program were in Chennai (Kuganantham 2004: 117). These were the Institute for Obstetrics and Gynecology (IOG), Chennai; Kasthurba Gandhi Hospital; and Rajah Sir Ramaswamy Mudaliar Hospital, all tertiary-care "Centres of Excellence" maternity hospitals with medical schools attached. After five years of "sentinel surveys"[10] (from 1995 to 1999) in Tamil Nadu, the pilot phase of the PPTCT program began in April 2000. It primarily used the antiretroviral zidovudine (AZT), comparing it with nevirapine. According to Dr. P. Kuganantham, who was in charge of the PPTCT program for TNSACS, this pilot study concluded that nevirapine "was more advantageous than AZT when used as a single dose for the mother and child" (Kuganantham 2004: 117). Nevirapine has therefore been used in the PPTCT program since that time. The PPTCT program was run through the auspices of NACO with technical support from UNICEF. SACSs, such as TNSACS, administered the program locally.

There are three ways that HIV can be transmitted from mother to baby: (1) during the prepartum period, when HIV can spread through the placenta to the fetus in the blood stream; (2) during delivery—the intrapartum period—when the baby may be exposed to the mother's blood during birth, especially through lesions in the mother's vagina; and (3) through breastfeeding in the postpartum period, when HIV can spread through the breast milk as well as through cracks in the nipples as a result of mastitis. Of these three paths the intrapartum period poses the greatest risk of transmission. Without any interventions, transmission rates can vary from 15% to 30% without breastfeeding and can be as high as 40% with breastfeeding up to 24 months (WHO 2002). Several strategies can be used to reduce this risk. The maximum protection involves the use of triple ART for the mother administered regularly during the second and third trimesters of pregnancy and during the postpartum period, combined with oral therapy for the infant at birth, an elective cesarean delivery, and the use of substitute feedings instead of breastfeeding for the infant. The use of all these things together is referred to as the "full package" of care to prevent HIV transmission from mother to child. HIV-positive mothers using the full package of interventions in the United States and Europe have been able to reduce the rate of transmission to less than 2% (WHO 2002).

Most women in the world, however, do not have the resources to use all these strategies. In addition, most governments and international aid organizations claim that they do not have the resources to provide all women with the means to use all these strategies together. Paul Farmer has vehemently critiqued this discourse of limited resources, pointing to the ways that it allows governments and international aid organizations to avoid the politically challenging task of equalizing the distribution of resources (Farmer 1999). This critique is more than warranted when we consider that only 0.7% of India's GDP went toward health care in 2004.[11] The Government of India and international donor groups have by and large accepted the logic of the discourse of limited resources. A compromise solution has therefore been made in India to give pregnant women living with HIV/AIDS a single dose of nevirapine at the time of delivery and a single dose of nevirapine syrup to the infant at birth. This treatment alone, without any other interventions, has been shown to reduce the risk of transmission to 8–10%.[12] Cesarean sections are not routinely performed for HIV-positive women through the government's PPTCT program, nor are replacement feedings provided free of cost.

At the time of my research in 2004, sixty-five hospitals in Tamil Nadu were participating in the PPTCT program. According to UNICEF, this meant that in 2004 approximately 20–25% of all pregnant women in Tamil Nadu were being covered by this program.[13] It is important to note that most women who attend public maternity hospitals in India come from low-income families, because women from the middle and upper classes (and even some from the lower class) typically go to private hospitals for obstetric care. The PPTCT program, therefore, both serves and targets women living in poverty who would not otherwise be able to afford these treatments.

Statistical Success of the PPTCT Program in Tamil Nadu

According to the TNSACS report for 2003 (published in 2004), the core components of the PPTCT program were counseling, informed consent, confidentiality, HIV testing, mother care, child care, family planning, and community networking. By the end of 2003 the program in Tamil Nadu had been rolled out in sixty-five centers (fourteen government medical college hospitals, six private medical college hospitals, twenty-eight district government headquarters hospitals, nine Corporation Health Posts, and eight private hospitals) (TNSACS 2004a: 4). The program covered 326,100 mothers in the state with HIV group counseling, gave HIV tests to 172,639 of these mothers, and identified 1,088 HIV-positive mothers through this program, indicating an infection rate of 0.6%. Seven hundred twenty-three (67%) of those HIV-positive mothers delivered their babies, of which 708 were live births. Eighty-five percent of those mothers with live-birth babies reported exclusive breastfeeding of their infants (TNSACS 2004a: 4). Overall, TNSACS reported an increase in mothers receiving prenatal counseling and testing over the course of the year in 2003 and also a marked increase in the number of mothers accepting HIV testing when they were coming directly to the hospital for delivery without having had any prior prenatal care at the hospital. HIV rates among these mothers coming for direct delivery were substantially higher than the rates among mothers tested during prenatal care (TNSACS 2004a: 6). TNSACS also noted that both pre-natal counseling and HIV testing rates were higher for urban mothers than for rural mothers: In July 2003 there were 32,224 urban mothers and 44,617 rural mothers registered in the PPTCT program. Ninety percent of the urban mothers received group counseling, as opposed to 78.2% of the rural mothers. In addition, 77.5% of the urban mothers received HIV testing, as opposed to 58.7% of the rural mothers (TNSACS 2004a: 7). Also, HIV prevalence rates across different districts within the state showed significant disparities, with Kanyakumari District recording a 0% rate for the PPTCT program on one side of the spectrum and the districts of Namakkal and Ariyalur reporting more than 2% (TNSACS 2004a: 8).

This was the statistical landscape at the onset of my ethnographic research in 2004. Since that time the PPTCT program has been officially implemented throughout India and has grown substantially. By 2009, 1.03 million pregnant women were covered under the PPTCT program in Tamil Nadu, and 91% of the mothers found to be HIV-positive through this program and their infants were given nevirapine.[14] For India as a whole, by 2008, 4.61 million women were counseled and tested for HIV during their prenatal care in government maternity hospitals; 21,483 pregnant women were found to be HIV-positive; and 10,494 mother-baby pairs were given a single dose of nevirapine (NACO 2009: 16).

As will be clear in Chapter 3 and throughout much of this book, the goal to achieve high numbers of women accepting HIV testing and accepting nevira-pine treatment if found to be HIV-positive propelled much of the PPTCT pro-gram. My ethnographic research examines the social processes and effects of this program and raises some issues beyond the public health arena indicated by these statistics. Based on my observations of prenatal HIV counseling and testing in some of the PPTCT centers in Chennai and on interviews with coun-selors and lab technicians at these public maternity hospitals, I found some discrepancies between the stated objectives of the prenatal HIV counseling and testing on the one hand and the actual implementation on the other.

3 "The HIV Test Is Like an Immunization"

Scenes from Prenatal HIV Counseling

AS IN MUCH OF THE WORLD, in Tamil Nadu HIV/AIDS is interpreted predominantly through the lens of the morality of sex. The prevailing view is that HIV/AIDS comes about as a result of *tahaada udaluravu*, a Tamil phrase that is most often translated into English as "illegal intercourse" or "illegal sex" and refers, not to law per se, but to all premarital and extramarital sexual relationships, both of which fall outside the prescribed norm in Tamil Nadu. Recent studies have revealed that sexual practice does not always conform to these normative ideals in India, and it is also well-known that an unstated double standard that tolerates men's premarital and extramarital sexual relations prevails (Goparaju 1998; Puri 1999; Jejeebhoy 2000; Verma et al. 2004). This is corroborated by comments from women I interviewed, as will be shown in Chapter 4. Nevertheless, the norms prevail. Thus, to be HIV-positive in Tamil Nadu is to be marked with a grave social transgression, and the disease is intensely stigmatized. Even when speaking in Tamil, the English translations of *tahaada udaluravu*, particularly the use of the English word *sex*, are used more often than the Tamil phrase. Stacy Pigg finds this to be the case in Nepal as well. Pigg argues that this kind of linguistic code switching provides a more neutral, safe way for people to discuss taboo topics while simultaneously marking the speaker as modern (Pigg 2001: 512–24). This explanation applies to the South Indian context as well.

Before the PPTCT program, HIV testing in Tamil Nadu was performed primarily in hospital wards designated for the treatment of STDs. This contributed to the stigmatization of people who might be seen going to have the test. According to women I met, if they did muster the courage to go in for the test, they sometimes faced derogatory statements from the medical staff administering the test. As one NGO community health worker in Chennai told me:

> One woman came to me and said very frankly, "My husband has connections [*sambandam*] with other women [i.e., sexual relations]. From what I have seen on the television, I think he has symptoms of HIV. I think I also have these symptoms." So I took her to the public hospital. There she was asked, "How many men do you entertain in a day?" This question upset her a lot. Instead of asking her how the infection came, they straightaway blamed her. We reported this to the head of our Health Post and they took up the complaint. Such incidents deter people who should be tested and who need health care from seeking it.[1]

In short, the overall stigma of being HIV-positive in one's family and community, the stigma of going to an STD ward, and the discrimination faced when getting tested all serve as deterrents to voluntary HIV testing.

In the United States since the mid-1980s, HIV counseling and testing centers have come to be viewed as a key component of HIV prevention in two respects. First, people found to be HIV-negative are provided with information about HIV transmission and prevention that, it is argued, will help them reduce their risks going forward and will therefore help them to remain HIV-negative. Similarly, those who receive an HIV-positive diagnosis receive counseling that, it is argued, will help them to take steps to avoid transmitting the virus to others. In short, as João Biehl and colleagues wrote, "The testing service became increasingly a preventive strategy under the banner of 'information dissemination on risk reduction and behavioral change' for both uninfected and infected clients. This intervention was based on a rational decision-making model, in which knowledge of the potential negative consequences of a person's behavior was seen as sufficient to influence his/her behavior" (Biehl et al. 2001: 106–107). Because such rational decision-making models are not accurate reflections or predictions of human practice, it is not surprising that social scientific studies have often found that the preventive impact of HIV counseling and testing is limited (Dawson et al. 1991; Higgins et al. 1991; Ickovics et al. 1994). Once antiretroviral treatments such as AZT were developed in the late 1980s, the focus of HIV testing in the United States shifted to being a gateway to treatment for HIV-positive people. But the earlier model, which viewed HIV counseling and testing centers as nodes for prevention, became a core component of global HIV/AIDS policy in other parts of the world, particularly in contexts where ARTs were unavailable or beyond the financial reach of most of those receiving an HIV-positive test result.

The Government of India established Voluntary Counselling and Testing Centres (VCTCs) in 1997 with voluntary, free walk-in services for anyone wanting to know his or her HIV status. The VCTCs were viewed as distinct from the PPTCT centers, but these two have now been programmatically combined and remodeled as the Integrated Counselling and Testing Centres (ICTCs) (NACO 2007b: iii). Because the Indian government did not roll out its ART program to treat HIV-positive people themselves (as opposed to the PPTCT program, which provides treatment for preventive purposes) until the middle of 2004, the VCTs and ICTCs were initially established for preventive measures alone, and prevention still remains a core goal of these centers today. In 2007 the NACO website stated:

> As of today, only 13 percent of HIV positive people in the country are aware of their status. The challenge before NACO is to make all HIV infected people in the country aware of their status so that they adopt a healthy lifestyle, access life-saving care and treatment, and help prevent further transmission of HIV. This counseling and testing are important components of prevention and control of HIV/AIDS in the country. (NACO 2007a)[2]

Unlike studies done by Biehl et al. (2001) in Brazil and Lupton et al. (1995) in Australia, in which the investigators discovered that large numbers of people who were not considered to be "at risk" were voluntarily coming to such centers for HIV testing, in India the VCTCs were underutilized. Thus, although the PPTCT program is aimed specifically at preventing HIV transmission from mother to child, it should also be viewed within the broader context of the drive to increase "voluntary" HIV testing in the general population. The assumption is that women living with HIV/AIDS and their partners who come to know of their status through this prenatal testing will take both preventive and palliative measures accordingly.

Based on my research, in this chapter I explore how counselors working in the PPTCT centers discursively negotiated the social and biological risks associated with HIV testing as they tried to encourage low-income pregnant women to undergo the test. I demonstrate that one approach was to circumvent the informed-consent process of HIV testing. Another tactic was to normalize the test as a basic part of prenatal care and to represent it as akin to prenatal immunizations. A third strategy was to emphasize the potential for "innocent" and "guilty" modes of transmission when motivating women to get tested and when getting them to convince their male partners to come in for testing. I argue that these strategies were used in part because of the pressure that the counselors felt to demonstrate statistical success in the numbers of women (and men) who undergo HIV testing; this is reminiscent of the target-based approach to the Family Planning program implemented in government maternity hospitals that I have documented previously (Van Hollen 1998, 2003a).

Official Structure of the PPTCT Program

The PPTCT program in Tamil Nadu was set up in such a way that when a woman came in for her first prenatal visit at a Government Hospital that had a PPTCT program, she would be registered as a patient with the hospital and then sent directly for group counseling with a PPTCT counselor. These counselors were employed by TNSACS and had been trained through one of two NGOs: the Chennai-based SIAAP or Gramodhaya. Counselors reported having taken six months of training to become PPTCT counselors. They had a range of backgrounds, mostly in social work and psychology rather than medical training. The minimum requirement to enroll in the training course was that the trainee must have completed the tenth standard. In her reflections on the relative success of SIAAP training in general (not just for PPTCT) over the years, Shyamala Natarajan, the SIAAP director, explained that initially SIAAP recruited people with postgraduate degrees. However, they found that, although these people were good educators, they did not always make the best counselors: "They had too many inhibitions about sex and sexual behaviour to be able to work with a truly non-judgmental attitude," and, because of the class differences between these postgraduates and most of their clients, these counselors tended to "sympathize" rather than "empathize" with their clients, leading to increased alienation (Natarajan 2004: 129–30). As a result, beginning in 1999 SIAAP changed its recruitment approach to try to include people who would be more comfortable discussing issues of sexuality and less judgmental about HIV/AIDS, such as people living with HIV/AIDS, homosexual and bisexual men, and sex workers. Overall, Natarajan concluded that "the optimum training group appears to be one that has a mix of people qualified in social work, psychology or sociology, PLHAs [people living with HIV/AIDS], and people with experience and understanding of sexuality-related issues such as MSMs and women in sex work" (Natarajan 2004: 133).

The PPTCT counseling was the first point of entry into maternal health care for these pregnant women. Counselors were expected to first provide women with group counseling about basic prenatal care and HIV prevention, particularly prevention of HIV transmission from mother to child, and then answer any questions the women might have. Following the group meeting, counselors were instructed to give individual counseling to pregnant mothers during which time they would try to ascertain their risk status for HIV, answer any personal questions the mothers might have, and try to motivate women to agree to have the HIV test. During the individual counseling, counselors were instructed to obtain written informed consent for HIV testing from mothers who voluntarily agreed to have the test before sending them to the lab for testing. Furthermore, counselors were instructed to try to get pregnant women to bring in their male partners for testing as well.

The ideal goal was to get the new mothers and their partners to agree to undergo HIV testing at the same time. There was both a public health and a sociocultural rationale for this. From a public health perspective it was possible that a woman whose husband was HIV-positive might in fact also be HIV-positive but, because of the window period, the woman's test result might read HIV-negative.[3] This situation was particularly possible if the couple was newly married, this was their first pregnancy, and the woman was fairly early on in her pregnancy. From a sociocultural perspective the concern was that if a wife tested HIV-positive, her husband might refuse to get tested and the stigma and blame would be placed squarely on the shoulders of the woman when, in fact, nine times out of ten, it was the husband who had infected the wife. It was because of these cultural issues that NACO chose to use the "prevention of *parent* to child transmission" appellation rather than adopt the internationally recognized "prevention of *mother* to child transmission" (PMTCT) terminology. The appellation and the recommendation to have partners tested at the same time were done in the interest of promoting gender equity. Some have argued that this appellation creates confusion and detracts from the program's aim to prevent transmission to the child and the biological fact that the transmission of the HIV virus to the child, which this program hopes to prevent, comes from the mother.[4]

The PPTCT Program in Tamil Nadu: The Practice

What in fact transpired in the patient-counselor interactions, how women interpreted the counselors' advice, and how women and their partners went about making decisions about HIV testing was much messier and more complex than what is spelled out in any guidelines. First, the extent to which informed consent was sought was uneven.

Informed Consent

In the first hospital where I observed HIV counseling and testing, counselors did follow the guidelines to the best of their abilities. They met with groups of five to ten women—typically accompanied by other female family members and children and sometimes also in the midst of a large waiting room with women seeking other prenatal care needs (to see the doctor, to get an ultrasound scan, etc.)—for group counseling, and then they did their best to provide individual counseling. However, providing individual counseling proved to be a nearly impossible task given the lack of private space in the hospital allotted to the PPTCT program. Typically these individual counseling sessions involved a counselor sitting in a chair across from a woman seated on the bench. They huddled together so that they could converse in whispers; the surrounding women stretched their necks and cocked their heads, straining to pick up whatever bits of this conversation they could. It is no wonder that counselors complained repeatedly about the constraints placed on their ability to successfully carry out the kind of individual counseling they had been taught to give through their training. As one counselor explained:

> Earlier we did the counseling in a separate room. But now we have been asked to counsel in the OP [outpatient] hall itself. This is a problem. The patient does not pay attention. We speak with them in the presence of many people. The place is noisy and people keep coming and going, and patients are reluctant to ask questions or to converse freely. When this point was raised in the hospital, we were told, "If you so wish, you can continue in the Health Post. If not, you can get transferred elsewhere. Furthermore, you are not indispensable. TNSACS pays you. If you wish, feel free to leave." We are threatened in this way.

The PPTCT program was negotiating with the maternity hospitals to get a separate space for the counseling sessions, but, given that space was already limited for these hospitals to carry out their other functions, it was not surprising that they were not able to provide private counseling rooms for the new PPTCT program.

Furthermore, there was discernible tension between the staff of the maternity hospitals, who seemed to want to defend their turf, and the staff of the PPTCT program, who were trying to establish themselves. It was clear that it would take some time to work out the kinks of inserting a new program into a preexisting one. I suspect that the staff of the maternity hospitals may have resented having to change the way they did things and give up space (both literally and figuratively) to the PPTCT staff, particularly given concerns that a disproportionate amount of international aid money was being allocated for HIV/AIDS, thereby crowding out other dire health needs, such as basic maternal-child health care (Shiffman 2006, 2008).

These resentments manifested themselves in a variety of ways, from the petty to the profound. For example, in one hospital a female counselor was on hand to counsel the pregnant women in the PPTCT program and a male counselor was down the hall for the VCTC program; his primary job was to counsel the partners of the women in the PPTCT program. The PPTCT program was administered through TNSACS, whereas the VCTC program was administered through the Corporation AIDS Prevention and Control Society (CAPACS). Both counselors complained that the nurses in the hospital incessantly teased and scolded them for talking to each other when they were both unmarried, accusing them of having a romantic relationship and saying that they should get married if they were going to carry on like that in public. This was particularly stressful for the female counselor, who said she did not know how much longer she could work in that kind of environment.

The lab technician for the PPTCT program at this hospital was asked by the hospital administration to pick up the lab work for the hospital's regular lab technician, who had gone on leave. The PPTCT lab technician agreed to do this, but when I met him, months had gone by and the hospital's own lab technician was still on leave and there was no indication of him returning anytime soon. When the PPTCT lab technician complained to TNSACS that he was doing two jobs, he was told to "adjust." Ultimately the PPTCT and VCTC staff members were at the mercy of the maternity staff, who held greater medical authority, and the administrators of TNSACS and CAPACS repeatedly told them that they had to learn to accommodate the hospital administration.

Counselors and lab technicians had other gripes about the lack of resources provided to adequately carry out the agenda of the PPTCT program. They complained that although they were aware of large sums of money having been transferred from TNSACS to the Corporation hospitals in which they were working to purchase such things as televisions, DVDs, and tables and chairs for the counseling, eight months later these objects had still not materialized. Furthermore, they said that they were not provided with syringes for the HIV testing, and the lab technician in one hospital said he was provided with only two sets of gloves per day so that he had to use one set to conduct all the HIV tests in the morning and the other set to test the samples in the afternoon. In addition, in one Corporation hospital that had been designated a PPTCT center, the counselors complained that they still had not received nevirapine doses, and so they had to refer the one mother whom they had found to be HIV-positive to the larger IOG–Egmore hospital for her delivery. Counselors were particularly frustrated by the shortage of resources because they believed that the government was receiving huge sums of money from foreign countries and organizations to fund this project and thought that the funds were not being used as they were intended to be. As one counselor put it, "There are lots of foreign funds coming in. But the funds don't seem to be reaching the common man. We counselors have to be silent and merely 'adjust.'" She saw me as someone who could help break this silence and asked me to please convey their complaints to the administrators at TNSACS. Another counselor used a Tamil proverb to express the same sentiment: "Having come in like an elephant, it happened like a cat." When I asked him to clarify the significance of this proverb to the situation at hand, he said [in English]: "It means that the money comes in huge sums at the top level and the expectations are very high, but only a small amount trickles down to the people who need it most and the end result is minimal."

Such allegations of corruption are a mainstay of the political discourse in India and cannot be taken as proof of any wrongdoing on the part of those people who were administering these programs through TNSACS and CAPACS. I brought up these concerns with the then director of the PPTCT program for TNSACS and with the UNICEF representative in charge of coordinating the program with TNSACS. They both acknowledged that they were still working out the kinks of initiating the PPTCT program in the smaller Corporation hospitals (Health Posts) versus the larger Government Hospitals, where they had been operating for a longer time period, and that they were trying to respond to the complaints as quickly as possible. Indeed, they said they were eager to hear from me about concerns voiced by counselors and patients so that they could respond to them. They explained that, because the PPTCT program was a vertical program and not fully integrated into the general maternity health care system, coordinating with other branches of the government so that the program functioned smoothly was a challenge. However, they assured me that the supplies of nevirapine would soon be delivered to all the designated PPTCT hospitals in Chennai. When I returned the following week to the hospital that had been waiting for its nevirapine, the supplies were in stock.

I return now to the earlier discussion about the best case scenario I observed in which PPTCT counselors in one hospital tried in earnest to provide group and individual counseling to the pregnant mothers, despite the constraints of space and privacy. These counselors would ask the mothers if they wanted to have the HIV test and, for those who were willing, they would give them a consent form to sign. Nonliterate women were asked to give a thumbprint.

In some of the other hospitals where I conducted observations, however, things ran quite differently. For example, in one hospital, after registering as prenatal patients, the pregnant women were ushered into a tiny waiting room in groups of ten or more and told to watch a video on a television screen. Like the group counseling sessions in the other hospitals, the video was designed to provide these women with general prenatal information as well as information about HIV prevention, the PPTCT program, and HIV testing during pregnancy. The video was thorough and informative, but in my observations many of the women did not watch it because they were either talking with other women (such as their mothers or mothers-in-law who had accompanied them) or tending to smaller children who had come with them. The room was typically quite noisy and active. All of this created a distraction for those women who were trying to watch the video. No counselors were present while the video was running, and there was no time for questions or discussion. After the video ended, the counselor returned to the room, passed out cards, and instructed the women to sign their names on the cards. The women would diligently follow the counselors' instructions. This constituted the informed-consent process for HIV testing in this hospital and was a marked difference from the painstaking efforts that counselors in the first hospital took to conduct group and individual counseling and request consent, all under difficult constraints.

Women interviewed in hospitals where informed-consent procedures were thorough spoke positively about the process. Women who did not receive proper informed-consent advice had mixed reactions. Some of the women I spoke to said that they did not want to be tested for HIV. For example, one woman said:

> When I came to the hospital for a check-up, I gave blood for other tests. They did not ask me if I wanted to take the tests. I did the test because everybody was doing it.
>
> My mother came with me when they did the test. I do not know if they did the HIV test. I spent nothing. No one in the hospital asked me to have the HIV test. Even though they talked about HIV on TV there, I am not interested. No one asked my husband to get tested. I do not talk about HIV even with my husband.

This woman's maternal-child health (MCH) record stated that she was HIV-negative, indicating that she had received HIV testing, even though she did not want it. Another woman said, "I am not aware that I have had any HIV test. I have given blood for testing. Nothing was said about what kind of test it was. If I am asked to have an HIV test, I will not take it." This woman's MCH record stated that she was HIV-negative, indicating that she too had received HIV testing without her consent. A third woman said, "They showed us a video, and that was useful because it talked about the benefits of breastfeeding. Then they told me that they were going to take a blood test for jaundice and diabetes. After the test, they said they had also tested for HIV and asked for my signature. I did not want the test but I signed because it had already been done."

The following two quotes similarly demonstrate incomplete informed consent, but in these cases it is clear that these women were inclined to accept the test and therefore did not feel that strict informed-consent procedures were necessary.

> Only the counselor advised me. It appealed to me and I accepted it in my mind. I had group counseling. They gave me a card and told me to sign it. I signed it. They asked everyone to have the test. They did not ask me if I wanted to have an HIV test. Neither do I feel that it was necessary for them to ask for my permission. I thought that I should know my HIV status.

> For the second child, when I went to the Government Hospital, they made a card for me. Then they counseled me. They asked me about my husband's habits. Then they tested me. They did not make me sign a consent form. It was compulsory. It is good to tell about HIV and then test.

In the WHO, UNAIDS, UNICEF, USAID, and CDC joint guidelines for pretest counseling during pregnancy in "resource poor" contexts, written informed consent was and continues to be considered imperative, and this measure has been adopted by the Government of India. The CDC policy recommendations on informed consent for the United States, however, were significantly altered in 2006, with a change away from "risk-based testing" to "screening" for pregnant women and a shift from pretest counseling (including prevention counseling) with written informed consent to a policy in which "patients should be informed orally or in writing that HIV testing will be performed unless they decline (opt-out screening)" (CDC 2006: 10). The nature of informed consent has thus been radically altered under the "opt-out screening" approach, the rationale being that this approach will increase HIV testing and improve the efficiency of clinical prenatal care. In the "Rationale for New Recommendations" section of the 2006 CDC report, the first rationale states:

> Since the 1980s, the demographics of the HIV/AIDS epidemic in the United States have changed; increasing populations of infected persons aged < 20 years, women, members of racial and ethnic minority populations, persons who reside outside metropolitan areas, and heterosexual men and women are

unaware that they are at risk for HIV. As a result, the effectiveness of using risk-based testing to identify HIV-infected persons has diminished. (CDC 2006: 5–6)

Thus, as prevention efforts in the United States have shifted from focusing on the more affluent gay white male community to the less affluent heterosexual female minority communities, domestic health policy for HIV testing is shifting from an individualistic human rights–based approach, which has been adopted within the global health policy framework, toward an approach that downplays the individual patient's fully informed decision in favor of the interests of a broader concept of public health, which resembles the local practices I encountered in Tamil Nadu. This raises an extremely controversial question: Are the individual rights of certain groups of people protected more than the individual rights of other groups of people? It remains to be seen how the shift in the U.S. policy will affect global health policy.

The women I interviewed in public hospitals who had also been to private hospitals (either for the same pregnancy or for a previous pregnancy) reported that there was no discussion about HIV whatsoever during their prenatal care in private hospitals; they were never asked for consent to get an HIV test, and they had no idea if an HIV test had been done. Some added that they did not see any problem with the possibility that they were tested without consent because they thought it was good for everyone to get tested. As one woman put it, "I did not get counseling when I was pregnant. They checked me before delivery. They did all tests for me. I was not consulted about having the test. But not asking is not an issue. Doing the test is good. I do not think prior permission to do the HIV test is necessary. There is no need for permission in my opinion." In my interviews with HIV-positive women who had received prenatal care in private hospitals, this lack of informed consent was a common theme. I heard of several cases in which the private medical institutions simply referred HIV-positive patients elsewhere without disclosing their HIV status. Some women living with HIV told me that private medical practitioners do not require informed consent because they consider HIV testing to be like other routine tests. Other women told me that the staff at some private hospitals fear that a patient may refuse to get tested given the option and that the hospital personnel will not treat anyone who is HIV-positive because of their fears of HIV transmission during medical treatment; they simply test without informed consent and refer any HIV-positive patients to private or public hospitals that are known to accept HIV patients, such as those with PPTCT services.

Kielmann and colleagues' study of the uncertainties that private practitioners in the North Indian city of Pune feel with respect to HIV testing and treatment corroborates this finding (Kielmann et al. 2005). In their interviews with private practitioners, Kielmann and colleagues found that often private medical practitioners would perform routine HIV tests for all patients "as a means to rule out their own fear and uncertainties about patients with recurrent infections rather than testing for the sake of the patient" (Kielmann et al. 2005: 1545). In addition, they found that obtaining consent for testing is rare because private practitioners "perceive their patient population to be of limited capacity for understanding the test and its implications" (1545). Furthermore, the doctors fear that patients will not return for follow-up if they know they are required to take an HIV test. Confirming the opinions of women in my study, the private practitioners in Kielmann's study admitted that they typically referred patients to other "specialists" without informing them of the HIV diagnosis (1546).

By pointing to this pattern of the uneven or nonexistent nature of informed consent in the context of HIV testing during prenatal visits at public and private hospitals, I do not mean to suggest that the informed-consent model is inherently the best policy in every case. It is certainly not fundamental to how health care has always been delivered in India. Many patients are understandably surprised and somewhat confused by having people involved in providing medical care asking them as patients to make a decision about what medical procedures they do or do not want. As some of the women stated, they do not see the need for the elaborate informed-consent practice required for HIV testing because it is not a requirement for most other prenatal tests. Indeed, the extent of the emphasis on informed consent for HIV testing has its roots in the gay activist framing of the response to the disease in the United States in the 1980s; activists viewed HIV/AIDS as an exceptional disease because of the intensity of the stigma attached to it, and therefore informed consent and confidentiality were of utmost importance, particularly in the days before ARTs were introduced. As discussed earlier, the U.S. practice has itself now shifted to the opt-out model of HIV testing as the epidemiology of the disease and the public health response to it have shifted away from the epicenter of the gay community.

Furthermore, some scholars have pointed out that the newfound emphasis on the ethics of informed consent within the global guidelines for all sorts of medical interventions is driven, in part, by the interest in providing legal protection for medical interventions that are increasingly being carried out for profit interests. Examples of these procedures are when women in India are asked to give consent to donate "spare embryos" in return for free in vitro fertilization treatments, which these women otherwise could not afford (Bharadwaj 2011), or when people are asked to give consent to participate in clinical trials in return for medical care that would otherwise not be available to them (Petryna 2009). In these instances we can see how ironically the bodies of certain populations, typically marginalized groups, are rendered "bioavailable" (L. Cohen 2005) precisely through the process of informed consent.

In short, I recognize these critical dimensions to the centrality of informed consent within the global and national guidelines for HIV testing, and I understand that such medical ethics should be interrogated as anthropological problems in and of themselves (Ong and Collier 2005). But my interest in this chapter is simply to point to the contradiction between the stated requirement for informed consent within these global and national guidelines on the one hand and the actual practice of prenatal HIV testing in India on the other. Expressing her frustration with the uneven practice of informed consent in the PPTCT program, Shyamala Natarajan wrote:

> If we wish to make it a policy to test all pregnant women under all conditions, then we need to be straightforward about it and acknowledge that informed consent may not be the most appropriate process for our situation. But we are currently making a mockery of the whole process, with everybody claiming to have received informed consent while, in reality, it is nothing of the sort. In our eagerness to follow international guidelines, we follow neither the prescribed process nor the practical one. Instead, we adopt a convenient mishmash that actually harms patients. (Natarajan 2004: 136)

In Chapter 7 I discuss how these practices in fact affected HIV-positive women as they tried to get access to obstetric care.

Making the HIV Test Palatable

Even in those instances where the PPTCT counselors closely followed the global and national policy guidelines by providing pretest counseling and soliciting informed consent before the test, they presented information in various ways to make the HIV test more appealing to the patients and to get them to accept the test and to get their partners to also accept. To appreciate this, we need to take a look at how information about HIV testing is conveyed to these pregnant women. Here is an excerpt from one PPTCT group counseling session, which is representative of other sessions I observed. In this case one PPTCT counselor is facing a group of eight pregnant women and the family members who accompanied them.

Counselor: Do you know why immunizations are given?
One pregnant woman in the group: It is so the child will be healthy.
Counselor: Yes. Do you know how many immunizations will be given during the pregnancy?

There was no reply to this question from the women.

Counselor: You will be given two. You must also eat nutritious food. You must drink milk and eat lots of greens. Similarly, do you know why various tests are conducted while you are pregnant?

There was no reply to this question from the women.

Counselor: The urine test is to find out the salt and sugar levels in the urine. If you have too much salt in the urine, your legs and hands will have swelling and the delivery will be difficult. If you find salt in the urine, you can reduce how much salt you are taking. Then the delivery pain will be less and the legs and hands will not swell.[5] "BP" [blood pressure] and the "scan" are also tests you have during pregnancy. Have you heard about HIV/AIDS? Do you know what it is?

There was no reply to this question from the women.

Counselor: HIV/AIDS is a "virus," a *kirumi*. If it enters the body, it cannot be removed. But it can be controlled. If it is inside us, our immune system reduces and then various diseases attack us. We cannot stop this disease. HIV/AIDS spreads in four ways only. First, "sex" without condom with various and unknown persons. Second, blood transfusion without HIV testing. Third, injections with unsterilized syringes used on various persons. And fourth, from the mother to the child. If the mother is "HIV-positive" during the pregnancy, medicines can be given to the mother and you can stop the transmission to the child. But this can only be stopped if the mother gets an HIV test during pregnancy. In that way, the HIV test is like an immunization.

The counselor then went on to discuss the importance of using condoms to prevent both unwanted pregnancies and HIV transmission. She told the patients that their husbands should use condoms if they have sex during the pregnancy to make sure that the baby is not infected with HIV. She then gave a demonstration of how to put on a condom using a real condom and a model penis, and she told the women that the condoms are available for free from the hospital. Next she discussed the importance of breastfeeding and said that breastfeeding was better than other feeding methods because the mother's milk would provide the baby with lots of immunities. She then closed the session by saying:

Counselor: It is also important for your husbands to get the HIV test. There is something called a "window period." It means that it is possible that even if you get a test and it is "negative," you might have the HIV *kirumi* but because of the "window period," it has not had enough time to show up in your blood. So the only way to know if that is so is if your husband is also tested. You should convince your husbands of this. They could have gotten HIV if they had *tahaada udaluravu* without telling you. But they could also have gotten it from a blood test, or they could have gotten it from donating blood. They need to know this. You need to tell them that they could have gotten HIV from having a blood test. Next time you come, be sure to bring your husbands with you for the test. Now, if any of you have any questions, you can ask me alone.

That marked the end of the group counseling session.

Several points can be made about this counseling session, but here I want to make three. First, we can see how counselors try to normalize HIV counseling and testing by integrating it into general prenatal care. Of course all these prenatal tests (urine tests, ultrasounds, etc.) can also be seen as routinized and as normalizing biomedicalized models of birth (Davis-Floyd 1992). What is interesting here is that, although the global health policy guidelines for HIV testing make the HIV test exceptional in terms of the process of informed consent, the counselors seem to being going out of their way to present the HIV test as being just like any other test in order to compel the women to give their consent.

Second, counselors deftly encourage patients to agree to get the HIV test by presenting the test itself as a form of immunization. As the counselor said, "The HIV test is like an immunization." In this first counseling session the social or medical consequences of a positive test are not discussed. Counselors told me that those are issues that come out in deeper one-on-one discussions in individual counseling with women. But the fact is that the counselor makes the one-on-one counseling an option, and many women do not pursue it. For many, if not most, the one-on-one session consists of the moment when the counselor asks the woman if she will take the test and asks her to sign the consent form. Medical anthropologists studying the use of other prenatal diagnostic tests in the United States, such as ultrasound and genetic testing, have similarly noted that, in the interest of compelling women to undergo testing, counselors tend to emphasize the reassuring nature of these tests following negative test results (i.e., negative in the biological sense) and to downplay the social and psychological trauma and physical suffering that may ensue with a positive test result (Browner and Press 1995; Taylor 1998; Rapp 2000).

Third, the counselors play into the innocent or guilty dichotomy of the HIV/AIDS blame discourse to make it easier for women to accept the test and convince their husbands to also get tested. On the one hand, all HIV-positive people get stigmatized and are viewed as tainted and morally bereft, particularly because HIV/AIDS is associated with sex and intravenous drug use and these two things are morally charged in most parts of the world today. On the other hand, we also see how societies categorize HIV-positive people as either innocent or guilty, often deeming children, receivers of blood transfusions, and increasingly "housewives" as innocent and lumping others—especially commercial sex workers (female and male), intravenous drug users, and "men who have sex with men"—together as guilty and somehow responsible for their fate. This discourse has been pronounced in India, as reported by the journalist Siddharth Dube (2000), who makes a plea to overcome this gross misrepresentation in India: "This prejudice is wrong, for every reason. As mortals, as people who are ourselves at risk of contracting HIV/AIDS (or suffering other tragedies), we must remember that every single person infected got it innocently, unwillingly, through no fault of theirs. Nobody deserves to die prematurely and with such suffering" (Dube 2000: 3). The counselor seems to allude to this innocent or guilty dichotomy when she said: "They could have gotten HIV if they had *tahaada udaluravu* without telling you. But they could also have gotten it from a blood test or . . . from donating blood [i.e., if these medical procedures were done using unsterilized, HIV-infected syringes]. They need to know this. You need to tell them that they could have gotten HIV from having a blood test." "They need to know this" seems to be a code to give women a comfortable way to broach this subject with their husbands—a way not only to justify to their husbands why they themselves are choosing to have the test but also a guilt-free way to invite their husbands to be tested. The irony that the counselors are highlighting the potential risks of medical blood tests in their attempt to encourage men and women to accept a blood test did not seem to register with either the counselors or the patients in these interactions.

Another example of the ways in which PPTCT staff members carefully choose their presentation of facts to encourage HIV testing can be seen in the interaction between the lab technician and the patients in the context of providing syringes for the test itself. Among other issues, the lab technician at one of the PPTCT hospitals complained to me that they were not provided with an adequate number of syringes to do the HIV tests. As a result, he was in the position of having to tell patients to go across the street to the pharmacy to purchase their own syringes and return for the test. In a private conversation with me he complained about how underresourced they were at the hospital and how he felt bad for having to send women off to buy their own syringes when it was a public hospital. He worried that women might not agree to get tested if they had to buy their own syringes. I expected the pregnant women to be equally indignant about this. But not at all. One woman who bought her own syringe had this typical response: "The lab technician explained to me that nowadays many hospitals ask people to buy needles from the pharmacy as a protection. They say it is good for us to get in the habit of buying our own syringes so that we will not get AIDS. This is not a problem for us. It is only 5 rupees. We think of this as protection for us. In this way, the people and the hospitals together are responsible for not spreading this disease." Here we see how Michel Foucault's notion of biopower (Foucault 1978) operates at the microlevel to ensure that individuals are exercising self-discipline over their bodies in such a way as to voluntarily act in accordance with the interests of the state and how this kind of governmentality is internalized in positive ways.

There is certainly nothing wrong with the government making public health recommendations and trying to encourage its citizenry to adopt certain practices that are deemed beneficial to them or to the public. But shouldn't citizens also be given full information before making choices about their health care? Why is all this duplicity—whether conscious or unconscious—necessary? To fully understand this, we must appreciate the pressures that counselors felt to increase the number of HIV tests for pregnant women and their partners.

Why the Duplicity?

During their training, counselors were told not to fixate only on getting immediate high acceptance rates for HIV testing. In fact, the program director of SIAAP told counselors that patient refusal of testing after the first counseling session is a sign of good counseling because the principle of counseling is to allow individuals to make their own decisions; thus refusal after the first session should be interpreted as a sign that the individuals want time to reflect on the pros and cons of testing and to discuss the issue with family members before returning to have the test done, preferably bringing their partner along for testing as well. [6]

Yet, based on my discussions with PPTCT counselors and on my observations of a three-day monthly review meeting organized by TNSACS and
UNICEF to evaluate counselors' job performance, it was apparent that counselors felt that they were being evaluated on the basis of the levels of acceptance of testing and treatment. For example, during the counselor evaluation
meeting, I observed one situation in which a counselor with low HIV-testing
acceptance rates was transferred from his city post to the rural hill station of
Kodaikanal. From the expression on this blue-jeaned urbanite's face, this was
clearly perceived as punishment. Counselors thought that there was a contradiction between what they felt was important for good counseling and what
was expected of them on the job. As one of the more disgruntled counselors
put it [in English]: "We are not doing counseling work. We are only doing
clerical work. We are clerks. The counseling idea from the West is good. But in
Tamil Nadu we have a way of turning everything into clerical work only. They
[TNSACS] are happy only if we keep good records and have good numbers.
They don't care about the counseling." Of course, prenatal HIV counseling in
the West is not always as comprehensive as this counselor seems to think. As
de Bruyn points out, there is a growing concern that the turn to the "opt out"
approach to prenatal HIV testing in some countries in the West may result in
insufficient information and questionable consent in prenatal care (de Bruyn
2005: 4–6).

The goal of the PPTCT program seemed at times to be to generate statistics that would demonstrate a high percentage rate of HIV testing and of
HIV-negative babies born to HIV-positive mothers. Counselors had to provide
reports to TNSACS, which in turn sent reports to NACO in Delhi. According to
SIAAP's program director, international aid organizations that provided funding for NACO and for the counselor training took these statistical reports into
consideration when allocating funds.[7] At the time, NACO was receiving funds
from the World Bank, the U.K. Department for International Development,
USAID, and the Canadian Development Agency (K. Jain 2002: 161). Thus the
PPTCT program seemed to operate within an unstated international, national,
and statewide targetlike approach that was the mainstay of the Family Planning program through 1996 (Van Hollen 1998, 2003a). Under these conditions
lower class pregnant women were not provided with complete and balanced
information about their reproductive health options. It is no accident that just
as the Family Planning program in India over time came to be integrated into
maternal health care to increase the number of family planning "acceptors" that
were demanded by international donors and government bodies, once again

the public maternity hospital had become the primary site for increasing HIV testing. In fact, one community health worker interviewed in Chennai went so far as to recommend that in order to increase HIV testing and prevent the spread of HIV/AIDS in India, the government should develop a monetary incentive scheme modeled after the earlier Family Planning target program. As she put it:

> It should be handled just like "family planning" was. . . . The government should give some monetary incentives for people to get tested. At first "family planning" was not accepted. There was great resistance. Now people practice "family planning" on their own initiative. Propaganda is the key. Remember how Indira Gandhi nearly forced "family planning" on people? In that way, HIV testing must become as routine as sugar tests [for diabetes].

Prevention of HIV transmission from mother to child is a critical public health measure in the battle against the spread of HIV. But poor, undereducated mothers deserve to know what they are subjecting their bodies to and what the potential consequences of their choices are. Sandra Hyde's work on HIV/AIDS prevention in China points to what Mary-Jo Good calls the aesthetics of statistics in public health (Good 1995 and 2001, cited in Hyde 2007: 37). Hyde rightly explains that "statistics allow governments to expand their moral and material authority over their citizens" (Hyde 2007: 38). My research on the experiences of women who test positive for HIV during pregnancy suggests that the bureaucrat's aesthetic can be the patient's worst enemy. The tyranny of large numbers has effects unforeseen by global health policy makers.

For most of the women the PPTCT counseling was the first prenatal advice they had ever received from a medical institution. Most prenatal mothers attending the hospitals with PPTCT programs were between the ages of 18 and 25 years old, were experiencing their first pregnancy, and had been married for less than five years (Kuganantham 2004: 119). HIV/AIDS counseling and testing was becoming the entry point for women's prenatal care, and HIV/AIDS was becoming a central and defining issue concerning prenatal care for these mothers, thereby further pathologizing pregnancy. Critical feminist anthropologists have argued that the biomedicalization of pregnancy and birth has pathologized reproductive processes, constructing them as inherently risky and necessitating biomedical intervention and thereby disempowering birthing mothers (Martin 1987; Davis-Floyd 1992). In this regard, foregrounding the risk of HIV transmission within the prenatal care provided to lower class women in India who attend the government maternity hospitals may have the effect of further pathologizing pregnancy. Although this can be a beneficial public health intervention, it is worth considering how this is affecting women's experiences of pregnancy and motherhood. How did the pregnant women attending these government maternity hospitals respond to the PPTCT program and make decisions about HIV testing during pregnancy? This is the question I pursue in the next chapter.

4

"I Don't Need My Husband's Permission"

Women's Views on HIV/AIDS and
Decisions About Prenatal Testing

IN CHAPTER 3 I DESCRIBED HOW COUNSELORS compelled pregnant women to get the
HIV test. In this chapter I explore pregnant women's own opinions about and
decision-making processes for prenatal HIV testing and partner testing. I also
address women's perceptions of the danger that HIV/AIDS poses to India, their
views about sexuality in India and its relation to the emergence of this disease,
and their opinions about recommendations regarding premarital HIV testing.
The information presented in this chapter is drawn from interviews conducted
with sixty-five randomly selected pregnant women during their prenatal checkups at government maternity hospitals with PPTCT programs in Chennai.
These women had sociocultural backgrounds similar to the backgrounds of
the HIV-positive women profiled in Chapter 1. They came from lower class and
lower caste communities and had low levels of education.

My interviews with these women reveal some trends that run counter to con-
ventional wisdom. Most significantly, whereas social scientists who study health
care decision-making processes in India often argue that women in India—
especially undereducated, unemployed, poor women—have little control over
the decision-making process surrounding reproductive health (P. Jeffrey and
Jeffrey 1997; Ramasubban and Jejeebhoy 2000), my interviews demonstrate that
women attending Government Hospitals in Chennai assert that they do in fact
take decisions into their own hands, and they are sometimes even offended by
the suggestion that their husbands should be included in decisions about their
prenatal care. Choosing to accept HIV testing of their own volition seemed to
be one way that women thought they could demonstrate their independence.
Ironically, this decision may contribute to the situation in which women are
increasingly being diagnosed as HIV-positive before their husbands are, and, as

the remainder of this book demonstrates, this often has negative consequences for HIV-positive women in their extended families.

Furthermore, contrary to the moral finger-pointing by such public figures as the former minister of health Sushma Swaraj and Dr. A. S. Paintal, who represented HIV/AIDS as a foreign disease wrought by immoral behaviors of "Westerners" and "Africans" that would not pose a threat to the majority of morally superior Indians, low-income women interviewed during their prenatal checkups perceived HIV/AIDS to be a serious threat to India but had no idea whether or not it was a problem elsewhere in the world. Some thought that the emergence of HIV/AIDS was revealing the long denied truths about people's sexual behavior in India. Others suggested that sexual practices in India had changed in recent times (especially among urban college students) as a result of foreign (i.e., Western) influence and that HIV/AIDS was the price to pay for this in India, but they did not view AIDS itself as a global problem.

When asked what they thought could be solutions to preventing the spread of HIV/AIDS, many women stated that they were not well educated and therefore were not in a position to make any recommendations. Most gave general responses, arguing that the government and the medical establishment needed to do more to find cures and provide information about preventing the spread of HIV or that the solution had to begin at home with each individual, that increased fear and self-induced discipline were required to reign in people's sexual practices and thereby stem the tide of HIV. Mandating premarital testing seemed like a good idea to most of the women interviewed in this context, although some doubted whether such a policy would be widely accepted within the Indian cultural context.

Women's Perceptions of HIV/AIDS

All the women interviewed for this portion of my study told me that before receiving counseling from the PPTCT counselors, their primary source of information about HIV/AIDS was the television. Some women said that in addition to television, they had also learned about HIV/AIDS from seeing banners and posters in public places or through dramas performed in their neighborhoods. These sources all represent media that TNSACS, in collaboration with other international donors, most notably USAID's APAC Project, used to disseminate its IEC materials about HIV/AIDS. A few women also told me that they had learned about HIV/AIDS in the tenth standard in school, but because the average level of education in this group was the eighth standard, most were never exposed to this material. Furthermore, for most of the interviewees who did complete their secondary school education, HIV/AIDS was not discussed in the curriculum. Although the Tamil Nadu government supported HIV/AIDS education in the context of sex education in schools, they faced a forceful opponent in the person of Sushma Swaraj, who was then the minister of health for India and was against condom promotion, which, she argued promoted promiscuity (Joshi 2003). Earlier, as the minister of information and broadcasting, she had banned sex education broadcasts, believing them to promote adultery (Gosh 2005: 494).

How had the women I met processed the information that they did obtain from these disparate sources? Interestingly, these women all believed that HIV/AIDS had become a serious threat to India, but they had no idea whether or not it was a problem in other countries. One woman did say that she thought people in Russia were also contending with the disease. Another thought HIV/AIDS was a problem faced by all of humanity. All the other women flatly stated that they did not know whether any other countries were dealing with this disease. This may seem surprising given what Paul Farmer refers to as the "geography of blame," in which other nations and whole continents (such as "Africa") and "others" within nations (such as gay men or Haitians in the United States) are discursively constructed as being the source of HIV/AIDS. As discussed earlier, the Indian government engaged in this sort of rhetoric in the early stages of the AIDS epidemic in the 1980s; they denied that AIDS was or could become a threat to the Indian population to the extent that it did in the United States and sub-Saharan Africa because Indians subscribed to a different set of cultural values (i.e., they did not engage in *tahaada udaluravu*) and therefore were not at risk as a nation. In that early stage the primary risk was thought to come from African students coming to India and from other Western visitors, and thus prevention was focused on mandatory testing of these groups of foreigners entering the country. Women in their late teens and 20s who participated in my study had not been exposed to that kind of nationalist discourse about HIV/AIDS and were unaware of the global impact of this disease.

The prevailing sense I got from my interviews was that, before the HIV counseling that they received through the PPTCT program, these women all believed that HIV/AIDS came about as a result of *tahaada udaluravu*. In short, they associated HIV/AIDS with immoral behavior, leading to its stigmatization. A typical explanation I heard went something like this comment from a 20-year-old woman: "If one is disciplined, if *penn* [women] are moral, it can be prevented. If women are not disciplined in 'sex,' it can come. Those women to whom it comes are *thevadiya* [prostitutes]." In Chapter 5 I further explore the gendering of stigma for HIV-positive people and the tendency to view this as a women's disease. For the most part, the women I interviewed rhetorically singled out female commercial sex workers as the source of HIV infection. This is not surprising given that the governmental and nongovernmental programs had been targeting this population in its prevention efforts. Only after pointing to the sex workers did the women in my study also say that HIV gets transmitted because men seek out sex with commercial sex workers.

Most of the women I interviewed said that if someone contracted HIV/AIDS, there was no cure and that person would die quickly. Many referred to HIV/AIDS as the *uyirkolli noi* (killer disease). The earlier IEC materials had used this phrase in campaigns aimed at changing behavior through fear. At the time of my research the IEC materials were no longer using this language because it was believed to perpetuate problems of stigma and discrimination for those living with HIV. Thus, although the walls of prenatal waiting rooms in the maternity hospitals displayed bright yellow and green pictures of happy mother-baby dyads to emphasize the successful prevention of mother-to-child transmission and "positive living," the closed room where the medical staff and counselors gathered in one of these hospitals still had a black and red "AIDS = Death" sticker prominently displayed.

Some women said that they had heard on television that medical treatments were now available to prolong the lives of HIV-positive people and that it was wrong to ostracize people who have this disease because they deserve as much care and support as anyone else. But others saw the connections between class, access to treatment, fear, and stigma. As one woman explained: "Educated people are not so scared of this disease, and they will be cared for by their families because they can afford to buy medicines to make them live longer. But for most of us, for the poor and the uneducated, these attitudes are just starting, but it is different for us because we cannot afford to buy those medicines." Recall that at that time there was no government program to provide ART free of cost.

A few women said that they had heard there was a cure for AIDS. Specifically they had heard that cures for AIDS were available through *nattu marundu* (country medicine) treatments, such as Ayurveda, Siddha, and homeopathy. Indeed, the HIV-positive women I met were well aware of doctors' claims to have Ayurvedic medicines that would cure AIDS. T. A. Majeed's clinic in Kochi, Kerala, was widely known among people living with HIV/AIDS. Families in Tamil Nadu spent large sums of their earnings to travel to Kerala to procure such treatments (Van Hollen 2005). I had visited Majeed's clinic and watched in horror as he told HIV-positive men that if they took his Immuno-QR pills for a specified length of time, they would convert from being HIV-positive to HIV-negative and they would no longer need to worry about using a condom when having sex with their wives and that if their pregnant wives took this medicine, there would be no need for them to use ART to prevent transmission of HIV to their babies. The networks for positive people, as well as the Lawyers Collective (a civil society organization headquartered in Mumbai), were actively working to prevent such practitioners from advertising claims of cures for HIV/AIDS and in some cases to prevent them from practicing altogether.

The women I interviewed in the government maternity hospitals told me that, although they had some vague ideas about HIV/AIDS, gleaned from various sources, most of what they knew about HIV/AIDS was what they had learned through the counseling they had received in the PPTCT program during their prenatal care. The consensus among the women interviewed at these PPTCT centers was that the prenatal HIV counseling they received provided them with valuable information and a deeper understanding about HIV/AIDS. It was through this counseling that many came to know for the first time that HIV could be transmitted from mother to baby and that the government was providing medicines that could help prevent this transmission. All agreed that this was a helpful new program, particularly for the poor who attended these Government Hospitals. As one woman said, "This scheme is important for poor people because poor mothers cannot afford to buy medicine themselves to protect their babies."

It was also during this prenatal pretest counseling that most of the interviewees learned that HIV could be transmitted through infected needles, not just in the case of intravenous drug use but also in everyday medical care if the medical practitioner was reusing an infected syringe. Furthermore, they said that during the prenatal counseling, they became aware that HIV could be transmitted through blood transfusions if the blood had not been properly screened for HIV. Some women said that they were vaguely aware of these things before the counseling but that during the counseling things became clearer and they became aware that even people who had not done anything morally wrong (*tappu*) and who had not engaged in *tahaada udaluravu* could get this disease. As discussed earlier, I suspect that these "innocent" modes of HIV transmission may have been overemphasized by counselors in the interest of getting women to accept HIV testing for themselves and to convince their husbands to get tested.

In short, to the extent that informed consent for HIV testing was in fact solicited from women during their prenatal care, the women were making their decisions on the basis of, first, the assumptions they had before counseling. These ımptions consisted of notions about HIV/AIDS that they had received from television and other media programs and from which they had come to view HIV/AIDS as a threat to India, something caused by *tahaada udaluravu*, and a killer disease. Second, the women were basing their decision on information conveyed by counselors in the PPTCT programs, which highlighted benefits of the prevention of mother-to-child transmission as well as nonsexual modes of transmission. It was from this vantage point that women were called on to decide for themselves whether or not to have an HIV test during pregnancy. Furthermore, because of their interest in also getting male partners tested for HIV at the same time as the women were, counselors often presented the decision-making process as one that ideally should be made in the context of a conversation between the woman and her husband. Again, this was motivated in part by the impetus to increase the number of people tested for HIV. It was also done in the interest of protecting women from being the only ones in the family to be tested and therefore singled out and discriminated against. It may have also been recommended in part because of a widespread assumption that Indian women typically do not make decisions about their health independent from their husbands and other family members.

Women's Decisions About HIV Testing During Pregnancy

What I found interesting was that the women themselves often seemed somewhat insulted by the suggestion that they should include their husbands in their decisions about whether to get the HIV test. Several women interpreted this to mean that counselors thought they should get permission from husbands to have the HIV test. When I too asked whether they had discussed HIV testing with their husbands, many interpreted this as a question about whether they got permission. Most were adamant that they did not need permission from their husbands or from anyone else to get the HIV test. One was a 20-year-old woman who had a ninth-standard education and described herself as being a member of a Scheduled Caste. Her husband was a tea master, and he earned approximately 2,800 rupees per month. She had come to the maternity hospital for her first prenatal checkup in the eighth month of her pregnancy, and she brought her 3-year-old daughter with her. I knew that she had had an HIV test and asked how she had decided to get the test and whether anyone else was involved in her decision to get tested. She replied:

> The counselors in this hospital told us about HIV, about how it comes, about how to prevent it from spreading from mother to child. And they gave advice

about getting a blood test for HIV. I accepted the counseling. I have just now had the blood test. This is the right decision for me. So I made my own decision and did the blood test. They said that I should discuss this with my husband and that he should get tested as well. But I don't need anybody's permission for this. I made this decision myself. I didn't need to get my husband's permission.

I heard a similar response from a 21-year-old woman coming for prenatal care in the eighth month of her pregnancy; she said she was a member of a Scheduled Caste and had studied through the seventh standard. She worked for an hourly wage at a catering company, and her husband had a job cleaning airplanes. Together they earned a total monthly income of 2,750 rupees. She said:

> They [the counselors] talked of many matters. I came to the hospital all by myself, and no one from my family was there for the counseling. I did not consult anyone in my family about whether or not to get the test. They [the counselors] told me to talk with my husband about this. But I didn't need to do that. I just went ahead and had the test. I told my husband that I had gotten myself tested only after I had the test. I didn't need to speak with him first.

Another woman's situation was slightly different because she did broach the topic of testing with her husband before getting tested. In essence, however, her story echoed that of the other women because she too voiced the opinion that this was her own decision to make. She was 23 years old and in the sixth month of her pregnancy. She was from the Mudaliar caste[1] and had studied through the tenth standard. Her husband was an electrician, and with the combined income of three men in their joint family (living with her parents-in-law and her husband's brother and his wife) she said they earned a total household income of 4,500 rupees per month. Here is what she said:

> My husband has come with me now. I asked my husband what he thought about the HIV test for me. He said it should be according to my wishes. He didn't have any second thought about it. I haven't yet had the test. I am going to do it today. . . . Up until now, he has not received any counseling. I received counseling for myself today only. Whether or not he gets tested is according to his wish. I don't know whether he will accept it or not. This is my decision. I am taking this test for my baby and for myself. Like this, he has to decide whether it's necessary or not. It's according to his liking. In my opinion, it would be good for him to be tested. I hope he will. He and I will always have a physical relationship, isn't that so? So I think it's a good idea.

These responses might not seem so surprising were it not for the fact that social science studies have often suggested that women in India by and large do not have much say when it comes to decisions about their reproductive health care. For example, Ramasubban and Jejeebhoy state in the introduction to their 2000 edited volume, *Women's Reproductive Health in India*:

> Good maternal health is also severely constrained by women's lack of authority to make health care decisions for themselves, seclusion practices that restrict their mobility, socialization that leads them to underplay their own health problems and bear them in silence, and lack of control over economic resources with which to seek health care. It is equally constrained by men's justification of the central role they play in health care choices for women. (Ramasubban and Jejeebhoy 2000: 21)

Several of the contributions to Ramasubban and Jejeebhoy's book echo the theme of Indian women's (and adolescent girls') lack of power in reproductive health decisions pertaining to such things as sexual activity, abortion, contraceptive use, pregnancy and delivery, and treatment of STDs.

In their book *Population, Gender, and Politics: Demographic Change in Rural North India*, Patricia Jeffery and Roger Jeffery point out that women in their study in North Indian rural communities "rarely decided to contracept themselves" (1997: 152); reproductive decision making about the number of children to have was typically a collective decision involving not only the wife and husband but also parents-in-law and parents. Nevertheless, Jeffery and Jeffery also argue that this does not imply that North Indian women have no agency when it comes to reproductive decision making, and they critique scholars such as Dyson and Moore (1983), whom they say make such assumptions based on a core cluster of structural determinants when comparing women's autonomy in North and South India. Jeffery and Jeffery suggest that the concept of women's agency (vs. autonomy) helps to better grasp women's active participation in reproductive decision making, and they find James Scott's concept of the "weapons of the weak" to be a useful tool for understanding the nature of women's agency in the context of reproduction in India (P. Jeffery and Jeffery 1997: 117–25).

I would argue that the statements women made about not needing their husbands' permission to make decisions about their prenatal health care represent such weapons of the weak. The decision to get the HIV test during pregnancy may have been one clear domain over which women felt they could assert control about reproductive decisions. My interviews can only represent what women say about decision making and do not capture what in fact transpired in practice. As such, these statements may tell us more about women's subjectivity and their desire to represent themselves as having autonomy over their reproductive decisions than about who, in fact, makes such decisions in private.

Similarly, Margaret Greene and Ann Biddlecom point out that, in their questionnaire-based studies from such disparate places as Egypt and the United States, men tend more often than women to assert that they have greater responsibility than their wives in reproductive decision making. This tendency may reflect "respondents' attempts to present a certain image to the interviewer" (Greene and Biddlecom 2000: 99) and cannot be assumed to represent the actual social practice of decision making. In short, men's assertion may be a reflection of the value of male dominance from the male perspective in various cultural contexts more than a window onto actual gender relations.

Some stories of HIV-positive women presented in other parts of this book indeed demonstrate the powerful role that husbands and other family members can and do play in women's reproductive decision making in Tamil Nadu. Nevertheless, these women's strong assertions that they alone make these decisions about HIV testing and that they do not need their husbands' permission to make decisions "for my baby and myself" are significant insofar as they defy stereotypes not only about women's potential role in reproductive decision making but also in terms of their subjectivity about their agency. It is interesting that the last woman quoted feels not only that she can make decisions for herself but also that, as a mother, she is in a position to make decisions "for my baby." Whereas the HIV-positive women in my study were mostly recruited from networks and therefore had already been exposed to a transnational feminist, human rights discourse about HIV/AIDS and reproductive health, the women interviewed in the government PPTCT hospitals were randomly selected. Perhaps this suggests that such individualistic subjectivities and reproductive-rights-based discourses are becoming more mainstream in Tamil Nadu.

Although in Chapter 3 I shed light on the structural factors of the PPTCT program that compel low-income pregnant women to undergo HIV testing, the comments presented in this chapter also show that these same women view themselves as having and asserting their agency within the arenas of both the medical encounter and their families. In Chapters 6–9 I similarly reveal ways in which HIV-positive women pragmatically use their agency as they navigate the myriad structures that constrain their reproductive decision making.

Women's Views on Partner HIV Testing

In the account of the last woman quoted, not only do we see how she felt about the issue of deciding whether she herself should get tested, but we also get insight into her thoughts on the issue of partner testing. Just as hospitals differed in the extent to which fully informed consent was obtained, my interviews suggested that the degree to which counselors, even within the same hospital, recommended that women bring their husbands in for testing also varied. Most of the women I met who were advised to bring their husbands in for testing thought that this was a good idea. Some in fact had gone home to discuss testing with their husbands and had returned with their husbands so that they could both be tested at the same time. But these cases were rare in my sample. Another woman told me that she had been tested and, although she tested HIV-negative, on the counselors' advice, she convinced her husband to also get tested because he had donated blood many times. She said that if a man and a woman had premarital sex with other partners, they should also get tested, but that was not the case for her and her husband, although how she knew this was unclear because she also said that they had never spoken about sexual experiences before their marriage, nor had they spoken of such things during their marriage.

Most women said that their husbands would agree to get the test and would think it was a good idea. However, they would go on to explain that, although they themselves had already been tested, their husbands had not because it was difficult for them to take time off from work to come in for the test. Many said that their husbands were wage laborers, and if they took time off to come in for the test, they would lose their wage for that day and that would create too much of a hardship on the family. Others said that their husbands were migrant laborers and frequently had to travel for work and therefore were not able to come to the maternity hospital for the test. Certainly the concerns about sacrificing wages are real, and indeed it is not uncommon to see people postponing much needed health care for these reasons. However, it is also possible that this gendered discourse about the nature of men's work can sometimes be used as a convenient excuse for men not to have to subject their bodies to the same kinds of interventions that women do. I have seen how this discourse operates in Tamil Nadu to justify why women are more likely to undergo sterilization than men (Van Hollen 2003a). Lawrence Cohen's work on organ donations has pushed my work on sterilization further, suggesting that in the globalized sites of the commodification of bodies and body parts, women's bodies have come to be viewed as being more available to medical operations, as having greater "operability" and "bioavailability," which serves the interests of both capital and the state (L. Cohen 2004, 2005). Women often buy into such discourses on the basis of normative assumptions about gendered divisions of labor and the value placed on men's versus women's labor; as a result, they do not think that it is appropriate to put too much pressure on their husbands to come to the hospital for testing.

In his ethnography about HIV/AIDS, caregiving, and dying in Botswana, Frederick Klaits found that, once antiretroviral medications became more widely available to the general population, women increasingly chose to get tested for HIV and to get their children tested, whereas men were reluctant to do so. Klaits explained that the health care workers in the Botswana clinics attributed this difference to the gendered differences in caregiving roles among women and men in Botswana and to "different conceptions of how anticipating their own respective deaths would affect their love and care for other people" (Klaits 2010: 243). Women thought that it was their responsibility to get tested so that they could get access to ARTs if they were HIV-positive; treatment would enable them to be healthy enough to take care of their children for as long as was necessary to bring them up to an age at which they could begin to take care of themselves. On the contrary, for a man, if he knew he was HIV-positive, he could become so emotionally disturbed by the prospect of his death that he might become suicidal and lose the "capacity to earn money, plan for the future, and act as a provider" (Klaits 2010: 243). Therefore women sought out HIV testing and men avoided it, although both did so to be good caregivers according to the gender norms of their society.

Klaits's study also suggested that in Botswana men did think that it was their responsibility to get tested when their partners were pregnant to protect their future children. Because my research was focused on women's perspectives, I do not know whether this kind of gendered perception of HIV testing also exists in India. Further studies could shed light on this. However, based on what women in my study reported, it seems that the situation is different in India because several HIV-positive women reported that their husbands in fact had been tested for HIV outside the context of pregnancy but had often kept that secret from their wives. In addition, when a woman was found to be HIV-positive through a prenatal test, many men tried to avoid getting tested, as I discuss in Chapter 7. Furthermore, apart from prenatal HIV testing and HIV testing done for women in my study who had a history of sex work, it does not appear that women are choosing to get an HIV test of their own accord so that they can be better nurturers. I suspect that the differences in gender patterns in India and Botswana with respect to HIV testing are probably due to the HIV prevalence rate in

Botswana being exponentially higher than that in India, the government's provision of ARTs in Botswana being more successful than it was in India during my research, and the greater stigma and discrimination faced by HIV-positive women in India than by HIV-positive men, as discussed in Chapter 5.

Most of the women I met during their prenatal care in the PPTCT center agreed with the counselors that even if they themselves were HIV-negative, it would be a good idea for their husbands to be tested because of the possible window period. Furthermore, several women thought that if both they and their husbands were tested, it would deepen their relationship, the assumption being that they would both be HIV-negative. As one woman put it, "If my husband also gets tested, it will strengthen our faith in each other." The counselors also used this idea to encourage women to bring their husbands in for testing. As we will see in the remaining chapters of this book, the stories of HIV-positive women and their relationships with their husbands after learning about their HIV status reveal how naïve this statement is in many cases. Medical anthropologists working in a variety of sociocultural contexts have reported on the use of the same kind of discourse used by counselors, technicians, and medical practitioners engaged in other forms of prenatal diagnostic testing; to motivate women to undergo prenatal tests, the counselors and medical personnel tend to emphasize the relief that mothers will feel from a "normal" outcome, and they underplay the social and psychological challenges the mothers could face if the result is out of the normal range (Browner and Press 1995; Taylor 1998; Rapp 2000).

However, not all responses reflected such perceived harmonious relations between husband and wife. One woman said that she wanted her husband to be tested to avoid his suspicions of her if she were to test HIV-positive. Another woman flatly stated that she wanted her husband to be tested right in front of her because she was suspicious of him. Furthermore, although most stated that they were certain their husbands would agree that it was a good idea for them to be tested, a few women had different responses. For example, one woman told me that her husband would consider it beneath his dignity to get tested. Another said her husband would beat her if she so much as suggested that he should get an HIV test.

Among the seventy HIV-positive women I interviewed, few learned of their HIV status at the same time as their husbands through couples testing in PPTCT programs. As I discuss later, several of these women were first tested after their husbands' illness or death resulting from AIDS. Some also learned of their HIV status as a result of their own health problems or the health problems of their children. Many did learn of their status through HIV testing during prenatal care, although for most of these women, their husbands were not tested until after the women themselves received a positive test result. Or, in some cases, such as Saraswati's (as described in the Prologue), husbands had previously gone for an HIV test but had done so secretly and had kept their HIV-positive diagnosis secret from their wives.

The number of women who reported having undergone couples testing during their pregnancy markedly increased between my 2004 interviews and my 2008 interviews. Based on some of my 2008 interviews it seems that in some hospitals the counselors were not simply urging women to get their husbands tested but were insisting that husbands get tested before either conducting tests or disclosing test results. For example, one woman told me that when she went for a prenatal care visit in a public hospital in 2008, the counselors recommended HIV testing but told her that they would not test her unless her husband came in for the test as well. When she brought him in on her next prenatal visit, her husband was tested first and found to be HIV-positive and then they tested her. She told me that the counselors were doing this because "sometimes the husbands will say, 'This is not my child so I do not need to get this test.'" Chellamma, another woman I interviewed in 2008, said that after she was tested, the counselors in the hospital refused to give her the test results until her husband had also come in to get tested. Once he had the test and was also found to be HIV-positive, they disclosed both HIV-positive test results and counseled both of them together. Because of a concern with stigma, Chellamma and her husband decided not to tell anyone else in their family. One and a half years later, when Chellamma's husband got very sick, his family took him to another hospital and he was once again tested and found to be HIV-positive. When the family learned of this, Chellamma's father-in-law (who was also her maternal uncle, following Dravidian kinship patterns, which I discuss later in this chapter) made her take the test in front of him and then he informed the rest of the family of her status. After that, she said the only person in her family who would talk to them and support them was her mother.

The Impact of HIV/AIDS on the Discourse and Practice of Sex

Because the women I interviewed saw HIV/AIDS as being primarily transmitted through "illegal sex" and thought AIDS posed a crisis for India as a country, this led to a discussion about the relationship between sexual mores and practice in India. When I asked the question, "Has HIV/AIDS changed the way people talk about sex or changed sexual practices?" the answers were animated.

First, women told me that the fact that HIV/AIDS had become a problem in India was in and of itself a clear indication that people were engaging in pre-marital and extramarital sexual relationships. In this sense the disease became a barometer for *tahaada udaluravu*. As one woman put it:

> They say that the sense of propriety [*murai*], duty [*kadamai*], and discipline [*kattupaadu*] are strong in India. But when we see the spread of HIV, it shows that this is not a fact. We must not have premarital sex like they practice in foreign countries. It will ruin our culture [*murai*].[2] But premarital sex has increased in India. Last week I went to a hospital near my house. I saw an un-married girl who was about thirteen years old. She was five months pregnant from her father's younger brother. The doctor did a scan and said that abor-tion was not possible. The girl's mother was weeping. This is our culture today.

Dravidian kinship systems prevail in Tamil Nadu, and for many families mari-tal relations between a woman and her maternal uncle are accepted and ap-proved of. Marriage alliances between a woman and her mother's brother's son or her father's sister's son are preferable. Because descent is reckoned through the patriline, none of these relationships are considered incestuous in this cul-tural context. However, sexual relations with one's father's brother (such as that mentioned in the passage just quoted) are considered incest (because they are part of the same patriline) and are not tolerated. Clearly this woman used that story to exemplify the depths to which society has sunk, and she viewed HIV as a sign of that depravity, which she associated with foreign countries. Others also associated sex outside marriage as something that may be acceptable to people in other countries but that is not suitable to Indians. As one woman said, "The spread of HIV has brought about some changes in matters of sex. More people are using Nirodh [a condom brand]. People use Nirodh because of the fear of HIV spreading. It is not good for us to indulge in premarital sex like they do in foreign lands. It will not suit us. The fear of HIV has reduced *tahaada udaluravu.*"

Another woman was also critical of sexual relationships outside marriage that she said prevailed even in the face of the AIDS epidemic: "No changes are apparent in sex matters. People have not changed. Usage of Nirodh has increased. But it is not good to have premarital sex. We are not as advanced as in your country. It is good for men and women to be friends. But it must not become a sexual connection. Premarital sex is common. It has not reduced. This is not good." It is interesting to note that this woman is critical of premari-tal sex while simultaneously being self-deprecating about this critique, as when she says, "We are not as advanced as in your country." Here, the implication again seems to be that this is suitable for foreigners (especially Americans) but not for Indians because India has not progressed to the same level of sexual liberation. Was she saying this for my benefit? Perhaps. For yet another woman, it was quite simple: "Young people are ruined from watching foreign movies." Thus, although these women had no idea whether HIV/AIDS was a problem elsewhere in the world and although they did not lay blame directly on foreigners for the actual spread of HIV/AIDS, as politicians had earlier, clearly they viewed the morality of foreigners, especially "Westerners," as the cause for what they considered changed behaviors that put Indians at risk for HIV/AIDS.

Others told me matter-of-factly that sexual relations outside marriage were common without lamenting this as the downfall of Indian culture or even criticizing it as inappropriate for Indians. As one woman put it, "There is a lot of discussion about HIV/AIDS on the television. But 'illegal sex' is still common in India. Men as well as women have premarital 'sex' and extramarital 'sex' is also prevalent. This has always been true, even though no one admits it. But people do not talk about 'sex.' That is kept secret. But AIDS is increasing so we cannot go on pretending that we do not have *tahaada udaluravu* in our country."

Whether women voiced an explicit critique of sex out of wedlock or spoke of it matter-of-factly, they did engage in a discourse that ascribed blame to particular categories of people, even though the finger was not always explicitly pointed at the "foreigner." In addition to prostitutes, the groups considered the most inclined to such sexual proclivities and intravenous drug use, putting them at risk for HIV/AIDS, were city dwellers, college students, and truck drivers. As one woman from Chennai said, "Women also have premarital sex. I know this happens in cities, but in villages people are more afraid of social condemnation and so premarital sex is less. Some neighbors of mine, the husband and wife separated and both started living with a new partner. Later, they both returned to each other. This happens in cities. Only in the city do people inject drugs. It is not there in villages. I have seen drug addicts only in the streets of Chennai."

For many others, it was not so much urbanites but "college students" who engaged in "risky" behavior, contributing to the rise of HIV/AIDS. For example, one woman who worked as a community health worker said, "College students are a big percentage of HIV-positive people due to drug addiction. And sexual control is lax among college students. College students come for abortions and we fit them with the 'loop' [an IUD]. Otherwise they come again for abortion. Parents don't know about this." Abortion rates among unmarried women are higher in Tamil Nadu than in other parts of India. Whether this reflects higher rates of premarital sex in Tamil Nadu or simply higher incidence of abortion for unmarried women who become pregnant in Tamil Nadu is difficult to assess. This woman seemed to be aware of the problem of denial that makes people naively believe that they are the pinnacle of morality while others fall short, leading people to shrug off the need for preventive practices. She mockingly mimicked the ways that women assume their husbands are beyond the pale of blame, saying, "People are resistant to discussing AIDS. Women will say, 'Oh, my husband is very honest. We don't need to worry.'" Ironically, however, when I asked her if HIV/AIDS was a problem in her community, she responded, "No, it is not a problem among my fishing community; it is a problem among 'lorry' drivers."

Had the media campaigns and public discussion of HIV/AIDS changed people's behaviors? This question met with a range of responses. All agreed that the primary effect was increased fear (*bayam*). As one woman explained:

> Because of HIV/AIDS there has been a change. Fear has come among the "gents." There is fear about whom one should have a relationship with. Not only that, even among the husband and wife, there should be fear. If a husband is going out and having a connection with anyone, the wife will be afraid that this disease will come to her. Moreover, because there are women who have affairs and deceive their husbands, this kind of fear of sex has come to the husband.

For the most part, this increased fear was viewed in a positive light if it also led to greater savvy (*ushaar*) or awareness, which could lead to preventive practices, either in terms of increased condom use or decreased sex outside marriage. Several women said they thought condom use had increased, but they added that they did not really know this for a fact and none of them reported ever having used a condom themselves. Another woman stated, "I don't see any changes. Changes are desirable. I don't think men use condoms more. If they did, how could HIV be increasing? Premarital sex has gone up; it has not come down." Some thought that sexual relationships outside marriage were declining as a result of the increased fear, or at least they thought this could be one beneficial result of such fears. As one woman put it, "Premarital sex is not good. Premarital sex is prevalent in India also. We must fear premarital sex. Awareness of the dangers of HIV must increase." Another woman revealed a draconian outlook about this issue.

> No cures should be found. Only then, the fear that there is no medicine for HIV will force people to stop their wrong habits. Since there is medicine, people think, "Oh, I will not die in six months. If I get HIV, I can take medi-

cines and I'll die only after fifteen years." During those fifteen years they go on engaging in wrong sexual habits since they think they can live up to a reasonable age, taking medicines for HIV. The fear of HIV will go. This is wrong. The fear must not go. Only the fear will force people to be disciplined.

The sad truth is that for someone like her—a *dalit* woman expecting her second baby whose husband was a "coolie" wage laborer and whose total monthly household income was 1,500 rupees (US$34)—antiretroviral drugs to prolong her life could have been nothing more than a chimera at that point in time in 2004. Yet another woman I met had a very different perspective on this issue: "Fear of HIV has not changed practice. It is good to have sex before you are married but you should marry that person. If you marry someone else but continue to have sex with your lover, that is bad." Many agreed that despite the fear and despite people's desire to control their sexual relationships more because of HIV/AIDS, in the end sexual behavior is extremely difficult to control. The need to control sexual desire within marriage was viewed as "a cruel discipline" (*kodumaiyaana kattupaadu*).

Views on Premarital HIV Testing

I wondered whether the HIV/AIDS media campaigns had led to an increase in comfort level for people to discuss sexuality and what effect that might have on premarital HIV testing. All but two women said that talking about sex was taboo in all contexts and that had not changed as a result of HIV/AIDS. One woman, however, said that husband and wife increasingly discuss sex openly with each other but that parents never discuss sex with their children. Another said, "I was not aware of many things before marriage. And I did not discuss these things at all with my husband before we were married. But now, having seen these programs about HIV on television, I talk freely to my husband. I do not know if everyone else talks freely about these matters like I do. I discuss these things freely with my mother. I will tell my daughter about HIV. I will do this when she becomes mature."

This woman's comment that she did not discuss anything about sexuality with her husband before marriage was common. Even though couples who have arranged marriages increasingly are given the opportunity to meet and correspond with each other so that they can have a say in the matter, women told me that sexuality typically is not a topic up for discussion. As I discuss in subsequent chapters, many of the HIV-positive women I met considered their lack of awareness of their husbands' premarital sexual relationships to be their greatest risk factor for contracting HIV, because they believed that their husbands had likely been infected before their marriage. This suspicion was often borne out by the fact that their husbands developed full-blown AIDS shortly after their marriage, many of them dying at a young age, leaving their young wives widowed. The HIV-positive women had strong, although not unanimous, opinions about premarital HIV testing, as will be discussed in Chapter 5. But what did these women, whom I met during their routine prenatal care checkups and who were either HIV-negative or did not yet know their status, have to say about premarital testing and whether it should be mandated? Opinions varied widely.

Some felt strongly that the government should make premarital HIV testing a law. One woman saw this as something much more worthwhile than a dowry: "Instead of asking for jewels, it is good to ask for this test. It is good to do it. But if they are scared, they won't go for testing. Both should agree. The government should make a law that HIV testing before the wedding is compulsory. Only then everyone will do it." The assumption for most was that if one partner (or both) was found to be HIV-positive, the wedding should not go forward. As one woman put it bluntly, "HIV-positive people should not marry." Another woman reported that both she and her husband did in fact get tested before their marriage. Her husband's first wife had died young, so the husband's sister insisted that the husband get tested and they also asked the bride-to-be to get tested. Both tested HIV-negative and were married. In addition, both agreed to get tested again together on the same day during her first pregnancy.

Others thought that, although premarital testing was a good idea in theory, "it will not be practical in our culture," because, even if it were a law, people would get angry if one family recommended an HIV test. It would be viewed as an insult to the other family. Some were flat out opposed to the idea, stating that it would ruin trust. One woman who had a love marriage thought that the best solution was to encourage love marriages: "Love marriage is good since each will know about the other's past." This sentiment, however, may lead to a false sense of security.

. . .

In this chapter I have provided a glimpse into what low-income women in Tamil Nadu thought about HIV/AIDS and how their opinions, combined with the institutional structures of the PPTCT program, informed their decisions about HIV testing during pregnancy. I have demonstrated that before PPTCT counseling most of these women were aware of HIV/AIDS primarily through television and other IEC campaigns, and their understanding of modes of transmission was typically restricted to unprotected sexual relationships outside marriage, which were deemed immoral. Upon entering the maternity hospitals with PPTCT programs, they received counseling about mother-to-child transmission and about other modes of transmission, such as blood tests and blood donations and transfusions, and they were either strongly advised to give consent to get tested or were tested without their full consent (as seen in Chapter 3).

Although counselors tried to encourage women to discuss the issue of HIV testing with their husbands before getting tested and to bring in their husbands to get tested at the same time they were tested, many women seemed somewhat offended by such recommendations; they felt as though the counselors were suggesting that they were not capable of making this decision on their own and that they needed their husband's permission before getting the test. As discussed, this response was particularly interesting because lower class Indian women are often depicted as not having an active say in reproductive health decisions; the response provides one example, among many others presented in this book, of the ways women use their agency to actively negotiate the structures that influence and constrain their choices about reproductive health care in the context of HIV/AIDS in India. Unfortunately, the result of women exerting their agency in this way in this particular case may in fact be detrimental to them if it means that their HIV status becomes known and disclosed to their spouses and then to their in-laws before the husband's status is disclosed. In fact, this was happening with greater frequency as an unintended consequence of a sound public health program to stem the spread of HIV from mother to child.

In the remaining chapters of this book I explore the social consequences for women who test positive for HIV and how their HIV-positive diagnosis affects their experiences during pregnancy, delivery, and the postpartum period. Before closely examining the intersections of HIV/AIDS and reproduction, however, in Chapter 5 I explore the relationships between gender, stigma, and HIV/AIDS more broadly from the perspective of HIV-positive women themselves. In the interest of encouraging women (and their partners) to get tested for HIV and in the interest of promoting the discourse of positive living, counselors in the pretest phase of the PPTCT program tend to downplay the issue of stigma and discrimination of HIV-positive people. In fact, however, my research shows that stigma and discrimination become perhaps the most salient aspects of the social lives of those women who test positive for HIV.

5 HIV/AIDS and the Gendering of Stigma

PULLI RAJA HAD BECOME A HOUSEHOLD NAME IN CHENNAI by the end of 2003. Like his Mumbai counterpart Balbir Pasha, Pulli Raja was a fictitious character created by Population Services International for their HIV-prevention media blitz campaign launched under the aegis of TNSACS in September 2003. This "self-risk perception" social marketing campaign, which targeted men between the ages of 18 and 34 from lower socioeconomic groups, began with what in media-speak is called a teaser, in this case an advertisement placed on giant billboards, posters, and television screens posing the question, "*Pulli Rajavukku AIDS varumaa?*" (Will Pulli Raja get AIDS?). This simple question created a stir: Who is Pulli Raja? Why might he get AIDS? Will he get AIDS? Follow-up ads provided further questions and finally information about abstinence, fidelity, and condom use with stylized, stereotyped images of female commercial sex workers hovering as the threat to married men and their wives. Members of some women's organizations in Chennai complained that these ads were sexist, that they portrayed women, particularly female sex workers, in a negative light, and that the ads served to perpetuate the social perception that ultimately women are to blame for the spread of HIV/AIDS in India (Majumdar 2004: 38). Studies have shown that HIV-prevention projects targeting female commercial sex workers have often resulted in further stigmatization of this vulnerable population in India (O'Neil et al. 2004).

By the time I arrived in Chennai in January 2004, I discovered that I had just missed the Pulli Raja ads because women's organizations had successfully put an end to the campaign. Although the Pulli Raja billboards had been painted over, the perception among members of some women's organizations (especially HIV-positive women's organizations) that women in India bore the brunt of the stigma and discrimination that crested in the wake of the HIV/AIDS epidemic was still palpable.

Gender ideologies and gendered social relationships are brought into sharp focus when examined through the lens of HIV/AIDS worldwide. This is of course glaringly apparent when we consider that HIV prevalence rates among women are now outstripping rates among men in most parts of the world. Since poverty puts people at risk for HIV globally, the global trend is for rates of HIV infection to become higher for women than for men, because women as a group are economically more vulnerable than men (Schoepf 1992; Obbo 1995; Farmer 1999; Majumdar 2004; Quinn and Overbaugh 2005). Furthermore, gender-based discrimination in the form of sexual violence and unequal access to nutrition, health care, and education also puts women at increased risk for HIV (MacNaughton 2004; Majumdar 2004). According to NACO, at the time of my research in 2004, 39% of all people living with HIV in India were women (NACO 2005).[1] In 2004 Dr. Suniti Solomon told me that, based on her clinical experience, the spread of HIV to women was increasing, and she predicted that HIV prevalence among women in India would soon catch up to and later exceed rates for men for the same reasons as just mentioned.[2] However, NACO's report from 2008–2009 suggests that the HIV adult prevalence rate among adult women (0.23%) still lags behind that of adult men (0.44%) in India (NACO 2009: 5).

Gender ideologies and gendered social relationships are also made apparent when we explore the gendering of stigma and discrimination of people living with HIV/AIDS. Like the women who were protesting the Pulli Raja ads in Chennai, scholars studying the social impact of HIV/AIDS globally have argued that women tend to be blamed for the spread of HIV/AIDS and, as a result, HIV-positive women face greater stigma and discrimination than HIV-positive men do (Bond et al. 2003: 9; Ogden and Nyblade 2005: 23). As I discuss later in this chapter, this condition is usually attributed to a double standard that prevails in most societies, including India, in which women are expected to be the bearers of morality, particularly in the realm of sexuality, while men are given greater license to breach norms of sexual morality. This is one of the primary reasons given to explain why NACO chose to use the term "*parent* to child transmission" rather than "*mother* to child transmission." It was hoped that fathers would undergo HIV testing during a woman's pregnancy to avoid having all the stigma placed on the woman alone and that men would be held accountable for their role in HIV transmission to their wives. But is it in fact always true that HIV-positive women experience more stigma and discrimination in society than HIV-positive men do? In this chapter I explore the nuanced ways in which HIV-positive women in Tamil Nadu themselves responded to this question.

Although much of my research supports this standard argument, my findings suggest that the gendering of stigma and discrimination in response to HIV/AIDS is more complex and context-specific. Many women living with HIV in Tamil Nadu told me that the nature of stigma and discrimination experienced by men and women varies depending on the social context. In particular, they pointed out that the gendering of stigma operates differently in the private and public spheres so that in fact in the public sphere, people are more sympathetic toward HIV-positive women than to HIV-positive men, but women do not necessarily appreciate this sympathy. Furthermore, my research also suggests that in Tamil Nadu the tendency to stigmatize women more than men is due in part to cultural constructions of gendered bodies and not just to a gendered double standard of sexual morality. Finally, I also suggest that even when a cultural argument about women's wayward sexuality is evoked to discriminate against women within the family, this rhetoric must be understood in part as a strategy to mask economically motivated responses rather than simply part of a sexist ideology per se. Thus in this chapter I reveal the complex ways in which gender, HIV/AIDS, and stigma are intermeshed in Tamil Nadu, South India.

Understanding how gender relates to HIV/AIDS-related stigma in a particular sociocultural context is not merely an exercise in cultural analysis for the sake of better understanding gender. It is also of critical importance for policy makers. They are the ones who develop programs not only for the care and treatment of HIV-positive people but also for HIV prevention, and stigma itself is known to be a major obstacle to prevention. Erving Goffman wrote that the discrimination resulting from stigma has the effect of reducing "life chances" for the stigmatized (Goffman 1963: 5). Studying stigma is therefore one way of understanding the unequal distribution of life chances. This is a key point to keep in mind, especially because the HIV/AIDS disease itself already reduces life chances without the added factor of stigma-based discrimination. The compounding of the effects of the disease and the stigma-based discrimination was particularly acute among the people involved in my study, because many of them were living in poverty and had little access to medical treatment for HIV/AIDS and little if any financial savings. Richard Parker and Peter Aggleton argue that most social scientists who study HIV/AIDS-related stigma tend to theorize stigma in overly individualistic, psychological ways and select those aspects of Goffman's work on stigma that support their approach. Instead, Parker and Aggleton suggest a different reading of Goffman and a joining of the work of

Goffman and Foucault to reconceptualize stigma as a social process that "plays a key role in producing and reproducing power and control. . . . Ultimately, therefore, stigma is linked to the workings of *social inequality*" (Parker and Aggleton 2003: 16). When we approach stigma in this way, they argue, "it becomes possible to understand stigma and stigmatization not merely as isolated phenomenon, or expressions of individual attitudes or of cultural values, but as central to the constitution of the social order" (Parker and Aggleton 2003: 17). Thus the study of gender and HIV/AIDS-related stigma must be situated at the center of social theory, in particular, at the center of theories of power.

Theorizing Stigma

Goffman's 1963 book, *Stigma: Notes on the Management of Spoiled Identity*, still stands as one of the most important theoretical analyses of the sociology of stigma. Goffman's work is arguably better known today than ever, as it is referenced not only by academic social scientists but also by the swelling number of individuals and institutions engaged in HIV/AIDS prevention and care programs around the globe. This is because the dominant social responses to HIV/AIDS documented globally have been accusation, stigma, and discrimination (Shilts 1988; Sontag 1989; Farmer 1992; Goldin 1994; Ogden and Nyblade 2005). Jonathan Mann, the director of the WHO's former Global Programme on AIDS, considered stigma itself an epidemic in need of controlling.[3]

Goffman defines stigma as a "social identity" (Goffman 1963: 2) and an "attribute that is deeply discrediting" (3) that emerges through social interactions. As he explains, when we interact with someone,

> evidence can arise of his possessing an attribute that makes him different from others in the category of persons available for him to be, and of a less desirable kind—in the extreme, a person who is quite thoroughly bad, or dangerous, or weak. He is thus reduced in our minds from a whole and usual person to a tainted, discounted one. Such an attribute is a stigma, especially when its discrediting effect is very extensive. (Goffman 1963: 2–3)

This discredited individual is differentiated from "normal" individuals: "We and those who do not depart negatively from the particular expectation at issue I shall call *normals*. . . . By definition, of course, we believe the person with the stigma is not quite human. On this assumption we exercise varieties of discrimination, through which we effectively, if often unthinkingly, reduce his life chances. We construct a stigma-theory, an ideology to explain his inferiority" (Goffman 1963: 5).

Goffman then provides a fine-tuned analysis of how "normal" individuals and stigmatized people manage their relationships with each other. As such, he views stigma as a fluid, contingent identity that is constantly created, recreated, resisted, and transformed through social practice. Reading Goffman through the lens of Parker and Aggleton (via Foucault), we can see the social negotiation of such interactions as a struggle over the power to determine the parameters of normalcy and thus of the social order. This is not to say that the stigmatized necessarily resist their stigmatization. In fact, Goffman clearly demonstrates how the stigmatized often internalize the stigma and thus participate in the reproduction of categories of normal and nonnormal, even to the detriment of their own lives. Parker and Aggleton argue that Pierre Bourdieu's notion of symbolic violence and Antonio Gramsci's concept of hegemony are both important theoretical concepts to help us understand this phenomenon by which individuals collude in their own stigmatization and thus their own oppression (Parker and Aggleton 2003: 18).

Goffman makes an important distinction between "discredited" and "discreditable" persons. Discredited people are individuals whose "differentness" is obvious through social interactions; discreditable people are those whose "differentness is not immediately apparent" (Goffman 1963: 42). HIV-positive people, particularly those who have not yet developed AIDS, typically belong to this category of discreditable people. For the discreditable, Goffman explains, "the issue is not that of managing tension generated during social contacts, but rather that of managing information about his failing. To display or not to display; to tell or not to tell; to let on or not to let on; to lie or not to lie; and to each case, to whom, how, when and where" (Goffman 1963: 42). In the ethnographic examples provided in this book, this constant concern about "managing information" is apparent.

Goffman addresses many conditions that give rise to stigma, including such physical traits as being blind, deaf, or crippled, as well as behaviors that are morally condemned by society, such as engaging in prostitution or being a criminal. The HIV/AIDS disease has proven to be a stigmatizing condition on both accounts, because of the (largely unfounded) fear of physical contagion associated with the disease and because of the moral issues that it evokes. Stigma has also been found to be more pronounced when it is associated with a condition that is incurable, such as HIV/AIDS (Ogden and Nyblade 2005). Because the modes of transmission of HIV include taboo topics and practices of sex and drug use, the moral accusations associated with this illness have been rampant around the globe and have been acute in India.

Despite Goffman's detailed analysis of the processes of managing stigma in social interactions, he does not address the fact that the experiences of stigma vary among people with the same condition, depending on various categories of social identity, such as gender, ethnicity, class, and sexuality. These differences can sometimes be pronounced, underscoring again the relationship between stigma and the production of social inequality.

As mentioned, scholars writing about gender and HIV/AIDS-related stigma in other parts of the world have reported that HIV-positive women carry a disproportionate stigma burden in relation to HIV-positive men. For example, based on a comparative analysis of HIV/AIDS-related stigma in Ethiopia, Tanzania, Zambia, and Vietnam, Jessica Ogden and Laura Nyblade found that "HIV-positive women tended to be more highly stigmatized than men" (Ogden and Nyblade 2005: 23). They explain, "Given the close associations between HIV and moral impropriety, the findings in all sites that the harshest stigma is reserved for those expected to uphold moral laws and the moral fabric of society should not be surprising. In all sites, for example, HIV-positive women tended to be more highly stigmatized than men" (Ogden and Nyblade 2005: 23).

In another study on HIV/AIDS-related stigma conducted in Zambia, Bond and colleagues found that "women are more susceptible to, and impacted by, HIV-related stigma" (Bond et al. 2003: 9). They argue that women living with HIV are stigmatized not only because of the association between HIV/AIDS and improper sexuality, which falls outside the acceptable cultural script for women, but also because the association renders women "everything they should not be." As they explain: "Women living with HIV and AIDS (or more often, suspected to be living with HIV and AIDS) are regarded as everything they should not be—sick and slim when they should be healthy; being cared for when they should be caring for others; sexually deviant when they should be sexually righteous. To be HIV-positive is not to be a proper woman" (Bond et al. 2003: 45).

During my research in Tamil Nadu, women members of the networks with which I was involved in Chennai, Namakkal, and Coimbatore frequently made the same argument. They explained to me that because of a double standard of sexual mores, women tended to be blamed for *tahaada udaluravu* more than men and that because HIV is assumed to result from "illegal sex," HIV-positive women often tended to face greater stigma and discrimination than HIV-positive men. I begin this chapter with an analysis of interviews with women who supported this viewpoint and then move on to a discussion of other perspectives presented to me in order to highlight the need to challenge this standard argument.

Before moving on to my case studies, though, it is useful to consider how Susan Seizer describes and interprets the gendered nature of stigma in Tamil Nadu, not as it applies to people living with HIV/AIDS but rather to people engaged in a particular form of theater in Tamil Nadu, known as Special Drama (Seizer 2005). Actors involved in Special Drama in Tamil Nadu explain that they are stigmatized because their lifestyle requires them to interact publicly with members of the opposite sex to whom they are not married, including traveling together and even touching each other on stage, and such behavior is considered inappropriate in Tamil culture. In addition, the roles that they play, particularly in comedy scenes, require them to publicly act out stereotyped characters who transgress social norms (enhancing the comical nature of the scene). As a result, the actors are said to "lack *murai*, a kind of propriety and sense of social order" (Seizer 2005: 31). Just as Bond and colleagues argue that HIV-positive women are viewed as being not "proper," the Special Drama actors too are said to lack propriety. Seizer explains that *murai* in fact comes to stand for Tamil culture itself: "Murai names a set of densely interconnected concepts regarding the norms of Tamil social organization. It defines a range of cultural expectations for the "normal" course of Tamil life" (Seizer 2005: 33). To view people as lacking in *murai*, or propriety, is thus to view them as lacking in culture. Within a Levi-Straussian analytic, this would then suggest that they are viewed as being nonhuman, and indeed this is precisely the point that Goffman was making when he wrote that the stigmatized are "not quite human" (Goffman 1963: 5).

Yet it is significant that among Seizer's informants, *murai* does not refer to culture in the generic sense but rather specifically to Tamil culture. In fact, in her conversations with actors about *murai* they clearly view *murai* in culturally relativistic terms, recognizing that what is considered proper and normal for Tamil culture is not universal and thus recognizing that the stigma actors experience is culturally relative—that the stigmatized behaviors that are considered inappropriate in Tamil society are perfectly acceptable in other societies. Such behaviors are referred to as "foreign" (read "Western"). They are seen as a threat to Tamil culture and are looked on with derogation. Stigma thus serves in this case to produce and reproduce Tamil ethnic (and even national) identity and to construct differences between the Tamil self and the foreign other.

Seizer's work clearly demonstrates that among Special Drama actors, women actors are much more severely stigmatized than male actors. As Ogden and Nyblade point out in their work on women and stigma, women in Seizer's study are blamed for breaching codes of culturally defined Tamil morality because the expectation is that women should be the bearers of morality and tradition within society. Other scholars revealed this tendency within anticolonial Indian nationalist discourses (Chatterjee 1989) and within Tamil nationalism (Lakshmi 1990; Ramaswamy 1997).

The existence of HIV-positive women threatens normative ideals of Tamil culture, ideals that are considered different from "foreign" culture. HIV/AIDS-related stigma is thus part of a process of defining, producing, and reproducing people's sense of their own culture, in this case, Tamil (or even Indian) culture. I argue that the spread of HIV not only threatens the lives of people living with HIV but also challenges preconceived normative Tamil or Indian ideas about such things as sexual practice. The spread of HIV itself makes the difference between cultural norms and social practice apparent. Recall the comment of the woman quoted in Chapter 4:

> They say that the sense of propriety [*murai*], duty [*kadamai*], and discipline [*kattupaadu*] are strong in India. But when we see the spread of HIV, it shows that this is not a fact. We must not have premarital sex like they practice in foreign countries. It will ruin our culture [*murai*]. But premarital sex has increased in India. . . . This is our culture today.

HIV-positive women can easily become targets for the anxiety that is produced when the cracks between norms and practice are made visible. As Seizer deftly demonstrates in her ethnographic account of female actresses, we must recognize that the processes of negotiating and managing this stigma can both reproduce and transform culture and social practice.

Engendering Stigma, Part 1: "Women Face Greater Stigma than Men"

One of the questions that I asked women during my interviews was, "Is there a difference between how society treats HIV-positive women vs. HIV-positive men? If so, what are those differences and why do you think such differences exist?" I analyze women's responses to this question while situating their responses within the context of their life histories, particularly as their life histories intersect with HIV/AIDS. My focus is therefore on HIV-positive women's own perceptions of this issue and trying to understand how their perceptions correspond to or depart from their own personal experiences.

Some women's responses clearly support the argument made by others, such as Ogden and Nyblade and Bond and colleagues, that HIV-positive women face greater stigma and discrimination than HIV-positive men do. For example, Vijaya, whose first husband died from AIDS and who discovered her

HIV-positive status when she became pregnant with her second husband's child, explained:

> Members of society will treat HIV-positive women worse than they treat HIV-positive men because if a woman is HIV-positive, they say that she is immoral [*tappu*] but they don't say that about men. For me, the fact that I got HIV from my first husband was demeaning. Now that I am HIV-positive and my new husband is HIV-negative it is impossible to explain that to the village without the other villagers thinking that I am immoral.

Following a Tamil cultural pattern of levirate kinship, after the death of her first husband, Vijaya's parents arranged a second marriage with the brother of her first husband. These two brothers were Vijaya's first cross-cousins (her father's sisters' sons). Her second husband was extremely supportive and caring toward Vijaya through the trauma of learning of her status and continuing with childbirth. She thought that perhaps her husband's unequivocal support for her was a result of the fact that he knew his brother had died from AIDS and he recognized that it was because of his own brother that she had contracted HIV. Although her husband was supportive, Vijaya thought that others in her village near Namakkal were not at all prepared to accept her situation; it was problematic enough to be an HIV-positive woman, but to be an HIV-positive woman married to an HIV-negative man could only bring scorn to her and to her family. Thus, to prevent anyone from knowing, she never informed either her own parents or her husbands' parents about her status. Such lack of communication with or awareness of both sets of parents about one's HIV status was an atypical, though not unique, situation in my research.

Like Vijaya, Angamma thought that HIV-positive women were stigmatized more than HIV-positive men. Her husband was a lorry driver in Namakkal, and she described him as a heavy drinker. She said that she knew without a doubt that he was having affairs with several women. When she saw posters about HIV/AIDS on the outside walls of a Government Hospital, she realized that she herself had many of the symptoms listed on the poster, including herpes and eczema, and she became worried, especially because she had two relatives who had died from AIDS.

She had visited a potter for treatment of the herpes, and the potter had smeared mud and chicken's blood on her body, but that had not cured her. Next she went to consult an allopathic doctor. The doctor would not treat her herpes unless she agreed to have an HIV test. The doctor said that if she treated Angamma and the herpes went away, Angamma would never come back for an

HIV test and it was critical to get tested. Angamma, however, was concerned that if she tested positive without having her husband being tested, her husband would blame her for the HIV. Her husband refused to get tested, and so Angamma's herpes went untreated for a while.

Eventually, Angamma's husband developed such severe sores in his mouth that he was unable to even eat. At that time Angamma and her husband were living with her husband's sister and brother-in-law, and they helped Angamma's husband get an HIV test, but they kept the positive test result secret from Angamma. When her husband stopped speaking to Angamma, and when his mother, his brother, and his brother's wife suddenly came to visit them for no apparent reason, she grew increasingly suspicious. One day, while her husband was sleeping, she saw what looked like a receipt sticking out of his pocket. She pulled out the piece of paper and saw the HIV-positive test result. After telling her husband that she knew of his HIV-positive status, she went back to the doctor and agreed to get tested herself. She also took their 2½-year-old son to get tested. Although she was positive, her son was HIV-negative.

Angamma's husband asked her to take their son, leave his house, and return to her parents' home. However, she was too ashamed to go back home, even though her parents knew about her HIV status and wanted her to come. Her husband drank more and more and became disruptive to the household. Finally his sister sent them away to live on their own. Angamma's husband became increasingly violent, and when her parents heard about this, they insisted that she come home and that they would take care of her and their grandson. Finally, with the acceptance of the village *panchayat*, she left her husband, returned to her parents' house, and filed for a divorce.

When I asked her whether society treats HIV-positive women differently from HIV-positive men, she replied:

> Society is more unkind to HIV-positive women. The women are condemned and blamed more. My parents-in-law never scold their son. But they often ask me, "In which inauspicious time did our son marry you?" [i.e., astrologically speaking] and say that I have brought HIV and all these problems into the family. Gossip is also much more focused on HIV-positive women than on positive men. People always say, "She was so good and so well once upon a time. But now look what has become of her."

Whereas Angamma's husband had asked her to leave the house upon learning of her HIV status and had harassed her at home when she refused to do so, the women I met said that they never felt as though they had the right to kick their husbands out of the home (particularly if they were living with their husbands' parents but also if they had their own home) or simply to leave on their own accord. As Shalini put it, "If a woman comes to know her husband is HIV-positive after marriage, she cannot leave him because people will say she is selfish." Furthermore, women with little education and measly job prospects express feelings of being trapped, without any options to separate, particularly if they have small children. As Geetha explained, "If we leave the man and go away because he has given us HIV, who is the sufferer? Only we and our children. Even if he did wrong, if a woman makes up her mind, she can live with this kind of person and make everything all right." This sentiment of forgiveness and reconciliation is laudable. Certainly I met women whose husbands had similar responses to learning of their wives' HIV status even when they themselves were sometimes HIV-negative. The problem arises when women are disproportionately expected and required to follow this script while men have more roles to choose from and when the unequal distribution of education and employment opportunities along gender lines justifies and reproduces this discrepancy.

In Saraswati's case she discovered that she was HIV-positive through prenatal testing when she was five months pregnant with her first child, and her husband tested positive shortly thereafter. When I asked if her in-laws had been supportive of her and her husband, she said, "They only created problems. They blamed me for having infected him. My husband would join his mother in accusing me. Once I tried to jump into a well. I climbed down the ladder steps of a well. I was going to jump in. But when I reached the last rung, at the last moment, I got scared and thought of my child in my womb." As mentioned in the Prologue, Saraswati herself had reason to believe that her husband knew of his HIV status even before their marriage because he had been taking ImmunoQR medication from the Majeed clinic in Kerala. However, Saraswati did not make this connection until after her HIV-positive diagnosis.

Although Saraswati and her husband were living with her in-laws, she temporarily moved back in with her own parents for the birth of her first child and stayed with them for a few months after the birth, as is customary in Tamil Nadu. Her parents and sister, who knew of her HIV-positive status, asked her to stay with them even longer so they could take care of her. But rather than remain with them, she thought that because of her HIV-positive status, she would be a liability to her family in their efforts to arrange a marriage for her younger sister. She returned to her in-laws' home, and even though her in-laws and her husband jointly made her life miserable by blaming her for having infected her husband, she resolved not to return home until her younger sister was married. In the end her husband died of AIDS before her sister was married, and her in-laws forced her to leave their home. She had no choice but to return to her parents' home with her son.

This case points to that fact that in-laws often blame the daughter-in-law for infecting their son (despite evidence to the contrary). Furthermore, it demonstrates the powerful way that stigma attaches itself not only to the individual who has the discrediting trait but also to others with whom one has close social connections. In this case we see how the stigma threatens to extend to Saraswati's sister, possibly preventing her parents from finding a suitable spouse. As Goffman writes, "In general, the tendency for a stigma to spread from the stigmatized individual to his close connections provides a reason why such relationships tend either to be avoided or to be terminated, where existing" (Goffman 1963: 30). It is interesting to see that in Saraswati's case it was she herself who seemed most concerned about avoiding contact with her sister, whereas the sister and her parents wanted Saraswati to stay with them so that they could take care of her. Goffman also points out that indeed it is often the stigmatized person who internalizes the stigma with the most vigor, leading to feelings of shame, self-hate, and self-derogation (Goffman 1963: 7).

Vasuthi's case also demonstrates this idea that stigma attaches itself to those people with whom one has close connections. Like Saraswati, Vasuthi thought her husband probably knew of his HIV-positive status before marriage and said that her suspicions were supported by her neighbors' reports that her husband had been frequently sick before he was married. When I asked if she thought premarital HIV testing was a good idea, she said, "Yes, it is a good idea. But there will be many problems. If the girl or boy tests HIV-positive, all the siblings will be under suspicion. If there are younger sisters or brothers, then their marriages will also get affected. The family name will suffer. So it is better not to test." Vasuthi contracted herpes soon after marriage but received treatment to control it. Three months after their marriage, in 2000 Vasuthi's husband received an HIV-positive test result from a private lab, and he took her there to get tested as well, although he never explained what she was getting tested for. Her test also came back positive, but even though her husband's parents and her own mother, sister, and sister's brother were informed about the HIV-positive status, Vasuthi herself would not come to know her status until a year and a half later, long after her husband had died from AIDS. Her husband died one month after having the test, just four months after they were married. She said that her parents kept the news secret from her for fear that she might commit suicide if she knew.

Soon after her husband's death, Vasuthi began having problems with her mother-in-law, so she returned to her mother's house and stayed there. Although she did not have formal nursing training, she was able to get a job doing nursing work for a doctor in a hospital. One day the doctor there told her that she had to get a blood test to determine her blood sugar levels. As it turned out, he was getting her tested for HIV, and when the result came back positive, he terminated her job and told her that she would die within a year or two. Eventually, she was able to get better counseling and treatment and joined a network for HIV-positive people; and because she had nursing experience, she was soon able to get a job as an outreach health worker with the network. It was through this job that she met and fell in love with a man who was working for an HIV/AIDS prevention NGO and, even though he was HIV-negative, they soon married. She said that they were planning to adopt children in the future.

When I asked Vasuthi if she thought there were differences in how society treats HIV-positive women and HIV-positive men, she explained, "In my own experience, this has not been the case. But in my fieldwork experience, I find that ninety percent of the time the family will blame the wife and say that it is because of the wife that HIV has come to the husband. Only in a few houses will people have pity [*paavam*] for the wife, saying that the husband gave HIV to the wife." When I asked her why she thought people had this reaction, she explained, "People usually say that HIV/AIDS is a *pombalai viyaadhi* [colloquialism for 'woman's disease']. They see that in advertisements. So maybe that's why people act and think like that. In many areas where I go, people will ask me about *pombalai viyaadhi*. People say that this disease comes because of the woman. That's what they think. They don't understand. Lots of people say that it comes when women have sex."

Vasuthi's comment that HIV/AIDS is considered a woman's disease was echoed by several people I met in Tamil Nadu. Women's bodies were always considered the original host for HIV/AIDS, and the disease was associated with sexually promiscuous women and particularly with prostitutes (*thevadiya* or *vilai maadu*).

Another Tamil phrase sometimes used to refer to the disease is *suga noi*, which literally means "disease of pleasure" and again connotes that HIV/AIDS is a disease that men get when they engage in sex with women purely for pleasure. The relationship between morality and the healthy body are announced through this term, serving both as a warning and a legitimation of the suffering that ensues from too much pleasure, particularly pleasure that does not serve a reproductive function. All STDs come to be viewed under this rubric of *suga noi* and, by extension, are considered by some ultimately to be *pombalai viyaadhi*.

Because HIV/AIDS is considered a *pombalai viyaadhi* and because *pombalai viyaadhi* is linked to *suga noi*, STDs, and prostitution, HIV-positive women are easily accused of improper sexuality and of being the original source of this *pombalai viyaadhi*, which has spread from a wayward woman (including a wife) to a husband. Thus this particular view of women's and men's bodies must be considered one reason for the unequal distribution of HIV-related stigma for HIV-positive women.

One would expect that because most HIV-positive husbands were dying long before their wives, it would be inconceivable that families would argue that the wife was responsible for spreading HIV to her husband. The evidence to the contrary seems incontrovertible from a biomedical framework. Although the average age of the HIV-positive women I interviewed was 28, 47% of them were already widows whose husbands had died from AIDS. It was typically while their husbands were on their deathbeds or after they had already passed away that the in-laws would blame these women and accuse them of having been promiscuous and of transmitting the disease to their sons. From a biomedical perspective on the relationship between HIV and AIDS and the relatively long incubation period in which HIV-positive people remain asymptomatic, it is likely that in most cases the reason the husbands died years before their wives even got sick was that the husbands contracted HIV long before their wives did and the virus therefore had more time to develop into AIDS.[4] But medical anthropologists have pointed out that people throughout the world often hold multiple systems of knowledge about illness and the body simultaneously and draw from these different knowledge systems to make sense of illness in a variety of contexts.

Indeed, some women I interviewed provided a different explanation for the earlier deaths of their husbands. According to these women, HIV/AIDS progresses much more slowly in women and is less damaging to women's health because women partially rid themselves of HIV every month through menstruation. Furthermore, I was told that when women give birth, they purge themselves of even more of the disease than through their monthly periods. This flow of women's blood is viewed as a ritually "polluting" process, and much has been written about this particular cultural construction of the body (Ferro-Luzzi 1974; P. Jeffery et al. 1989; McGilvray 1994). But, whereas anthropologists writing about menstrual and childbirth blood typically focus on the polluting nature of this bodily process while it is occurring, the comments of these HIV-positive women points to the view that, although the blood is "polluting" during the time of the flow, the end result is that women are purified through this process and that their regular bleeding brings with it the possibility of restored health.

This idea of purification is supported by studies by Mark Nichter and Mimi Nichter, anthropologists working in South India and Sri Lanka. They write that women are perceived as being most "pure" immediately following menstruation (Nichter and Nichter 1996: 5). Adhitya Bharadwaj's research shows that this idea has textual basis in the Hindu *Laws of Manu*, as exemplified in the following quote from this text: "Women (possess) an unequaled means of purification; they never become (entirely) foul. For month by month their temporary uncleanness removes their sins" (cited in Bharadwaj 2013: 143). According to Wendy Doniger O'Flaherty, in Hindu mythology, in order to expiate himself of the sin of having killed a Brahmin, Lord Indra transfers that sin in three portions in the form of boons transferred along with sin. One third is transferred to the soil of the earth, one third to the trees, and one third to women. For the women the boon of this transfer comes in their ability to "enjoy intercourse right up to the birth of their children," whereas the "guilt became their garments stained (with menstrual blood)" (O'Flaherty 1976: 157). Further, O'Flaherty explains that there is a secondary transfer of sin away from the three recipients (earth, trees, women); in the case of the women this secondary transfer of the sin occurs when it "flows out of women in their monthly period" (O'Flaherty 1976: 158).

Interestingly, this idea finds parallels in Victorian American conceptions of menstruation, described by Carol Smith-Rosenberg, in which menstruation is considered to promote health through purging. In that case the emphasis is on the purging of the contagion of the blood, which in Judeo-Christian folklore is said to be women's punishment for Eve's sins (Smith-Rosenberg 1985: 189). Emily Martin notes a historical shift away from a view of menstruation as beneficial to women's health, because of its role in releasing heat and balancing hot-cold properties of the body in premodern Europe, to a view of menstruation as pathological in the industrialized West, culminating in the medicalization of premenstrual syndrome (Martin 1987).

Despite the general similarities about the beneficial role of menstruation in maintaining women's health, the perspectives of HIV-positive women in Tamil Nadu differ from these earlier European and American cultural constructs insofar as the Tamil women are suggesting that some amount of the disease itself exits the body with each flow. During educational presentations by counselors in hospitals and in network support group meetings, I frequently heard HIV referred to as "HIV-*kirumi.*" *Kirumi* can be literally translated as "worm" or "maggot" (Winslow 1979), but it is also a term used in colloquial medical conversations to refer to what could be glossed as "germs" or even "microbes" (*Dictionary of Contemporary Tamil* 1992). Through blood flow, women are thought to be able to flush out some of this HIV-*kirumi.* Men's bodies, however, do not have such a mechanism, and consequently HIV-positive women are thought to outlive their male counterparts. Because of this cultural construction of gendered bodies, the earlier deaths of the husbands is not necessarily thought to prove anything about the direction of HIV transmission within the family.

One of my interviews suggests that some people in Tamil Nadu may have similar (though not identical) ideas about health benefits of sex and ejaculation for HIV-positive men. During my interview with Maliga, she repeatedly complained about her husband's incessant demands for unprotected sex. She explained that even though they were both HIV-positive, their doctor had warned them that too much sex could compromise their immune systems and that they should have protected sex using a condom because it was possible that they had different strains of the HIV virus and they would not want to infect each other with yet another strain. The husband, however, did not heed the doctor's warnings. As Maliga explained:

> My husband needed sex everyday. I would refuse sometimes but would agree on some days. He would often not use condoms. I became scared when my CD4 count was 365 so I did not have sex for twenty-three days. But I could not hold out much longer. Yesterday I agreed to his demand for sex. His CD4 count is only 136.
>
> The doctor says we must eat well. My husband eats fruits when his body heat goes up. We must eat nutritiously, be clean, and we must not have too much sex. This is the advice of doctors. But my husband told me that frequent sex boosts his immune power [*ethirppu sakti*] and raises his CD4 count.

In Chapter 8 I provide further analysis of the use of the term *ethirppu sakti* in the context of HIV/AIDS and breastfeeding.

Lawrence Cohen notes that HIV/AIDS prevention studies in India have represented Indian men, particularly truck drivers, as doubly at risk for HIV transmission because of a cultural belief that truck drivers' bodies become overheated and that they must therefore engage in more sex to restore the proper hot-cold balance in their body. Cohen remarks that these studies seem diametrically opposed to the anthropological fascination with the value of semen retention and its ties to the Hindu notion of *brahmacharya* and celibacy as both spiritually and physically fortifying in South Asia (Alter 1992, 1997). Social science studies have also been conducted to determine how the "culture bound syndrome" of the fear of semen loss can affect HIV intervention projects (Lakhani et al. 2001). Ultimately, Cohen warns that both approaches have the effect of constructing South Asian men as exotic "others" who seem to want to engage in either too little or too much sex, compared with the unstated white Western norm (L. Cohen 1997).

By quoting Maliga, I certainly do not want to fall into such Orientalizing tropes. The fact that Maliga found her husband's demands to be excessive itself points to the lack of normativity in this case, and none of the other women I met made precisely the same comments about their husbands. Nevertheless, if it is in fact the case that Maliga's husband thinks that sex will help his CD4 count to increase, thus reflecting an idea that for men sex can boost the immune system, and if he is not alone in this thinking, then this should be addressed in prevention efforts. My research only points to this as a possibility, but further studies would need to be done to determine how prevalent such beliefs are and what their consequences might be.

The opinions of HIV-positive women in Tamil Nadu given here support widely held assumptions that HIV-positive women face greater stigma and discrimination than HIV-positive men—that as a result of prevailing gender ideologies about sexuality, HIV-positive women tend to be blamed for spreading HIV to their husbands. Yet these accounts also suggest that in addition to a double standard of sexuality in gender ideologies, we need to take seriously the fact that cultural constructions of the gendered body also play an important role in the production of disproportionate HIV-related stigma for women. Of course gender ideologies about appropriate sexual practice (among other things) inform cultural constructions of the body, disease, and medicine, as feminist analyses of the biomedicalization have so powerfully demonstrated (e.g., Martin 1987; Davis-Floyd 1992; Ginsburg and Rapp 1995; Davis-Floyd and Sargent 1997). Nevertheless, we must appreciate how knowledge systems about the body are often assumed to be "culture free" by people who participate in those knowledge systems. In this case we must acknowledge that the idea that HIV/AIDS is a *pombalai viyaadhi* and that women with HIV live longer than men do because of menstruation and childbirth is considered an embodied explanation and legitimation for the unequal blame and stigma attached to HIV-positive women.

Engendering Stigma, Part 2:
"Stigma Affects Men and Women Differently"

Unlike the cases discussed in the previous section, the responses of several other HIV-positive women challenge presuppositions about gender, stigma, and HIV/AIDS. These women make a distinction between the gendering of stigma for HIV-positive people within the family and outside the family, a distinction between private and public, the home and the world. The similarities of these responses are striking. In short, the women argue that society (*samudaayam*) supports the married woman but blames the married man. The implicit assumption is of a triad, with a married woman and a prostitute at either end of the innocent-guilty spectrum and a married man situated in between, at the mean. But in comparing a married woman and a married man as a dyad, these women say that society places innocent women in opposition to guilty men. On the other hand, the family—more specifically, the husband's family with whom these women frequently live after marriage—torments the women and protects the men.

As Gayathri succinctly explained: "In society [*samudaayam*] people look at HIV-positive women with pity [*paavam*], but they will say that the man is to be blamed for getting HIV and spreading it to his wife. But in the family it is different. In the family, the parents-in-law will say, 'It's only because of you that our son got the disease.'" It seems that Gayathri is speaking based on her experiences as an outreach health worker for a network more than from her own personal experience, because her account of her husband's experience with social contacts outside the family does not support her argument. Gayathri's husband was a lorry driver, and when he became too sick to work, he had to leave his job and pawn all of Gayathri's jewels to make ends meet. But his fellow lorry drivers and even his own boss were supportive of him, providing him first with (poorly informed) advice about Majeed's medical treatment to cure AIDS in Kerala and later with advice about treatment through YRG Care in Chennai, and they provided constant reminders about adhering to a healthy diet. Gayathri and other people I met in Namakkal District suggested that lorry drivers tended to be more supportive of HIV-positive people within the public sphere because they had been severely stigmatized as a group. Gayathri said that the response from her husband's workplace is atypical of responses to HIV-positive men in most work environments.

Gayathri's own experience also diverges from her general statement about stigma in the family, because, unlike the parents of Angamma's or Saraswati's husbands, Gayathri's husband's parents were far from supportive of him.

When they learned of his HIV status, they informed him that he would not receive a share of the family property, saying that because he and his wife had HIV/AIDS, they would die soon and Gayathri's son, who was then 1½ years old, would also die soon (even though the son was later found to be HIV-negative). His parents said that if they gave him a share of the property, it would only end up in the hands of Gayathri's family, so they refused. Shortly thereafter, Gayathri's husband committed suicide by poisoning himself. The in-laws then sent Gayathri and her son back to her parents' home, giving her only 25% of her rightful share in cash and saying that her son might be able to have access to a greater share only after he turned 18 years of age. The *panchayat* agreed to this arrangement. Despite these personal experiences, Gayathri's work with other HIV-positive people led her to hold a clear perception that, in general, HIV-positive men are blamed by the public but supported within the family.

Leelavathi, who was also working for a network in Namakkal, held the same view when I interviewed her on a separate occasion. As she put it: "Society [*samudaayam*] sympathizes with HIV-positive women since they have the idea that the women got HIV from their husbands. Society blames the men who get HIV. But the in-law's family [*maamiaar viidu*] always blames the woman." Like Gayathri, Leelavathi's own experience contradicts this statement, but only to a degree and only as it pertained to the lack of support that a woman receives from her in-laws. Leelavathi's case was unique compared to the vast majority of women I met. She described a pronounced discrepancy in the treatment that she received from different in-laws. After the early death of her husband as a result of AIDS, she found her father-in-law to be one of her closest allies, advisers, and confidants in her battle against her mother-in-law and brother-in-law, despite the fact that they all lived together. She explained:

> My parents-in-law were very supportive of my husband and took care of him while he was sick. I also had to sell off my jewels that were given to me at marriage in order to pay for my husband's medical expenses. My own parents and my neighbors have been very supportive of me and my husband. They supported me after my husband's death. The only place that I have faced discrimination as a result of my status has been in my husband's family. My mother-in-law is not at all supportive of me. After my husband died, she said that neither I nor my two sons [both HIV-negative] would receive any share of the family property. But my father-in-law was good to me. He has three sons and he gave me my rightful share in the family property after my

husband died. Since he knew there would be trouble from my mother-in-law, my father-in-law said: "Write up a document saying that you have lent money to me so that that money will now be entitled to you and I will sign it." In that way, I was able to inherit the house that my husband and I were living in separately. But my mother-in-law is still contesting this, and my husband's younger brother doesn't let me make use of the property. That brother came and damaged the property. He took off the roof. The "advocate" [lawyer] whom I just met today said that I could sue since I have the will.

The lawyer whom Leelavathi is referring to was working for the High Court in Chennai and had come to Namakkal with the positive people's networks to provide free legal aid to HIV-positive women. Although Leelavathi's story stood out as unique compared with other accounts that I heard about the in-laws of HIV-positive women, especially widows, it does remind us that people do not necessarily follow their expected social scripts.

It is also interesting to note that the term that Leelavathi used for her in-law's family is *maamiaar viidu*, which translates as "mother-in-law's house." Although it might seem that Leelavathi used this term specifically to single out her unsupportive mother-in-law, this expression is in fact typical of the way that women refer to their in-laws' family. Despite the tendency to define the Indian family as patriarchal, the use of the term *maamiaar viidu* itself speaks volumes about the powerful position that mothers-in-law wield within the extended family system in Tamil Nadu, and Leelavathi's mother-in-law, who holds her own against the father-in-law, appears to be no exception in this respect. Indeed women in positions of power within the families can often be the staunchest supporters of patriarchy when they stand to gain from it.

Another HIV-positive widow who worked for a network gave a similar response to my question about gender and stigma. Jayanthi, the mother of two HIV-negative children, said: "In the society [*samudaayam*] they will blame the husband, saying, 'You would have gone to some other woman and got this disease. You spoiled the life of this innocent woman.' So the society will always take the side of the woman. But the in-laws would say, 'You spread this to our son.'" Jayanthi said that she had seen this scenario played out repeatedly in the families of people she counseled, although she said that this attitude did not apply to her own parents-in-law. After the death of her husband, she and her children returned to live with her parents and, because her father was unemployed and her mother earned a measly income as an *ayah* (maid) at a village school, she had been forced to get a job in a positive people's network to support the household. She reported that all of her in-laws were emotionally supportive of her, that they would come to visit her and the children, that she was free to take her children and visit her in-laws, and that they never blamed her for transmitting HIV to their deceased son. When I asked her if she was able to receive a share of her husband's property, she said that her husband's family owned no property at all and they had no savings, so there was no question of inheritance. I suspect that the absence of such a property dispute was an important factor explaining why none of Jayanthi's in-laws blamed her for spreading HIV to their son, as was the case in many other families.

Pushpa echoed the comments about different kinds of stigma in different social spheres. She added that the private sphere of the home is a place where gossip percolates and spreads and that because women are typically staying at home, particularly newly married women with children, they are constantly subjected to this gossip, including gossip about their HIV status, and they have no choice but to put up with it. She explained that this kind and level of gossip was not common in the public working world of men and therefore that men living with HIV had greater peace of mind because they did not have to tolerate such gossip. On the other hand, she acknowledged that precisely because men do have to work, they are extremely vulnerable should others learn of their HIV status. Her own husband was a cook who made biryani rice dishes for special occasions, such as weddings. When a young boy with whom he worked somehow learned of or suspected his HIV status and told others, the orders for Pushpa's husband's biryani came to a screeching halt. It was not until he convinced people not to believe the words of a foolish young boy over his own assertions that he was not HIV-positive that the orders resumed. Convincing people that HIV does not spread through food or cooking utensils was clearly not a battle he thought he could win.

These stories raise an important point about the need for a nuanced interpretation of the gendering of stigma and the tendency for the husband's family to blame the incoming wife for bringing HIV to their son. The tendency to blame the incoming wife is clearly due in part to the moral guilt associated with HIV/AIDS more broadly and the desire for parents to absolve their children of moral approbation and protect the reputation of the family lineage, including the reputation of any unmarried siblings. It may also be due in part to the cultural construction of HIV/AIDS as a woman's disease and therefore possible to write off as a problem introduced by the wife. But what struck me in my meetings with HIV-positive women was that this blame seemed to be the most intense *after* the death of the son, when a woman became a widow.

This can be partly explained as an emotional response to the premature loss of a son. Furthermore, it reflects what is considered to be a widespread Hindu view with textual basis that widows are inherently responsible for the deaths of their husbands—particularly premature deaths—and widowhood is therefore tinged with sin and is itself stigmatized (Lamb 2000).

Yet it seems that the blame meted out to the HIV-positive widows in these instances was most acute when the issue of inheritance came into play. Thus it seems that the use of a gendered ideology about the wayward sexuality of women to blame HIV-positive widows for the death of their husbands may at times serve to mask a desperate attempt by families to hold onto whatever property they have and to absolve themselves of the financial responsibility of supporting a daughter-in-law and grandchildren. This financial burden is perceived to be particularly acute, given the relatively low levels of education and therefore limited employment opportunities of their daughters-in-law and given the fact that the families expect the HIV-positive daughter-in-laws to soon require substantial sums of money for medical expenses. In addition, they expect the children to either require expensive medical treatment if they are HIV-positive or to become orphaned, requiring full financial support from other family members. These are problems faced by widows more generally in Indian society, but because HIV/AIDS is spreading in India, women are increasingly becoming widowed at a young age. And because HIV/AIDS is already associated with "illegal sex," it may be convenient to place blame on a widow to exempt the family from financial responsibility.

Although in 2004 no ARTs were available free of cost, AIDS patients did seek out treatments from unlicensed doctors and other more legitimate practitioners to "cure" this disease or to deal with opportunistic infections. Often such practitioners charged HIV-positive people more for services than they did HIV-negative people, and this put families into deep debt. Given that many of these families were already severely strapped financially, the added economic burden of caring for these widows and their children may have seemed simply impossible to manage. The discourse of women's improper sexuality and the discourses of gendered bodies and women's diseases can be viewed as a means of justifying a decision made in the face of the specter of financial ruin for the husband's family.

Just as some of the women I met noted different degrees of stigma in public versus private spheres of life, Goffman also argues that the degree of stigma expressed in more anonymous public spheres may be different from the degree expressed in more intimate private spheres; in addition, under some circumstances stigma may be more pronounced in the public sphere, whereas in other instances it may be more pronounced in the private sphere.

> There is a popular notion that although impersonal contacts between strangers are particularly subject to stereotypical responses, as persons come to be on closer terms with each other this categoric approach recedes and gradually sympathy, understanding, and a realistic assessment of personal qualities take its place. The area of stigma management, then, might be seen as something that pertains mainly to public life, to contact between strangers or mere acquaintances, to one end of a continuum whose other pole is intimacy. (Goffman 1963: 51)

Yet Goffman suggests that this "popular notion" is not always accurate: "In spite of this evidence for everyday beliefs about stigma and familiarity, one must go on to see that familiarity need not reduce contempt. . . . There are sure to be cases where those who are not required to share the individual's stigma or spend much time exerting tact and care in regard to it may find it easier to accept him, just because of this, than do those who are obliged to be in full time contact with him" (Goffman 1963: 53). Those HIV-positive women who suggested that stigma varies based on the public-private divide would appreciate Goffman's understanding of the challenges they face in their intimate familiar relationships. His counterpoint about the possibility of less stigma in the public sphere, however, suggests that the greater acceptance that HIV-positive women sometimes receive from society might have less to do with genuine sympathy and more to do with the fact that strangers are absolved from responsibility for caring, whereas the expectation is that the family will care. The burden of care thus can exacerbate stigma, as suggested by the fact that it is often only after the death of their husbands that HIV-positive women in Tamil Nadu have to contend with the most extreme forms of blame and have to face the greatest stigma and discrimination.

The women who stated that the gendering of stigma varied in public and private spheres typically used the term *paavam* (pity) to refer to society's response to HIV-positive women. Outside the in-laws' family, society was said to take pity on women, both because of the perception that it is usually the husbands who spread HIV to their wives and because of the recognition that the wives are (often wrongly) blamed by the in-laws' families and have limited means to defend themselves or to make claims to their rightful share of property after their husbands' deaths.

Some women I met took comfort in the pity and sympathy that society provided. In fact, many women commented that, as women, they were able to receive more support from NGOs and networks working for HIV-positive people than men were. Some men I met said that they felt more alienated than HIV-positive women because they had fewer options for support in public forums.[5] Yet Vijaya, who was HIV-positive while her husband was HIV-negative, thought that she was at a distinct disadvantage because, even though her second husband was supportive of her, it was difficult for her to be identified as innocent and receive sympathy from society as a result of the nature of the HIV discordance within her marriage. She would have welcomed some pity.

But not all women appreciated the pity. Some women said that pity served to reinforce their feelings of vulnerability and helplessness. Angamma told me:

> Women who are HIV-positive are also given sympathy and viewed with pity [*paavam*]. We do not like that. Since women cannot talk back to others who make comments about how sad it is that we are HIV-positive, it gives people the license to discuss this and say whatever they want to a woman. But people will not speak this way to men, pointing out how terrible it is that men have HIV, because the men will speak back to them. We do not like it when people pity us. It makes us feel helpless.

Pity calls attention to the perception of abnormality for the pitied and the normality of the one who pities. As such, pity is an expression of stigma. For some women I met pity was a welcome response, even though it reproduced social inequality. Women like Angamma, on the other hand, who resisted the unequal power that pity enacts, bristled in response.

Rather than accept others' pity, some women I met seemed quite comfortable expressing their anger directly. Kaliamman from Madurai was a good example. Her marriage had been arranged when she was 26 years old to a man who was then 35. She became pregnant right away and tested HIV-positive through a prenatal test in a private hospital. Without informing her of the test result, the hospital referred her to a Government Hospital for the delivery, and it was not until after the birth of this child that she came to know about her HIV status. The hospital counselors recommended that her husband also get tested, whereupon he admitted to her father that he already knew that he was HIV-positive and had known for the past ten years and had been taking tablets for it. A fight between her parents and his parents ensued. His parents said, "You have given us *this* kind of girl" (i.e., HIV-positive and therefore promiscuous), while her mother was chasing his mother down the street, shouting, "You have cheated my daughter! Even if he had been a man without a house or anything she would have been better off. Even if she had only had rice porridge [*kanji*] and simple foods, she would have been better off. How could you do this to our girl?" Kaliamman herself was angry at all parties concerned. When her husband died of AIDS shortly thereafter and then her first child died at the age of 1, her anger turned from her husband to other family members. As she said, "At that time I was very angry at my parents for arranging this marriage and told them that even if I had married a beggar with no disease, I would have had a happy life." About her in-laws she said, "When I asked them, 'Why did you do this to me?' they said their son never told them that he had this disease. But I know they are liars." By the time I met her, Kaliamman was saying, "Now I have accepted that this is my fate and so I keep quiet." Although she may have accepted this fate, she had also clearly not let it cripple her own agency. After her husband died, Kaliamman remarried another HIV-positive man against her parents' will, and they were expecting a baby of their own and receiving care from YRG Care when I met her.

Despite her anger toward her parents and in-laws about the marriage arrangement with her first husband, surprisingly Kaliamman did not believe that premarital HIV testing should be mandatory. This differs from the opinion of most of the women I met whose husbands had clearly already been infected at the time of their marriage. For example, although Shalini's comments about her disappointment with her marriage were similar to those of Kaliamman, she strongly endorsed mandatory premarital testing. As she stated,

> To stop the spread of HIV in India, I suggest that people should have the test before marriage itself. Out of one hundred percent, I would say that ninety percent of the people are making mistakes [*tappu*] and having sexual relations before marriage. The moment a young man sees a "female," he goes and tells her that he likes her; he tells her that he loves her and spoils her heart. Finally they have "sex." Those girls will also have "sex" with men. Then, because they are afraid to admit this and are afraid that others will find out, they do not say anything and they marry someone else. Even if they don't bring wealth, at least men should leave women with health. I got HIV through my husband only because of his mistakes before we were married. I would not have married him if he had been tested at the time of our marriage arrangements. If everyone was required to get tested before marriage, I would be happier.

The statements about society's sympathetic reaction to HIV-positive women and condemnation of HIV-positive men provide a clear example of the discourse of guilt and innocence that haunts social responses to HIV/AIDS worldwide. In Chapter 3 I discussed how this discourse was leveraged by the

CT counselors to encourage women to accept HIV testing and to convince their husbands to agree to accept the test. When I observed support group meetings and other special events of the networks that catered specifically to HIV-positive women, I sometimes thought that in their efforts to overcome the internalized feelings of guilt and shame held by many HIV-positive women, members of these women's networks veered uncomfortably close to shifting the blame onto the shoulders of HIV-positive men, thus following the deeply rutted tracks of the discourse on innocent versus guilty people living with HIV/ AIDS. In so doing, they made their stated goal of promoting stigma-free positive living unattainable. When I asked members of these organizations about this, they acknowledged that this was a dilemma but said that there is such a strong tendency to view women living with HIV/AIDS as "bad women" that women feel an intense desire to absolve themselves of guilt, and the network organizers feel the need to educate women about the cultural construction of gender in order to denaturalize women's shame.

Finally, several women commented that, as women living with HIV, they suffered more than their male counterparts, not so much because of the stigma they faced but because of their challenging roles as mothers. For example, Kaliamman said that HIV-positive women suffer more than HIV-positive men because their bodies are weaker as a result of giving birth and taking care of babies. This makes it harder for women to fight off infections that come from a weakened immune system.

Chitra also focused on women's roles as mothers when she said that HIV-positive men do not have to worry about their future as much as HIV-positive women do because they do not feel the same level of responsibility toward their children so they just keep on doing whatever they were doing in the past. She said that they are not as concerned about their mortality because they are not the primary nurturers of their children. On the other hand, she also said that HIV-positive men have an advantage because they do not hesitate to go to the hospital on their own, whereas HIV-positive women are shy about going to the hospital by themselves. The end result is that men may be better positioned to ward off mortality because of their privileged position in a gendered hierarchy. Like many of the comments from women I interviewed, Chitra's comments are based partly on speculation and partly on experience because in her case her husband was HIV-negative and she said that he was extremely supportive of her. He was convinced that she had contracted HIV several years ago when, as young, unmarried lovers, they had been forced to resort to a secret abortion at an off-the-beaten track "hospital," which he thought probably did not take necessary precautions to avoid HIV transmission from patient to patient.

Given that rates of suicide are reported to be relatively high among HIV-positive people in India, one way of gauging the role that gender plays in divergent concerns about mortality would be to see whether more HIV-positive fathers commit suicide upon learning of their status than HIV-positive mothers. Recall Gayatri, whose husband committed suicide (when his parents shunned him), leaving Gayatri to fend for herself with their young son. Shoba also had to cope with her husband's suicide. She had been married at the age of 25 to a 40-year-old husband. She first learned of her HIV status in 2008 through prenatal testing in the fourth month of her pregnancy (only six months after she was married). Before disclosing the results of the test, the counselors told her to bring in her husband for testing as well. After both had been tested, and the results were positive for both, the counselors informed them together. The next day, her husband took a bus to Chennai, where he bought some poison and drank it before boarding the bus back home. He collapsed and died on the road while walking back to his house from the bus stop. When I met Shoba, she was in the ninth month of her pregnancy and still living with her in-laws, who were recommending that she consider getting remarried. She said she had no interest in ever marrying again. Contrast Gayatri's and Shoba's stories with that of Saraswati, who was on the verge of committing suicide by jumping into a well when thoughts of her child drew her back to life. Could it be that mothers feel a stronger sense of responsibility and moral obligation for the future welfare of their children and that this leads them to ultimately protect their own lives when it matters most? Klaits's study in Botswana suggests that men may avoid HIV testing because of their concern that if they test positive, they may be driven to commit suicide, and they want to avoid this to ensure that they live up to their expected role as providers for the family. Women in Botswana, it seems, do not have the same worries that knowing their HIV status will drive them to suicide; rather, they want to know their status to access needed medications, which will enable them to be better caretakers of their children (Klaits 2010: 237–45). This kind of nuanced study should be undertaken to better understand the relationships between gender, HIV/AIDS, and suicide in the Indian context as well.

Maheswari echoed Chitra's perception that husbands are less concerned about their mortality. But whereas Chitra viewed this as something that gave men greater freedom, Maheswari viewed it as the ultimate sign of sacrifice on the part of men. In her own life situation Maheswari and her husband and their

4-year-old son were all HIV-positive and she was pregnant with another child. She repeatedly stressed that they were financially severely stretched and struggling to feed themselves. As she said, "If we have the money, we will buy rice and make rice porridge. Otherwise, we will starve only." Because of this, they had placed their first son in a hostel (a boarding house for orphans)[6] so that he would be fed and cared for. She told me that often her husband would make sure that she ate and received proper medicine, while he sacrificed his daily meals and medication because, "He says he can die but I should be healthy to take care of my child who will soon be born." In short, this is hardly an abnegation of responsibility. Does the difference between Chitra's and Maheswari's perceptions lie in the fact that one is speculative, whereas the other is not? Or does it lie in different personalities and life circumstances of the men and women involved? I suspect the answer lies somewhere in the mix of these two possibilities.

. . .

Although the combination of blame, stigma, and discrimination has been a universal (though by no means exclusive) response to the HIV/AIDS pandemic, the nature of this response varies depending on local context. HIV-related stigma and discrimination refract gender ideologies and gendered social relationships. Because gender varies cross-culturally, the gendering of stigma also varies. In this chapter I have examined some of the ways in which constructions of gender in Tamil Nadu result in different meanings attributed to HIV-positive women and HIV-positive men and consequently different social responses to HIV-positive women and men.

The argument made by researchers working in disparate parts of the globe that HIV-positive women face greater stigma and discrimination than men—because women are expected to uphold social norms of morality and HIV is viewed as a symbol of the transgression of morality—is certainly supported by many of the HIV-positive Tamil women I met. But I have also demonstrated that the gendering of stigma in Tamil Nadu is more complex than that in several ways. First, some women thought that it was specifically in the context of interactions with their in-laws in the private sphere that they faced disproportionate stigma and blame, whereas in the public sphere they encountered more sympathy and pity than men. Second, even when they were blamed for transmitting HIV to their husbands, this was not simply due to a double standard of sexual morality; it was also rationalized through constructions of gendered bodies, including both the fact that HIV/AIDS is viewed as a *pombalai viyaadhi* and the fact that HIV-positive women are often said to outlive their spouses not because their spouses contracted HIV first and transmitted it to them but because women's menstrual and childbirth blood purges them of some amount of the HIV-*kirumi*. Finally, the use of the discourse of blaming women for being promiscuous was most pronounced after the husband's death, suggesting that this discourse may be strategically deployed to justify and mask an underlying motivation to exempt the husband's family from financial responsibility for these widows and their children.

These responses to HIV/AIDS in Tamil Nadu thus reflect specific systems of knowledge and social practices of gender, kinship, and the body. Although social responses to HIV/AIDS follow the grooves of normativity (indeed Goffman [1963] and Parker and Aggleton [2003] suggest that stigma serves to assert and reproduce normativity), at the same time, people living with HIV/AIDS actively negotiate these social responses to best serve their own interests in whatever ways are possible. This is evident in the critiques embedded in the accounts of the HIV-positive women I have discussed. Such critiques suggest that the responses to the gendering of stigma may not be simply reproducing gender, kinship, and cultural constructions of the body but also transforming them, as I discuss in subsequent chapters.

Although stigma and discrimination play a huge role in the lives of HIV-positive women and men, more immediately, women receiving an HIV-positive diagnosis during their pregnancy must make quick decisions about whether or not to continue with their pregnancy and give birth. Concerns about stigma and discrimination do not factor heavily into these decisions in part because this issue is not emphasized in counseling and in part because other factors take precedence at this vulnerable time in women's lives. In the next chapter I examine how women navigate the complex web of factors that go into this decision-making process.

To Birth or Not to Birth?

Constraints and Pragmatics in HIV-Positive Women's
Childbearing Decisions

*If I had known I was HIV-positive when I was pregnant, I would have aborted
the babies.*

—HIV-positive widow, age 39; mother of six children,
four of whom are HIV-positive

*If it [HIV test] is positive, it will be difficult for me to the extent that I will die; I
will kill myself. There would be quarrels in the family. There would be no peace
of mind. My husband would leave the house. Keeping the children, I would
suffer, wondering whether I would live or die. I would not have the child.*

—Twenty-year-old mother with a 3-year-old daughter, in the eighth month of her
second pregnancy. She had just given blood for an HIV test in a Chennai public
hospital and had not received the results.

*If a pregnant woman is HIV-positive, it is good to abort the baby. It is a "waste"
if the child is born. And the mother will also get a bad name.*

—Twenty-one-year-old pregnant woman in her eighth month of pregnancy who
had just received her HIV-negative test result at a Chennai public hospital

Speculations about how one would respond to an HIV-positive diagnosis in
pregnancy may lead to decisive statements such as those made by the three
quoted women, whom I interviewed. One of the women was HIV-positive, and
I interviewed the other two women during their prenatal care in PPTCT centers.
In the minds of these three women there is no question that they would choose
not to continue with the pregnancy and birth. Studies suggest that this opinion prevailed in India at the beginning of the twenty-first century (Yadav 2001;
Ananth and Koopman 2003). Yet reality is more complicated and fraught with
ambiguity. In fact, many poor women in Tamil Nadu do continue with childbearing despite a positive HIV test, and this trend was increasing at the time
of my research. By the end of 2003, TNSACS reported that 67% of the women
in Tamil Nadu who had been diagnosed as HIV-positive through the PPTCT
program went on to deliver their babies, and this rate has increased consider-

ably since that time (TNSACS 2004a: 4). In this chapter I examine how women living with HIV navigate decisions about pregnancy and birth and demonstrate that this decision is influenced by a complex web of sociocultural factors.

Of the seventy HIV-positive women I met, thirty-two found themselves in the situation of knowing that they were HIV-positive while they were pregnant. All these women opted to continue with childbearing. Their decision was informed by (1) institutional interests of the government (both central and state), NGOs, and international aid donors (in terms of the structures of maternity health services available and the government's PPTCT program); (2) cultural constructions of gender and of the self, particularly the centrality of motherhood, expressed by women themselves and also by members of their extended families (especially husbands, in-laws, and parents); (3) Christian-based organizations in Tamil Nadu that cater to lower class and lower caste communities; and (4) the networks for people living with HIV/AIDS. Women's decisions to continue with childbearing were not made by favoring one factor over another but emerged through each woman's own synthesis of coexisting structures and discourses, which sometimes converged on the same conclusion despite differences in their underlying logics. In this chapter I demonstrate how women assert their agency as they make their way through a web of interlocking structures.

Some structures provide women with the possibility of making reproductive decisions that they find to be more enabling[1] and thus more satisfying than others. I argue that of the four main structural factors listed—all of which contributed to HIV-positive women deciding to continue with pregnancy—it was the influence of the networks for people living with HIV/AIDS that women found to be the most enabling. Unlike the other factors, the influence of the networks allowed women to make decisions that they thought would lead to beneficial outcomes for their futures (without having to sacrifice core aspects of their identity, such as their religious identity).

Context for Discovering HIV-Positive Status Among Mothers

Twenty-two of the thirty-two women who knew they were HIV-positive during their pregnancy first learned of their status through HIV testing as part of their prenatal care, either in Government Hospitals with PPTCT programs that required informed consent (although as seen in Chapter 3 informed consent was not always operationalized) or in private clinics where testing was done routinely, often without informed consent. Six women learned of their HIV status because their husbands were sick or had recently died and they learned that the husband's illness was a result of AIDS; therefore they themselves had also been tested. In some cases testing occurred while the women were pregnant, even though it was not a result of routine prenatal testing. Two of the twelve women learned their HIV-positive status, not in the context of prenatal care but rather as a result of their first child's illness and subsequent HIV-positive diagnosis. One such woman, Amaldevi, was already pregnant with another child when she learned that she and her first child were HIV-positive. The other woman, Punitha, came to know of her HIV-positive status while her first child was dying, but she chose to become pregnant and give birth to a second child anyway. Two women were first tested as a result of their own illness. For example, because she had a history as a commercial sex worker, Karpagam was tested for HIV when she went to see a doctor about a health problem she was having. Even knowing her HIV-positive status, she and her husband chose to conceive and give birth to two children. Finally, two women tested positive during prenatal care in a private hospital but were not informed of their status until after the baby was born.

Social Responses to HIV Status: The Story of Punitha

How these women responded to discovering their HIV-positive status and how others responded to them reflect the dominant social responses to HIV/AIDS that have been documented globally: accusation, stigma, and discrimination (Shilts 1988; Sontag 1989; Farmer 1992; Goldin 1994). Specifically their HIV status was perceived as a scarlet letter, a badge of shame, marking them as *tappu* (immoral) and thus inciting them to place blame on another. As discussed in Chapter 5, because of a double standard of sexual mores, women tend to be blamed for "illegal sex" more than men and HIV-positive women often face greater stigma and discrimination than men within their families, the predominant domain within which their HIV status is known. Because many women discover their HIV-positive status only after the death of their husbands, they are blamed for these deaths, and the stigma of their HIV-positive status is exacerbated by the stigma of being a widow in the Indian cultural context, in which widows are commonly viewed as responsible for the deaths of their husbands and are therefore deemed inauspicious (Lamb 2000).

Many poor HIV-positive women in India become widows at a young age; in my sample of seventy HIV-positive women, 47% were widows, even though the average age of all seventy women was only 28. These HIV-positive widows faced extreme difficulties supporting themselves because of poverty and low levels of education, which prevented them from finding employment opportunities and from seeking legal recourse to rights to their husbands' property. Their difficulties were compounded as a result of the stigma of HIV/AIDS, which shut them out of jobs and homes, denied them and their children access to medical care, and led to the expulsion of their children from school. It is because of such extreme cases of stigma and discrimination that reports of HIV-positive women contemplating suicide are not uncommon.

Yet women also engage in a discourse of blame. When discussing their life stories, the women I interviewed invariably began by blaming someone else for infecting them, thereby exempting themselves from responsibility. The need to blame is clearly a symptom of the intensity of the stigma attached to having HIV. The most extreme manifestations of this were a couple of cases in which women flatly denied (to family members and to me) that they were HIV-positive, despite the claims of medical personnel that they had tested HIV-positive.

The story of Punitha provides a window into understanding the ways in which gender and class place women at risk for HIV. It illustrates the multiple layers of blame, stigma, and discrimination against women that result from discovering their HIV-positive status and the complex, pragmatic decision making that follows when a woman is faced with an HIV-positive diagnosis. Punitha was an only child, born and raised in Chennai. Her father died of tuberculosis when she was 5 years old. When Punitha came of age, her mother was eager to arrange a marriage as soon as possible because she was worried that it would be difficult to arrange a marriage without a father; people would suspect that the family would not be able to provide an adequate dowry.

Punitha discontinued her education after completing the eighth standard, and a marriage was arranged when she was 16. She was married to a 26-year-old man. Punitha was opposed to the marriage. She told me, "When he came to see me, I did not like his appearance. I told this to my mother. He was very thin and had ulcers and sores in his mouth. But my mother went ahead with the engagement." Based on this description, it is possible that Punitha's husband was already suffering from opportunistic infections associated with HIV/AIDS. Indeed, several women I met believed that their husbands knew of their HIV status before marriage.

Following the patrilocal tradition, Punitha went to live with her husband's family. Within three months she got pregnant and gave birth to a girl. Her baby was constantly sick, and finally a doctor told her to take her husband and daughter to a Government Hospital for blood tests. All three of them received a blood test, but they did not know what they were being tested for. All three were diagnosed as HIV-positive. Punitha said that there was no process of informed consent before taking the test and that they did not receive counseling after getting the results. The only thing she remembers being told at that time in the late 1990s was that they would all die within four to five months. Although she and her husband have lived much longer, the baby died soon thereafter.

Within Punitha's family the response to the HIV-positive status was a layering of blame and counterblame and of assumptions and accusations of improper sexual behavior. The first person to know of their status was Punitha's father-in-law, because the doctor informed him directly (breaching codes of confidentiality). The father-in-law's response was to make sexual advances on Punitha, saying that she must have been promiscuous and that since she was dying anyway, she had nothing to lose from having sex with him.

Punitha and her husband fled the advances of the father-in-law and went to live with Punitha's mother in Chennai. Punitha was quick to blame her husband: "Until today, he has not accepted responsibility for having infected me." Punitha's husband blamed Punitha's father, saying that her father must have been HIV-positive and contracted tuberculosis as a result. He then claimed that Punitha's father must have transmitted HIV to Punitha's mother, who then transmitted it to Punitha at birth, who in turn transmitted it to him. When I first met Punitha, she suggested that this was ludicrous because, according to her, her mother was not HIV-positive.

When I attended the next PWN+ support group meeting, Punitha's mother, Manjula, was there. I first assumed that she had come to accompany her daughter, but I soon discovered that she was herself a member of the network; she too was HIV-positive. When I interviewed Manjula in their home, she had her own theories of blame that seemed to come tumbling out in a heap, even though I never asked her how she got infected with HIV.

> My son-in-law used to visit often before he married my daughter. He wanted to marry her but Punitha refused. In an argument he bit my hand.

> My son-in-law cut his hand with a blade, and I held it tight to stop the bleeding.

> I was washing my daughter's cloth sanitary pads after she had her baby, and I must have gotten it through that blood.

As always, the goal seemed to be to exempt oneself of blame, even if, as in this case, it meant implicating one's own daughter.

Manjula's neighbors soon came to know that members of the family had AIDS. They were ostracized and forced to leave their home. So they fled once again, this time to the far southern outskirts of Chennai where a new, treeless government housing development had been built to relocate squatters from the city. Punitha, her husband, her mother, and her second child, who survived, were living in a one-room apartment when I met them, trying to keep their HIV status secret from their new neighbors.

How to Decide Whether to Continue with Childbearing

Despite the intense stigma and discrimination women faced on discovering their HIV-positive status, these women decided to continue with childbearing. Punitha herself became pregnant again following the death of her first child, and she decided to give birth to the second child. Lisa Richey's study of HIV/AIDS and reproductive health in South Africa suggests that in that context women like Punitha who become pregnant after receiving an HIV-positive diagnosis without explicit authorization from the medical personnel treating them for HIV/AIDS are criticized for having an "adherence problem" with respect to the counselors' recommendations to use condoms, even within their marriages (Richey 2011). Although Richey finds Vinh-Kim Nguyen's concept of therapeutic citizenship (Nguyen 2010) useful for understanding this situation, she argues that cases such as this demonstrate the need to add a gender dimension to such theories to "gender the therapeutic citizen" (Richey 2011: 80). Unlike Punitha, most of the other women in my study discovered their HIV status for the first time during their pregnancy. In the remainder of this chapter I explore the factors that are involved in women's decisions regarding childbirth following a prenatal HIV diagnosis. Because of the PPTCT program, prenatal testing is increasingly becoming the primary context for women in India to discover their HIV-positive status. Therefore the criticism about HIV-positive pregnant women having an adherence problem with respect to condom use is not widespread. As more women in India elect to become pregnant following an HIV diagnosis, this discursive kind of regulation of the therapeutic state could very well emerge in India as well.

I am not suggesting that the unanimous decision among the women I interviewed to continue with childbearing is representative of all women living with HIV in Tamil Nadu. Obviously, my recruiting methods tilted my data in this direction. Nine of the thirty-two informants were selected through networks promoting positive living. I met three through hospitals with PPTCT programs, and such women may be more inclined to continue with childbearing than others. And the twenty women that I interviewed through YRG Care were all coming to YRG for either prenatal or postnatal care. Nevertheless, the trend for women living with HIV to continue with childbearing is on the rise, at least in Tamil Nadu. Therefore a close examination of the complex decision-making processes of these women who do choose to continue with childbearing could benefit those engaged in HIV/AIDS prevention and treatment efforts, whether they are policy makers, health care providers, or social workers. Ultimately, such an understanding could benefit other HIV-positive women in the future insofar as it can contribute to policies that enable women to make fully informed decisions.

Detecting HIV Late in Pregnancy

Twenty of the women I interviewed got their first HIV test and were informed of the diagnosis at a late stage in their pregnancy—two in the ninth month, two in the eighth month, four in the seventh month, four in the sixth month, five in the fifth month, and three in the fourth month.[2] As seen in Chapter 3, typically hospitals that provide HIV testing do so during the first prenatal visit, and my research on prenatal HIV testing suggests that most women do undergo testing on their first or second prenatal visit. The late stage at which these women detected their HIV status, therefore, supports the already documented fact that poor women in Tamil Nadu who attend government maternity hospitals often do not seek prenatal care until late in their pregnancy (Zurbrigg 1984). According to Dr. V. L. Srilata of UNICEF, for approximately 40% of Government Hospital deliveries in Tamil Nadu, the woman's first visit to the hospital was at the time of delivery.[3] This is because, when family resources are limited, women's health does not become a priority, especially when seeking health care involves time away from paid labor or needed housework and involves transportation costs—problems that are most pronounced in rural areas with fewer medical facilities. Fifty percent of the women in my sample came from rural village areas, even though they were getting maternal health care in towns or cities. Women receiving care from YRG Care were often traveling extremely long distances to receive prenatal, delivery, and postnatal care. Furthermore, based on evidence from my previous research, some women might put off seeking prenatal care in Government Hospitals in part due to concerns that because of their class and caste status, they might be mistreated by medical staff or pressured into accepting family planning procedures that they may not want (Van Hollen 2003a).

In short, cultural constructions of gender and inadequate public health resources for women's reproductive health combined with the government's stepped up efforts to screen for HIV during pregnancy seem to lead to a situation in which women are increasingly learning about their HIV-positive status late in their pregnancy.

Diagnosis of an HIV-positive status late in pregnancy was usually perceived by women as precluding the option of having an abortion. Abortion, referred to as MTP (medical termination of pregnancy), is legal in India under certain conditions. According to Indian law, abortion in the first trimester is legal with one doctor's certificate and does not require consent of a family member. During the first trimester of pregnancy (months 1–3), it is relatively easy to get the medical certificate, and the state's interest in family planning renders this unproblematic. In the second trimester (months 4–6), abortion is legal with two doctors' certificates and requires consent of a family member. For a doctor to certify an abortion in the second trimester there must be a medical reason (relating either to the mother's health or to the health of the fetus). These certificates are also relatively easy to procure. Abortion is legal in the third trimester (months 7–9) only if it is deemed medically necessary to save the mother's life. These certificates are more difficult but not impossible to obtain.

It is important to note that in 1996 UNAIDS and the UN High Commissioner for Human Rights jointly issued what were referred to as the international guidelines on the topic of human rights for people living with HIV/AIDS. These guidelines included rights to access to medical care and required that "HIV-positive women have the option of legal, safe abortion" (Cook and Dickens 2002: 61). In particular, these guidelines stipulated that "where laws accommodate legal access to abortion when pregnancy endangers women's life or health . . . HIV positivity renders abortion lawful" because the combination of HIV infection and pregnancy were deemed to make "women particularly vulnerable to life- or health-endangering infections" (Cook and Dickens 2002: 61). Because India is a member of the United Nations, women who thought they were being denied such an option in a late stage of their pregnancy could, in theory, demand this as a human right. Neither the HIV-positive women nor the counselors or medical practitioners in my study referred to these international guidelines.

Studies have shown that in India many unlicensed practitioners perform abortions illegally, and such abortions have been associated with maternal morbidity and mortality (Ganatra 2000). Ganatra's review of studies of abortion in India indicates that most abortions occur in the first trimester and that women who delay abortion until the second trimester tend to be adolescents and unmarried women and increasingly women seeking sex-selective abortions (Ganatra 2000: 207). Her review of the literature does not include discussion of third-trimester abortion.

Most of the women in my study stated that they could not consider an abortion because of the late stage of the pregnancy. It is interesting to note that even those women who were in the fourth and fifth month (second trimester) of their pregnancy stated that they could not consider an abortion because it was "too late" and therefore "nothing can be done." Women did not elaborate on what precisely they meant when they said it was too late, but I believe they were responding to a combination of the perception of the illegality and of social stigma associated with later stage abortion. Further studies could clarify this issue. For some, statements that it was too late may have been used to buttress other reasons for wanting to continue with childbearing, as discussed later in this chapter. Several women said that it was the doctors who had told them it was too late to consider an abortion.

The Role of the PPTCT Program

In the past medical personnel encouraged abortions for poor HIV-positive women and this was previously the path endorsed by and pursued by most women in India (Yadav 2001; Ananth and Koopman 2003), but starting in 2002, thanks to the government's PPTCT program, poor women could have the option of pursuing childbearing at reduced risk. The presence of the program itself was clearly a critical factor in this decision, providing poor HIV-positive women with more options than they previously had. However, the role of the PPTCT program in these decisions was more complex than that.

PPTCT counselors often (though not always) glossed over abortion in pretest counseling, and rather than discussing probabilities, some stated that with medication HIV would not be passed to the baby. In fact, at the time, statistics indicated that a single dose of nevirapine alone could reduce transmission rates only to 8–10%. This is demonstrated in the following three quotes from counselors speaking to patients in pretest counseling sessions that I observed in public hospitals.

> If one gets the HIV test, just like one has other blood tests, HIV will be prevented from passing on to the child. [There was no mention of medication in this session.]

> By giving medicine to the mother before the child is born, HIV will be prevented from passing to the child. It comes to the child through the umbilical cord, during childbirth, and by breastfeeding. This is prevented by medicine. So it is good to get tested for HIV.

> If the mother is "HIV-positive" during the pregnancy, medicines can be given to the mother and you can stop the transmission to the child. But this can only be stopped if the mother gets an HIV test during pregnancy. In that way, the HIV test is like an immunization.

Counselors avoided discussing stigma in pretest counseling, and as late as mid-2004 counselors did not explain that there was—at that time—no government provision of antiretroviral medication for the sake of the mother's health. In 2004 the Indian government (as well as the CDC and WHO) did not recommend prescribing antiretroviral treatments until a patient's CD4 count dipped to at least 200. It usually takes several years after HIV infection before the CD4 count falls to that level. Therefore, because most women in Tamil Nadu have children soon after marriage, assuming that they were infected after marriage, their CD4 counts were not likely to be so low at the time of giving birth that they would have been eligible for ART themselves, even if it were available. However, decisions about whether to continue with childbearing often include consideration of one's long-term ability to care for one's future children. Failure to mention abortion, discrimination, and the lack of long-term availability of medical treatments for the mothers themselves thus seemed to encourage women to get tested during pregnancy and to continue with childbearing if they were found to be HIV-positive. By not providing women with full information about the consequences of this decision, the structure of these counseling sessions tended to foreclose the possibility of women exercising their agency. A 2005 report by the Center for Reproductive Rights states:

> As programs to prevent mother-to-child transmission of HIV become increasingly available, there is a strong incentive to raise enrollment in those programs by scaling up HIV testing of pregnant women. Expanding women's access to HIV testing during pregnancy is a necessary component of any campaign to prevent mother-to-child transmission. It is crucial, however, that efforts to increase testing be complemented by similar commitments to pretest counseling. (Center for Reproductive Rights 2005: 6)

My research underscores the need to heed this advice in the Indian context, emphasizing the importance of the quality of the counseling. MacNaughton's analysis of women's health care and HIV/AIDS globally suggests that lack of fully informed consent for HIV testing in pregnancy is a widespread problem in many parts of the world and one that needs to be addressed as a human rights issue (MacNaughton 2004).

As discussed earlier, the PPTCT program seemed to operate within an unstated international, national, and statewide target-based approach to increase HIV testing during pregnancy and to increase the use of nevirapine treatments for those women who test HIV-positive during pregnancy and for their newborns. Under these conditions pregnant women were not provided with complete and balanced information about their reproductive health options. Other studies have pointed out that President George W. Bush's policy of not funding international organizations that provide abortion counseling or services—known by critics as the global gag rule—which was then policy, also influenced HIV counseling and services for pregnant women worldwide (de Bruyn 2002: 18). This may have been a contributing factor in the PPTCT counseling, although no one stated that directly.

PPTCT counselors may have thought they had a stake in dissuading HIV-positive women from opting for an abortion. Evidence of this is supported by statements made by two women who discovered their status in the second trimester and thought that abortion was not an option. For example, Amaldevi said, "I was five months pregnant when I tested HIV-positive so I couldn't abort. The counselors said that there was medicine in the hospital to stop HIV from passing to the baby." Saroja, who discovered her HIV-positive status in the fourth month of her pregnancy, said, "I asked if my baby will get HIV. They [the counselors] said that they will give medicines so that this will not happen and that anyway it was too late to consider an abortion. I felt reassured. So I decided to continue my pregnancy. My husband also agreed." In these statements we see how the factor of HIV diagnosis late in the pregnancy and the nature of the PPTCT counseling become neatly linked in such a way as to close off perceived options for women in their decision making. It is difficult to know whether the counselors spoke with such absolute confidence about preventing the spread of HIV as these statements suggest, and I was unable to observe post-test counseling of HIV-positive patients, so I cannot corroborate these statements. It is possible that mothers remembered what they wanted to hear. However, given the certainty with which counselors discussed the effectiveness of nevirapine in the pretest counseling, it seems highly possible that this was the position presented during post-test counseling as well. What is evident from these statements is that counselors were not highlighting the abortion option, despite the fact that both these women were in the second trimester of their pregnancy.

I want to stress that I am not suggesting that HIV-positive pregnant women should opt for an abortion or that counselors should steer them in that direction. Such suggestions would be a violation of human rights for people living with HIV/AIDS (de Bruyn 2005: 7–8) just as much as denying an HIV-positive woman access to abortion when legal would be a violation of an internationally recognized human right. De Bruyn suggests that movements to designate HIV/AIDS as a specific indication for legal abortion could lead to the further stigmatizing of HIV-positive women and could even lead to coerced abortions for these women. Instead, she recommends that "it could be better to advocate for the full reproductive rights of WHA [women living with HIV/AIDS] and to advocate for the passage and implementation of laws that permit abortion for 'chronic conditions that may endanger a woman's health,' without naming HIV/AIDS specifically" (de Bruyn 2002: 22). I agree with de Bruyn that women should be presented with all reproductive options so that they can make the best decisions for themselves within the law. Tamil Nadu has the highest incidence of abortion in India at a rate of 5.2% of all pregnancies, as opposed to the national rate of 1.7% (Anandhi 2005). According to ethnographic research on abortion in Tamil Nadu, abortion is practiced among married and unmarried women both as a family planning method and as a tool to negotiate domestic violence and other oppressive social conditions (Anandhi 2005). Despite criminalization and widespread opposition to the practice, abortion has also been used for sex selection in a sociocultural context that increasingly favors male children (Bumiller 1990).

Given the context that most HIV-positive women are living in poverty, widowed at a young age, and unable to find employment or remarry because of the triple stigma of being HIV-positive, an HIV-positive *woman*, and a widow, women must be provided with full disclosure of their reproductive options and of the medical, social, and psychological benefits and risks of all those options.

Although almost all the women in my study said that they did not consider abortion once they were diagnosed as HIV-positive because it was too late and/or because the doctors and counselors had assured them that the treatment to prevent HIV transmission would be successful, that did not mean that abortion was something they would never contemplate. Some had either considered having an abortion before learning of their HIV status or had had an abortion or had attempted to get an abortion at some point. For example, when Nagalakshmi became pregnant with her third child, she wanted to have an abortion early in the pregnancy, but her husband had said no and so she followed her husband's request. By the time she tested HIV-positive, she was in the sixth month of that same pregnancy, and so she said it was too late to consider an abortion. Following her diagnosis, her husband and their first two children were tested. Although her 5-year-old tested HIV-negative, her husband and 3-year-old tested HIV-positive. She was getting excellent care and treatment for free through YRG Care, but her husband was not seeking medical care because he said he could not afford to take off any time from work to go to the doctor. He was a wage laborer on construction sites and would not get paid for any time missed from work. Instead, he was simply going to the medical shop and self-medicating for various ailments. If he continued on this trajectory, it was likely that Nagalakshmi would become an AIDS widow, raising three children on her own with uncertain prospects of access to treatments for herself and her second child once she was no longer enrolled in the YRG scheme for pregnant women (which I discuss in Chapter 7).

Fatima, one of only two Muslim women in my study, had not only contemplated an abortion before learning of her HIV status but had in fact actively tried to abort. She reported visiting several "doctors," getting numerous injections and consuming countless pills to try to abort. She wanted an abortion because she already had four children and did not know how her husband could support another child since he was a part-time worker at a tea stall, earning 100 rupees per day, sometimes working five days a week, sometimes not. Along the way, she spent 1,000 rupees on these abortion treatments. Her husband and others in her family also encouraged her to seek an abortion because they said she was already weak and would not have the strength to take care of a fifth child. Despite spending 1,000 rupees on various treatments, all her attempts to abort were in vain. "I decided this baby wanted to live," although she worried about the effects of all those injections and pills on the development of the fetus. By the time she tested HIV-positive in the fifth month of that pregnancy, she said, "Now nothing can be done," and she said that the counselors in the hospital told her that she could not abort at that stage in her pregnancy. Her husband and all four of her children tested HIV-negative. Although it was fortunate that her husband was HIV-negative, being an HIV-positive woman in a "discordant" couple in which it is the man who is HIV-negative can be particularly challenging from the perspective of social stigma, and such women often face harsh treatment from their husbands, who suspect them of being unfaithful. In her own marriage Fatima said that her husband did not accuse her of any wrongdoing and was trying to be supportive, but he did not want her to share food and water with their children and he was afraid of coming to YRG Care, where Fatima was receiving treatment during her pregnancy, or bringing the other children to YRG Care because he was anxious about coming into contact with so many HIV-positive patients. Because they were keeping this news secret from other family members, this meant that Fatima had to travel alone all the way from Nagapattinam (almost six hours by bus) for all of her doctor's visits. Although Fatima said that her husband was supportive, she also thought that being a Muslim woman in a discordant couple was particularly precarious, because in her mind the Muslim community stigmatizes HIV-positive people, especially HIV-positive women, with greater intensity than Hindus or Christians.

Such a comment can be read as a critique of one's own religious community, but it can also be interpreted as an indirect way of suggesting that Muslims have higher moral standards than others.

Chitra, a Hindu, was also an HIV-positive woman in a discordant couple, but her husband did not blame her. Rather, he was convinced that she had gotten HIV through an abortion that she had had before they were married. She was 17 at that time and was in love. When she got pregnant, both she and her husband (who was then her boyfriend) agreed that she should get an abortion in the second month of the pregnancy. She confided only in her grandmother, who secretly took her to a small private hospital in Chennai. Chitra said that she suspects she got HIV there because lots of young, unmarried women were coming to that hospital for abortions. Her implication was that because HIV is associated with sex out of wedlock, it stands to reason that it could spread through medical procedures when many such women are receiving abortions in the same place. Three years later, she and her boyfriend entered into a love marriage. She was tested for HIV in her second pregnancy and found to be HIV-positive, whereas her husband and 2-year-old child were both HIV-negative.

Finally, I met one Hindu woman who did have an abortion after getting pregnant while aware of her HIV status. After the abortion, however, she immediately got pregnant again. This was Tamilarisi. When she 20 years old, her marriage to her father's sister's 30-year-old son was arranged. Soon thereafter, they had a child, who died at the age of 2. Her husband then fell ill and learned that he was HIV-positive. Another test revealed that she too was positive. When I inquired whether she thought the child had died as a result of HIV, she was adamant that this was not the cause. Rather, she explained, a gecko had fallen into a cup of warm milk and the child had unknowingly drunk the milk, which poisoned the child.

A Siddha doctor in Tiruchirappalli, which was the closest city to their village, sold Siddha medications to Tamilarisi and her husband, claiming that these would cure both of them of HIV. But after some time, when her husband's health was clearly not improving, someone referred him to YRG Care in Chennai, seven and a half hours away by bus. At YRG Care she and her husband were both put on ART. It was at that time that Tamilarisi found herself pregnant again. Because she had been getting treatment at YRG Care, she knew that they had a program to provide care for HIV-positive women. But, she said that when she went to YRG Care for her prenatal care, the medical staff told her that if she wanted to participate in the scheme for free treatment from YRG Care, she would have to first undergo an abortion and then, if she got pregnant again, they would accept her into the scheme. She had an abortion in the fourth month of her pregnancy, got pregnant again, and then was included in the YRG program. This was confusing to me, and I kept asking her to explain why they had asked her to first have an abortion and then get pregnant again. She was unable to come up with an explanation and simply said, "The doctor told me it was necessary." I later asked the primary doctor in charge of obstetrics and gynecology for YRG Care why such advice would have been given. She explained that it was because Tamilarisi had been taking efavirenz, an antiretroviral medication that was thought to cause birth defects; they had urged the abortion so that they could then change her medication and re-enroll her in their program with another pregnancy. The doctor explained that since that time the recommendations have changed; women taking efavirenz are no longer urged to abort, but their medication is immediately changed.

Tamilarisi also told me that the doctors recommended that she have a tubectomy at the time of the cesarean birth, and she concurred that that was what she wanted as well. Her husband, however, refused, saying that he wanted another child after this one, and she felt that she could not act against his will. As she said, "I cannot make any decisions. He must sign. Then only can I sign." This is an example of a woman whose body seems caught between the dictates of the medical establishment and those of her husband with little room for her own agency. It is women like Tamilarisi whom social scientists seem to have in mind when claiming that Indian women do not have control over their own reproductive decision making. As seen in Chapter 4, as well as in other stories throughout this book, this lack of agency around reproductive health issues is certainly not representative of all women in India.

The Parental Mandate

For some women the cultural imperative to be a mother weighs heavily on their decision. Similar tensions between fears of transmitting HIV to a child and anxiety surrounding the failure to bear children have been found in other cultural settings throughout the globe (e.g., Mill and Anarfi 2002; Doyal and Anderson 2005). For example, Kirshenbaum and colleagues' study of four major cities in the United States found that the presence or absence of children before HIV diagnosis was the primary factor determining whether women would have children following their HIV-positive diagnosis (Kirshenbaum et al. 2004). They found that this factor significantly influenced women's perceptions of the efficacy of medications to prevent HIV transmission from mother to child. Women who already had children had concerns about the efficacy of this treatment, whereas women who had not borne children were confident that these medications would effectively prevent transmission (Kirshenbaum et al. 2004). The HIV-positive women I met who became widows as a result of AIDS before they ever conceived went through an intense period of grieving, not only for their husbands but also for their chance to become mothers. For a woman to be married and not produce a child would lead not only to a sense of personal loss but also to a feeling of public shame. In Tamil Nadu a woman is expected to conceive within the first year of marriage, and if this does not happen, it can sometimes be grounds for the husband's family to seek a new wife, the assumption being that the woman (and not the man) must be infertile. This assumption is legitimated by cultural notions that the woman's body is like a field, which is impregnated by the husband's seed; the field may be barren, but a seed is never considered to be inactive.

Maliga, whose husband, mother, and brother all encouraged her to abort the fetus even though she was eight months pregnant, explained it to me this way: "Some said there was a ten percent chance that the baby would be HIV-positive. So they felt it would be better to abort. For me . . . I am a woman . . . there is no reason to live if I do that. For a complete family you need a baby. Otherwise I shouldn't live." In this case it is clear that Maliga had not been told that the nevirapine would guarantee an HIV-negative child but rather that it would substantially reduce that possibility. According to Dr. Suniti Solomon at YRG Care, this imperative to be a mother was so strong that HIV-negative women sometimes knowingly put themselves at risk of infection by their HIV-positive husbands so that they could become mothers.[4] Because of this, YRG Care was engaged in a clinical trial to give ART to the HIV-positive person in a discordant couple to prevent transmission to the HIV-negative partner. Dr. Solomon believed that this was particularly important for women because women would put themselves at risk of getting HIV in the hopes of conceiving.

Punitha's story (discussed earlier) provides another example of the parental mandate. One month after the death of her first child, Punitha, pregnant again, was determined to keep the baby, even though her husband and her mother were opposed and wanted her to get an abortion. In this case Punitha's mother said that Punitha was determined to have another child to please her in-laws and reconcile a broken family.

The case of Vijaya (discussed in Chapter 5) also demonstrates a woman's agency in her choice to keep a baby, despite the fact that, as with Punitha, Vijaya's motivation can be viewed within a broader patrilineal and patriarchal context. Vijaya, who came from a village in Namakkal District, was 34 years old when I met her. When she discovered her HIV-positive status in her pregnancy, she already had a 7-year-old child from her first marriage and so she did not feel that it was critical to have another child. She explained to me that she wanted to keep the baby, not for herself but for her husband and his family. Recall that after Vijaya's first husband had died, she had married her husband's brother and both were her cross-cousins.

Vijaya knew that her first husband had been HIV-positive and had died as a result of AIDS, but she did not come to know about her own HIV status until she had remarried and was in the ninth month of pregnancy with her second husband's child. At that time she was tested during her prenatal checkup at a PPTCT center. She tested HIV-positive and VDRL-positive (a positive syphilis test).[5] Vijaya explained that although she was aware that she herself could have contracted HIV from her first husband, she did not know that there was a possibility that she could transmit HIV to her baby or to her second husband. She said that if she had known that earlier, she would not have agreed to get married again.

Vijaya's second husband, who tested HIV-negative, had not been married before and did not have any children. Vijaya was worried that her child from her first marriage would not treat her second husband like a father. She was concerned that her child would not take care of her second husband in his old age or if he got ill. This was particularly worrisome because she imagined that she herself would die before her husband, due to her HIV status. Therefore she believed that it was important to have another child with her second husband so the child would have a strong bond with the father and she could die in peace knowing that he would be cared for. Furthermore, although she already had a child, she thought that it was important for her husband to have his own child to carry on the family lineage and that this was important for her husband's family as well. Although his family did already have a grandchild (Vijaya's daughter), they did not yet have a grandson, and because a son is important to carry on the family lineage, she thought that she should give birth to this child in the hopes that it would be a boy. Along with the love and affection that Vijaya expressed for her second husband, her decision was also influenced by structures of kinship and patriarchy.

This imperative to bear children and to continue the family lineage, despite one's HIV status, is not surprising in a cultural context where demands for infertility treatments are intense and where adoption is rarely sought (Bharadwaj 2002). People in India seek out multiple modes of fertility treatments, ranging from in vitro fertilization to Ayurvedic and Siddha remedies to vows and prayers made to deities (as evidenced, for example, by the tiny cloth cradles hanging from the branches of trees at many Hindu temples in Tamil Nadu). For HIV-positive men who can afford it, sperm washing before in vitro fertilization is one method increasingly sought by couples in India longing for a biological child.

The fact that women would make the decision to bear children for the sake of their in-laws or their husbands is also not surprising in a cultural context in which the conception of the self is said to be more sociocentric, or "dividual," as opposed to the egocentric, individual conception of the self that is more normative in the Euro-American cultural context (Dumont 1970; Marriott 1976). Anthropologists have described this Indian conception of the self as "fluid," pointing to the notion that person-substance flows from one individual to another through multiple social interactions, from the most intimate sharing of body substance between mother and child or husband and wife to the more intermediate sharing of food to the more remote transference of person-substance through touching the same object (Daniel 1984; Lamb 2000). In this context not only are women's reproductive decisions influenced by social factors such as patriarchy and class, but also their decisions are based on a keen sense of being socially, emotionally, and substantially connected to a broader kinship community.

Sometimes the incentive to bear a child comes not from the pressure to be a mother or the desire to continue the male lineage but simply, as Suguna put it, "because we want a child to support us in the future." In the absence of any system of Social Security, in India children are expected to be the caretakers of their parents when they grow old. There is an assumed system of reciprocity at work here, as has been poignantly described in Sarah Lamb's ethnography, *White Saris and Sweet Mangoes* (2000). Within the context of partilineal, patrilocal kinship systems, this is one of the primary reasons for son preference in India.

For Suguna and her husband, however, making the decision to bear a child for their future security came at the expense of familial support in the present. Suguna had married her maternal uncle when she was 17 years old. They had a baby, who died after nine months, and the next year her husband died of AIDS, just two years after their marriage. Widowed and childless at age 19, Suguna moved back in with her parents. She remained there until she was 27 years old, when she married an HIV-positive man whom she met at YRG Care, where she was receiving treatment. Both families accepted the marriage, and Suguna moved into her in-laws' home. They had never intended to have a baby and were vigilant about using condoms for birth control. But the doctors at YRG Care told them that they could participate in a scheme for pregnant women free of cost and could be virtually guaranteed that the baby would be HIV-negative, and they were convinced because they would be provided with the full package of PMTCT care. Thus, knowing that they were both HIV-positive, they chose to conceive. When the couple announced to the family that Suguna was pregnant and that they intended to have the baby, her in-laws vehemently disapproved and made them leave the home to live on their own. When I met Suguna, she was completing the sixth month of pregnancy, and she hoped that once the baby was born, her in-laws would have a change of heart and welcome them back into the family home.

The Role of Christianity

Nine of the thirty-two women I met considered their Christian faith an important factor in their decision to continue with their pregnancy following an HIV-positive diagnosis. These were all cases of lower caste women who had converted to Christianity, reflecting a broader trend of lower caste conversion in Tamil Nadu that began in the colonial era and continues to the present. Christianity, of course, is an enormously broad category, encompassing a wide range of denominations, theological perspectives, and practices. Nevertheless, the women I interviewed did not identify themselves with particular Christian denominations but rather stated simply that they were Christian. When I asked them to clarify or whether they were Protestant or Catholic, they did not know how to respond. When I asked if they were Pentecostal, they would nod affirmatively, which was not surprising, given the rising popularity of the Pentecostal church in Tamil Nadu. All nine said they had converted to Christianity after having learned of their HIV-positive diagnosis. Those women who claimed that their Christian faith was an important factor in their decision to continue with childbearing told me that abortion was not problematic for Hindus but was unacceptable for Christians.

For example, Maliga went against her Hindu husband's wishes for an abortion. As she put it, "I was against abortion. Hindus do not see abortion as a sin, but Christians do. I have turned Christian. It was only Bible reading that prevented me from committing suicide [after discovering her HIV status]. The Bible gave me strength and hope. My husband tried his best to abort the child." It is important to note that not only did Maliga make a reproductive decision that went against her own husband's decision but she also made the decision to convert from Hinduism to Christianity independent of her husband. This reflects a particularly high degree of autonomy and agency for this woman when we take into consideration that in the predominantly patrilineal Indian cultural context, a wife is expected to adopt her husband's family's religious identity and practices (if she does not already belong to the same religious group, as is expected in arranged marriages). Maliga was born into a Hindu *dalit* caste, and her marriage was arranged when she was 26. Maliga adopted the Christian faith only as a result of her interactions with a Christian Ayurvedic doctor who was treating her for HIV/AIDS. When I met this doctor in Maliga's apartment, he claimed that his Ayurvedic treatments could cure HIV/AIDS.

Maheswari's story also demonstrates an independent streak in an HIV-positive woman who was comfortable asserting her choice of religion, even though it led to conflict with her husband. She had been born Hindu and married a Hindu man, but she chose to convert to Christianity after learning of her HIV status and becoming affiliated with the Community Health Education Society, an NGO. However, her husband, who was also HIV-positive, remained Hindu, and this created some conflict between them. As she stated,

> I am now a Christian. Every day I read the Bible. My husband has no faith.
> He usually says, "What's the use of reading the Bible? We have this disease.
> Do you think we are going to get better by praying?" But I would tell him: "As
> long as we are alive, we have to live for our children. God only created us. He
> knows the good and bad. Can we live without God and without trusting God?"
> Still, my husband will scold God and he will break the picture of Jesus in my
> home. He is a Hindu and I am Christian. Whenever I find time, I go to church.
> Otherwise, I read my Bible at home, but he will tell me not to read the Bible.
> If I read the Bible, I will have peace in my heart. When I read the Bible, I feel
> consoled and comfortable and I have the feeling that I am not sick.

Maliga's earlier statement that "Hindus do not see abortion as a sin" was echoed by others, but this statement begs for clarification. Attempts to uncover a "Hindu perspective" on the topic of abortion above all reveal the absence of a homogeneous Hindu viewpoint. The different perspectives seem to reflect the researchers' own political and moral positions on the topic. On the one hand, some scholars provide evidence from ancient Hindu texts (including the Vedas, Upanishads, Dharmasastras, and the medical treatises of the *Caraka Samhita* and *Susruta Samhita*) to argue that, according to Hindu belief, abortion is antithetical to Hindu notions of ahimsa (nonviolence) and that it is a heinous crime, a *mahapataka* equal to killing one's own parents or to killing a Brahmin (Thandaveswara 1972; Lipner 1989). These scholars point to the fact that Hindus believe that the soul joins matter at the moment of conception and that this soul moves through a series of incarnations, each of which is determined by the karma of the previous life, toward the goal of liberation (moksha). In this light, abortion is viewed as thwarting the unfolding of karma and the soul's movement toward moksha, particularly because incarnation as a human being indicates the soul's proximity to moksha.

On the other hand, Sandhya Jain argues that, although it is true that abortion is considered a *mahapataka* in some of the classical texts, Hinduism also rejects absolutism. She points out that the ancient Ayurvedic medicoreligious texts, such as the *Caraka Samhita* and the *Susruta Samhita*, tolerate abortion to save a mother's life and even recommend abortion if a fetus is said to be "defective" and that these texts prescribe methods for abortion (S. Jain 2003). Furthermore, Jain argues that Hindu notions of dharma (proper conduct) encourage flexibility by accommodating individual circumstances and accommodating social changes through time.

> In such a radically changed environment, it stands to reason that the demands of dharma must be appropriate to the demands of the time in which we live. The stability of the social order now necessitates adoption of the small-family norm, and dharma includes the notion of public duty and public responsibility. Hence, the small-family norm, achievable through contraception and family planning methods (including abortion in rare or necessary cases), is entirely consistent with, and in no way opposed to, the Hindu concept of dharma. (S. Jain 2003: 139)

In her ethnographically based research in predominantly Hindu communities in Tamil Nadu, S. Anandhi suggests that previously abortion was considered shameful, not because the procedure itself was viewed as a sin but because it pointed to one's sexuality. Anandhi found that among the younger generation, women believed that having a large family or being pregnant relatively late in life was much more shameful than having an abortion (Anandhi 2005). Anandhi also reports that pregnant women commonly consult with "the local priest (*samiyar*) or persons who are 'possessed'" to determine whether or not to have an abortion (Anandhi 2005: 17). She quotes one woman as saying that a local village priest insisted that she abort in the seventh month of her pregnancy because he felt that the fetus was possessed by a ghost and would harm the male members of the family if it were born (Anandhi 2005). It is interesting to note that in this particular example, the advice of the priest legitimated the pregnant woman's own desires, which she had been unable to act on independently because her husband and mother-in-law were against the abortion. According to this woman, once the priest issued the warning and sanctioned the abortion, the husband too "insisted on the abortion" (Anandhi 2005: 17–18).

Regardless of the debates about the Hindu perspective on abortion, abortion was legalized in India in 1971 under the Medical Termination of Pregnancy Act. It is practiced by members of all religious communities and has not been politicized to the degree that it has in other parts of the world, in large part because of overarching state concerns with family planning and population reduction (Van Hollen 2003a; Anandhi 2005). The use of abortion for sex selection, however, has been condemned and criminalized. The rhetoric of Maliga that "Hindus do not see abortion as a sin, but Christians do," which was also voiced by other women I met who had recently converted to Christianity, may be indicative of an attempt among anti-abortion groups to make this a religiously charged political issue, but such a claim would require further research and documentation.

One and a half years after her baby was born and was officially declared HIV-negative, Maliga became pregnant again. Although she claimed that her Christian faith's opposition to abortion was her primary reason for having given birth to her other child, when she became pregnant this time, her husband once again wanted her to get an abortion and she consented. She described the event:

> When I became pregnant a third time [her first pregnancy had resulted in a stillbirth], my husband took me out of the city to his sister's place. His sister knew a doctor who would perform an abortion. At that time I had to attend a housewarming function. So I decided to go for an abortion after the function. I don't think I will conceive again. We calculate safe dates. My husband doesn't want another child, but he is against permanent sterilization. My mother too is against it since I am weak. But he will not agree to get himself sterilized. He thinks his sexual potency [*veeriyam*][6] will go down.

This was the same husband who, as mentioned earlier, insisted on frequent sex to boost his CD4 count (see Chapter 5), so perhaps his concern about losing his sexual potency was not only reflective of normative ideas about masculinity that deter men from undergoing vasectomies in India (and elsewhere) but also tied to his understanding of the relationship between sex and the immune system. Maliga's story suggests to me that it was the need to become a mother more than her Christian opposition to abortion that was the strongest factor in her decision to keep her baby after discovering her HIV status during pregnancy. Her Christian faith seems to have served to bolster her argument in favor of keeping the earlier baby. With a healthy baby boy in her arms, however, she was willing to concede to her husband's wishes to abort the baby the next time around.

The women I met who were converting to Christianity all did so after discovering their HIV-positive status. Most converted as a result of their association with World Vision. World Vision is one of the largest Christian relief and development organizations in the world. Founded in 1950, World Vision is a private Christian organization. It is structured as a global partnership with no formal affiliations to a particular denomination and works primarily in the area of children's emergency relief and development in ninety-nine countries.[7] World Vision is associated with Protestant groups worldwide and has been described by one scholar as being among the most influential forces in the rise of the post–World War II evangelical coalition (Carpenter 1998: 823) and by another as having "link[s] with Protestant groups in the United States that emphasize religious conversion" (Cruz 1999: 381–82). Yet in the "Frequently Asked Questions" section on the World Vision website, the answer to the question, "Is evangelism a part of World Vision's projects?" is:

> Educational activities based on Christian values are included in World Vision projects if appropriate and desired by the community. However, World Vision respects the religious beliefs and practices in countries where it operates, and seeks mutual understanding with people of all faiths. World Vision does not proselytise. We do not coerce nor demand that people hear any religious message or convert to Christianity before, during or after receiving assistance.[8]

Punitha was one of the women I met who converted to Christianity after learning that she was HIV-positive and coming into contact with members of World Vision. She recounted:

> I have changed from being a Hindu to being a Christian. My husband observed a fast after he knew his HIV status and went to Sabarimalai [a Hindu pilgrimage site]. He became very sick on his return. The doctor said that he had jaundice. They gave up on him, saying that he was dying, and he was sent home. He became bedridden. A neighbor came and prayed every day for his recovery. That lady was a Pentecost. She told us about World Vision. We too started praying and developed faith in Christianity. He improved slowly. We were baptized after that.

This account suggests that Punitha believed that the Hindu god at Sabarimalai was not as capable of healing as the Christian god. In addition to the neighbor's daily prayers, World Vision began to provide her husband with free ART. Punitha and her daughter also received free medical treatment from World Vision.

Similarly, Amaldevi, who discovered that her 2-year-old child and she were HIV-positive when she was pregnant, was put in touch with World Vision, which provided her child with ART. She told me, "The government has not done anything for HIV-positive people. People must not reject them. I prayed to Jesus that my son must walk and become free of HIV. I vowed that if he could walk, I would become a Christian. Jesus takes care of me. He gave me courage. Now my son has strength to stand up. Jesus gave me hope to have the second baby so I didn't want an abortion."

Renukha discovered her HIV-positive status while pregnant, and she too was put in touch with World Vision at that time. She said, "When the child was in the womb, we would pray for its welfare. I became a Christian. Among Hindus, an HIV-positive lady is rejected. Neither my mother and father nor my husband's family have helped me. They are all Hindus." Renukha told me that she was opposed to the idea of abortion and that, as a Christian, if she prayed to God, her baby would be saved. Renukha and her HIV-positive husband were also receiving medical support from World Vision, and Renukha was earning about 50 rupees per day selling oil for World Vision.

Karpagam, who began attending World Vision meetings and receiving medicines for free when she was seven months pregnant, said, "Before, I was a Hindu. But then I vowed to Jesus that I would get baptized if my child lived. I prayed to him to save my children from HIV. The first boy was saved, but the second was HIV-positive. This was because I breast-fed the second baby." World Vision was providing ART for the second child.

None of the women I met who were affiliated with World Vision stated unequivocally that World Vision was opposed to abortion or that abortion was not permissible according to their new religion. However, as Amaldevi stated, these women believed that putting their faith in Jesus was preferable to pursuing an abortion. The World Vision website does not include an official statement on abortion, and my phone calls for interviews with World Vision representatives in Chennai were not returned, so I do not know with certainty whether World Vision in Tamil Nadu has a particular position on abortion. Through an Internet search on the issue, I did locate a World Vision "Topic Sheet" titled "Population and Poverty: What's the Connection?" published in 1998; this document supports family planning but states, "As a Christian organization, World Vision highly values life, and does not support abortion as a means of family planning" (World Vision 1998).

The HIV-positive women I met who had stayed in the World Vision hostel at different points in time had all converted to Christianity during their stay. Those who were interviewed while they were living at the World Vision hostel or living in housing subsidized by World Vision said that they had chosen to convert freely. But Devi, who had previously lived in the hostel but was living with her husband in a thatch house when I met her and was still receiving medical treatment from World Vision for herself and her children, said, "World Vision asked me to become a Christian and I did. I think Jesus saved my son. They allowed me to stay in that hostel only because I agreed to become a Christian. World Vision gives my son ART. Before taking ART, my son weighed only four kilograms. Now he is ten kilograms [within eight months]. Now he does not get ill so often."

The decision to continue with childbearing in these cases evokes a sense of hope and of the possibility for these women to take matters into their own hands to make their own reproductive decisions, independent of their families (husbands, mothers, mothers-in-law, etc.). However, these decisions also suggest a complex web of factors that tend to limit women's options, compelling them to continue with childbearing. The comments of these women suggest that (1) they needed a place to live and/or medical treatment for themselves and their children, and they thought that because the government was not providing for those needs, World Vision would; (2) they felt that they were stigmatized by their Hindu community but that the Christian community offered through World Vision would provide them with psychological and spiritual support; and (3) through their association with World Vision they articulated their new identities as Christians by being opposed to abortion and by putting faith in Jesus to provide them with healthy babies. The fact that these women's conversions under these circumstances fostered an anti-Hindu sentiment and a sense of the superiority of Christianity is particularly problematic when we take into consideration that World Vision was founded in the United States and much of its funding comes from the West. I am not claiming that World Vision is explicitly engaged in a process of proselytizing by providing treatment and care contingent on conversion. I do not have evidence to prove such a claim. Clearly, however, World Vision does not appear to have actively attempted to prevent women like Devi from having that perception and making such strong claims to the contrary.

Positive Networks: Positive Living

Finally, some women living with HIV explained that they opted to give birth because they thought they could be good mothers, regardless of their HIV status, and that their children could lead satisfying lives whether they were born with HIV or not. Women who made such statements were all affiliated with the networks for HIV-positive people. Women I met who attended support group meetings at PWN+ in Chennai, SPMD in Coimbatore, and the HUNS network in Namakkal came to know more about the PPTCT programs, and this information itself influenced their decision to continue with childbearing. More important, through talking and interacting with other HIV-positive women and children, these women were exposed to the possibility that HIV-positive mothers and children could live positively.

For most people in Tamil Nadu living positively was a novel concept because initially most of the HIV/AIDS prevention campaigns had been aimed at instilling fear into people in the hopes of dissuading them from engaging in risky behavior and because, as seen earlier, most people believed that HIV/AIDS was a prescription for sudden death, an *uyirkolli noi* (killer disease). But by 2004 brightly colored posters covered the walls of the hospitals with PPTCT programs; they admonished against stigmatizing HIV-positive people and advocated positive living. HIV-positive women attending the network support group meetings came to understand that an HIV diagnosis did not necessarily mean an imminent death.

This was the situation for Punitha. Although motivated to keep her baby for her in-laws and because of her new-found Christian faith, Punitha said that the most important factor for her was that she had been actively attending the PWN+ support group meetings. When she became pregnant and went for her prenatal consultation with her doctor, she had already made up her mind to continue with the pregnancy, despite her family's wish for her to abort. As she said, "When the doctor first explained to me that even with the medicine to prevent transmission of HIV, there was still a chance that the baby could be HIV-positive, I told the doctor that I could live a happy life myself even with the HIV virus, and I told him that I knew how to raise a baby whether the baby was HIV-positive or HIV-negative."

Like Punitha, Renukha also opposed family pressure to abort based on her confidence about being an HIV-positive mother. Renukha was in her second marriage and pregnant for the first time when she discovered her HIV-positive status. Her first marriage had been arranged when she was 19 years old. She said that her first husband turned out to have bad habits (*mosamaana pazhakangal*). According to her, he was a drunkard, smoked ganja, and visited sex workers (*vilaipengalidam poradu*). So she left her first husband and married her older sister's husband (while he was still married to her older sister). He already had two children with his first wife (Renukha's sister).

Polygyny is not commonly practiced in Tamil Nadu, particularly not among Hindus (Renukha and her new husband were Hindu when they were married but converted to Christianity after discovering their HIV-positive status). However, the DMK political party started the tradition of the *swayam maryada kalyanam* (marriage of self-respect), which eschews the official sanctity of court marriages or priestly presence and requires only the tying of the *tali* (a special necklace placed around the neck of a woman at the time of marriage; the necklace is never removed as long as she is married). Although the Hindu Marriage Act of 1955 legally recognizes marriage between only one couple at a time, a loophole exists that makes this possible without punishment, and the *swayam maryada kalyanam* tradition makes it possible to take advantage of that loophole. As Anuradha Raman explains, "In fact, there is one loophole in the Hindu Marriage Act that does make two wives possible. For a specific charge of bigamy, the aggrieved party—in this case, the first wife—has to approach the court. But instances of women approaching the judiciary for redressal are rare; in most cases, they just resign themselves to the new arrangement" (Raman 2009).

Although legal loopholes may allow a man to have more than one wife and this does happen, a man marrying two sisters simultaneously is certainly highly unusual and not normative behavior in Tamil Nadu. On the contrary, Renukha described this second marriage as an exceptional act of empathy and concern for her well-being on the part of her second husband and her sister because she had suffered so much while married to her first husband.

Renukha became pregnant soon after the second marriage and discovered that she was HIV-positive through prenatal HIV testing in the seventh month of her pregnancy. Her new husband was then tested, and he too was found to be HIV-positive, but her sister and sister's children were HIV-negative. Initially Renukha's sister was angry with Renukha and blamed her for passing HIV to their mutual husband, but Renukha blamed her first husband for his bad "character."[9] She did believe that she had transmitted HIV to her second husband, and she felt a sense of remorse for this and a sense of humiliation that her first marriage had failed. In her mind the blame and culpability could be placed squarely on her first husband's shoulders.

Renukha decided to continue with the birth of her first child and received zidovudine treatments under the PPTCT pilot project. Five months after her first baby was born, she found herself pregnant again. She and her husband recounted that moment.

Renukha: I became pregnant a second time just five months after my first delivery. My parents as well as my husband wanted to end the pregnancy. We even quarreled over this.

Husband: My wife was not well informed about HIV at that time. Why should we
have another child when we ourselves are going to die soon?

Renukha: I was strong in my decision that I wanted this baby and that I would not
have an abortion. But my husband took me to the hospital for an abortion. I
told the doctor that I didn't want an abortion. I told him: "Why should I have
an abortion when my first child had been born without a problem?" This doctor asked me to go to the same hospital where my first baby was born. Doctors
used to take good care in those days, but now they do not. Now they ask me to
sit separately and do not touch me. Actually, we people who have HIV do not
need counseling. It is the doctors who need counseling! Society rejects HIV-
positive people. Doctors also do this.

Renukha delivered her second child in a PPTCT Government Hospital in Chennai. Renukha said that PWN+ support group meetings had made her aware of
the problem of stigma. She was not going to be cowed by fear of such stigma;
she refused to let this deter her from having the children she wanted.

In rare instances couples entered into a marriage knowing that they were
both HIV-positive. This trend was increasing and was facilitated by organizations such as YRG Care, the support group networks, and even through Internet discussion groups such as AIDS-INDIA and SAATHII. I met seven women
in such marriages, five of whom had gone on to have children with their new
spouses and thought that they could live positively as HIV-positive parents.

. . .

As stated earlier, it is often assumed that poor women in India have little or no
control over their own reproductive decisions. The stories shared by the women
involved in my study, however, provide a quite different impression of women's
roles in making decisions about their reproductive health. Although I have demonstrated that these women's decisions were constrained by patriarchal factors,
limited by their class and caste position, and pressured by the demands of the
international, national, and state-based targetlike approach of the PPTCT program and by the interests of evangelical Christian organizations, nevertheless we
can see clearly how women pragmatically negotiated these varied structures. In
several instances we even see women making decisions that went against the will
of their husbands, their parents, and their in-laws.

Of all the factors contributing to these decisions, the role of the networks with
their discourse of positive living can be categorized as the most enabling. Women
who couched their decision within this framework were choosing to continue
with childbearing because it would lead to a fulfilling life for themselves and their

future children. This factor was not driven by a sense that childbirth and motherhood were their only viable options but rather by the contention that they were just as entitled to motherhood as any other woman and that their children should have the opportunity to live just as satisfying lives as any other children. In addition, the positive living factor was not dependent on changing one's religious identity or denigrating another religious community.

None of these women, however, stated that their decisions were made based solely on one factor alone. Instead, their comments point to a complex configuration of competing influences and underscore that these decisions reflect the kind of ambivalence coupled with pragmatism that Margaret Lock and Patricia Kaufert (1998) describe as characteristic of women's engagement with the medicalization of reproduction. For example, Maliga and Amaldevi claimed that they essentially had no choice but to continue with childbearing because they learned of their HIV status late in their pregnancies. Yet both women felt compelled to rationalize their decision by drawing on other explanatory logics.

Maliga was in the eighth month of her pregnancy when she discovered her HIV status. Even though she was in her third trimester, her husband, mother, and brother were encouraging her to have an abortion, but the late stage in the pregnancy was not the only factor she had to contend with in making her decision to keep the baby. She also drew on her new-found Christian faith to take a stance against abortion and, in so doing, she constructed herself as morally superior to her Hindu husband, who wanted her to abort. She also drew on the cultural construction of motherhood as the defining characteristic of being a woman to formulate her argument against her family's wishes for her to abort. When we consider that she later willingly agreed to an abortion in her next pregnancy, the pragmatics of her use of the Christian anti-abortion rhetoric for the earlier pregnancy become apparent.

Amaldevi was five months pregnant with her second child when she received her HIV diagnosis. Although she believed that abortion was not an option at this stage in her pregnancy and although she seemed to have been convinced by the PPTCT counselors that medication could guarantee that HIV would not pass to her baby, she also felt compelled to justify her childbearing decision along religious lines. Critical of a government that she thought "has not done anything for HIV-positive people," she found support only with World Vision, converted to Christianity, and claimed that "Jesus gave me hope to have the second baby so I didn't want an abortion."

For Maliga and Amaldevi the late-term HIV diagnosis was in and of itself not the sole deterrent precluding the abortion option. Similarly, for Renukha and Punitha their strident confidence in positive living did not stand alone in their explanations of their decisions. In addition to Punitha's confidence about positive living that enabled her to defy her husband's and mother's wishes for her to abort and emboldened her to stand up to her doctor, telling him "I know how to raise a baby," she also stressed the importance of prayer and her new-found faith in Christianity as a factor that gave her the strength to continue with childbearing. Her mother pointed out that Punitha's motivation to have the baby was to regain respect from her parents-in-law, who had spurned and harassed her after she and her husband were found to be HIV-positive.

Likewise, Renukha drew from the positive living discourse of the networks when she made the cutting remark that "we people who have HIV do not need counseling. It is the doctors who need counseling!" when recounting her confrontation with her husband and doctor in her decision not to abort and to continue with childbearing. The human rights–based positive living discourse was not the only factor that she cited as informing her decision, however. Feeling cast off by her own Hindu parents and her in-laws because "among Hindus, an HIV-positive lady is rejected," she found support within the Christian World Vision community and said that, as a Christian, she was opposed to abortion.

The fact that these women drew on multiple logics to explain their childbearing decisions points to their ambivalence coupled with pragmatism. Multiple explanations were developed as pragmatic strategic responses to the competing and varied opinions of family members, medical personnel, religious organizations, and networks with whom these women interacted as they navigated the decision-making process. On the other hand, the multiple explanations may also have been a sign of the ambivalence that these women continued to feel about the decision they had already made. Such ambivalence is not surprising, given that many people in Tamil Nadu—like the three women quoted at the beginning of this chapter—believe that HIV-positive women should not bear children. Such ambivalence is also not surprising given that these women and their children face an uncertain future.

Once these women decided to continue with their pregnancies following an HIV-positive diagnosis, what was the actual birth experience like? In the following chapter I revisit the social and medical context within which pregnant women first discover their HIV-positive status, and I then discuss the social context and consequences of their deliveries as HIV-positive women. Here again the pragmatism that women use within the boundaries of sociocultural structures will be evident.

7 HIV-Positive Women Give Birth
Deception and Determination

IN THIS CHAPTER I FURTHER EXAMINE the social context within which pregnant women discover their HIV-positive status and the ensuing birthing experiences of those women. In doing so, I vividly demonstrate how local social practices of medicine are linked to local social practices of kinship and marriage for women with HIV who are seeking reproductive health care in Tamil Nadu. This is evident both in the context of receiving an HIV-positive diagnosis and in the context of birth itself and demonstrates how global health guidelines for the prevention of mother-to-child transmission can become localized. Janet Carsten suggests that, after a period of hibernation in the 1970s and 1980s, kinship, or the study of "relatedness," is reclaiming a central role in anthropological analysis, albeit in radically different ways than it did in the early days of our own anthropological kin, such as Lewis Henry Morgan and Claude Lévi-Strauss (Carsten 2000, 2004). In my study I did not set out to discover the role of kinship in the social practice of medicine; it was simply impossible to ignore because of its centrality.

I am not arguing that the disjuncture between global policies designed by international planners and local realities results in "needless barriers," as Whiteford and Manderson (2000: 1–2) suggest (see Chapter 1). Rather, it appears that certain aspects of global (and national) policies, such as informed consent and confidentiality, are at times sidestepped or go unacknowledged or are reinterpreted. Although I do point out the obstacles that women living with HIV faced in accessing basic obstetric care, following Lock and Kaufert (1998), in this chapter I once again illustrate the pragmatic strategies that these women used as they navigated the institutions of both medicine and family.

As in Chapter 6, in this chapter I draw from the experiences of the thirty-two HIV-positive women I met who were aware of their status before giving birth. The births of all thirty-two women were hospital births that took place in Tamil Nadu. This is representative of broader trends toward hospitalized births throughout Tamil Nadu; rates of hospitalized births in Tamil Nadu are much higher than the national average (Van Hollen 2003a). Furthermore, women who come to know that they are HIV-positive are more likely to seek hospital care for delivery, particularly in hospitals that have PPTCT programs.[1] All but one of these thirty-two women had given birth to their babies while knowing their HIV status after 2000. The year 2000 was a watershed year for mother-to-child transmission programs in India because it was in 2000 that NACO and UNICEF piloted the PPTCT program.

In this chapter I focus on four case studies of women from Namakkal District who gave birth in 2000, 2002, 2004, and 2008. These cases allow us to see both continuity and change through time in this district, which has gained international notoriety for having one of the highest HIV prevalence rates in India, a fact attributed to Namakkal's position as the major hub of the trucking industry in South India.

I begin by returning to the case of Saraswati, not because it is representative of all the birth experiences but because her story includes many of the key themes that emerge in other women's stories: the lack of informed consent, the duplicity and pragmatism of both medical personnel and family members in the process of HIV testing, and the stigmatization of and discrimination against HIV-positive women in maternity hospitals coupled with private acts of resistance against such discrimination. Some elements of Saraswati's story that were introduced in the Prologue are included once again here to flesh out the details of her narrative more fully.

Saraswati Gives Birth: 2000

I met Saraswati in a hotel in Namakkal in 2004. She had come to the hotel along with a group of other women living with HIV to attend a meeting organized by INP+, PWN+, and the HUNS network. The purpose of the meeting was to educate women about the sex and gender framework, to inform them of their rights under the United Nations Convention on the Elimination of All Forms of Discrimination Against Women (CEDAW), and to provide free legal counseling with the lawyer from the High Court in Chennai who was doing pro bono work for women living with HIV. Based on interviews with nine of the women who attended this workshop, it was apparent that they found the legal aid that was provided for their individual cases to be more beneficial than the more generalized international human rights education because they did not clearly see how they could deploy the human rights critique using CEDAW in such a way that might actually benefit them. Pursuing their grievances through the courts, however, was perceived as being potentially more effective than relying on the police, which had previously been the practice.

After the meeting Saraswati came to my hotel room for an interview, and she shared her story about the birth of her son in 2000. At the time of the interview Saraswati's son was 4 years old and HIV-negative. She recounted the experiences of her pregnancy and birth.

> I first learned of my HIV status when I was five months pregnant when I went for my first prenatal checkup with a private doctor. Since my husband was a "lorry driver," they did an HIV test without saying anything and without asking my permission. And then they told me that I was HIV-positive. After that I got tested in at least ten other places just to be sure that I really was HIV-positive. My parents had to borrow money from the moneylender to pay for the tests. It cost 10,000 rupees just for all those tests. My parents and my mother's younger brother were the only ones who knew about my status at first.

Here we see echoes of two points made earlier. First, we are reminded that in Tamil Nadu women like Saraswati often do not get any prenatal care until well into their pregnancy, often precluding or problematizing the possibility of abortion. Second, we see that Saraswati's HIV test was carried out without informed consent, a phenomenon that was reportedly common in private hospitals. As discussed earlier, many HIV-positive women told me that the staff in some private hospitals routinely tested for HIV without informed consent because they feared that patients would refuse to get tested given the option, but the private hospitals wanted to know about the HIV status so that they could refer those patients elsewhere.

Saraswati continued her account.

> My husband was on the road for his work when I found out about the HIV. I realized at that point that my husband must have had HIV even before we were married because before our marriage he was taking medicines from Majeed's clinic in Kerala. When I had asked him about those medicines at the time of our marriage, he had told me that it was for some other minor illness. After I learned about my HIV status, I told my parents about the Majeed medicines, and my parents and I decided that if my husband had been keeping this a secret, he would not agree to get tested now. So when he came back home, we took him to the hospital and got him tested on some other pretense

without his knowledge. He wouldn't have agreed otherwise. We didn't tell him that I had tested HIV-positive. My doctor had cheated me, so I cheated my husband [she said, laughing].

This passage points to the multiple levels of duplicity that emerge in response to an HIV-positive diagnosis and affect marital relationships and broader kin and community relationships as well as the doctor-patient relationship. The secrecy surrounding testing and the disclosure of an HIV diagnosis is a result of the stigmatization of HIV in medical settings and within the confines of the family; at times members of these two arenas are adversaries, and at other times they are collaborators in schemes of deceit. The kinship and marriage fault lines along which such schemes were played out were by no means predictable.

As mentioned, many of the HIV-positive women I met believed that their husbands were aware of their HIV-positive status before the women themselves were tested and that their husbands had kept their HIV status secret to avoid blame and conflict within the family. This perception among women emerged particularly within the context of the support group networks for HIV-positive women, such as PWN+, which highlighted gender-based forms of discrimination in their efforts to redress violations against people living with HIV/AIDS within a human rights–based discourse. In fact, many women told me that they believed their husbands had known of their HIV status even before marriage. Yet it was increasingly women's HIV status that became known to other family members first because women were being tested for HIV during their pregnancy. In these situations men could continue to avoid moral blame by refusing to get tested, and the moral stigma could in this way attach only to the woman and, by extension, other members of her natal kin. As a result, within the context of marriage and kinship relations, women were often blamed by their in-laws for bringing HIV into the family. It was due to the prescience of this that Saraswati and her own parents sought to get her husband tested without his knowledge.

The Indian government also foresaw this possibility, as evidenced by their calling their policy the Prevention of Parent to Child Transmission program (vs. mother to child transmission) and by their encouraging simultaneous partner testing. This is one example of the ways in which global policies are mediated through national policy. The tendency to place HIV testing and counseling squarely within a set of kinship and marriage relationships not only is a policy move on the part of the government but also reflects the social and cultural understanding of HIV/AIDS and reproduction for the women, families, and medical personnel.

It is clear from Saraswati's comments that the medical personnel colluded with Saraswati and her parents to test her husband without his knowledge. This demonstrates that a concern with protecting themselves from HIV in the medical setting is not the only factor leading medical staff to bypass informed consent. Another reason is that HIV is not viewed as a private, individual issue so much as it is seen as a social issue and, in particular, a family issue that may warrant the abnegation of individual rights.

Saraswati's account also demonstrates that stigma within medical settings resulting from fears of transmission through medical interventions was clearly intense in 2000.

> After I tested HIV-positive, my doctor told me that she could not attend to my delivery. I saw two or three other doctors who also told me very openly that they would not attend my delivery. I didn't receive any medical care during my pregnancy at all after that. I wasn't even given iron tablets. Those doctors told me that I should have my delivery in a public hospital in Erode [the neighboring district], where HIV patients are cared for. I went to that hospital in Erode, and the doctor there said that he would care for me during my delivery.

Although it is easy to fault medical institutions and personnel for violations of human rights in discriminating against HIV-positive patients, it should also be noted that in some medical institutions, guaranteeing "universal precautions" may not be so simple.[2] For example, not all public hospitals have an adequate supply of sterilized disposable gloves to use with each patient. As mentioned earlier, in one public maternity hospital in Chennai where I conducted ethnographic research, the lab technician told me that he had a supply of only two pairs of gloves per day; he had to use one pair for all the HIV blood tests that he did in the morning and a second pair when he did the laboratory analysis of the tests in the afternoon.[3] Patients coming to this same hospital were expected to bring their own syringes for HIV testing, as noted earlier. Furthermore, in many cases hospitals are not air-conditioned, and wearing latex gloves and caps in the hot season can be extremely unpleasant for medical personnel. One doctor told me that the biggest problem in this respect is footwear. Disposable medical foot coverings are hard to come by, and medical practitioners are advised to wear heavy knee-high rubber boots. But wearing such boots in extremely hot and humid conditions is exceptionally uncomfortable, so many doctors resort to wearing rubber flip-flops and washing off any blood that may have gotten on their feet.[4] This poses risks for HIV transmission because blood can be transferred through cracks in the doctors' feet. It is also

...... to point out that, from the perspective of the medical personnel, vaginal childbirth deliveries pose one of the greatest risks for HIV transmission of all medical procedures—more than surgery—because bodily fluids (blood and amniotic fluid) flow uncontrollably and can easily splatter whoever is assisting with the delivery, thus posing an increased risk for HIV infection for medical personnel who do not have appropriate protective wear. Finally, training programs for medical personnel to handle HIV-positive cases have been uneven and were not universally carried out throughout Tamil Nadu, particularly not in rural districts, at the time of Saraswati's delivery in 2000.

I met women who had similar stories to tell about the prenatal and obstetric care they had received in 2000 elsewhere in Tamil Nadu. For example, Shalini came from a village in Perambalur District near Tiruchirapalli and had gone to a private hospital when she was pregnant with her first baby in 2000. When she tested HIV-positive there, they told her that they could not treat her and that she would have to go to the Government Hospital for her prenatal care and delivery. She said that, although she understood that she had an infection, she did not fully comprehend the nature of HIV and therefore did not believe that it was necessary for her to go to the Government Hospital. She explained that because Government Hospitals have a reputation for not providing optimum care, when she was in labor, she presented once again at the private hospital, whereupon they transferred her to the Government Hospital in the middle of labor because they said they could not handle HIV-positive cases. Once in the Government Hospital, she ended up having a cesarean section, which Shalini said was done because there was "not enough water in my uterus." That baby died four days after the birth, and she attributed the death to AIDS.

Returning to Saraswati, after she complained about her lack of medical care during her pregnancy, she qualified her point.

> There was one allopathic doctor who was treating me and my husband for HIV/AIDS while I was pregnant. He gave us injections. We were both supposed to have thirty injections on alternate days, and he said this would cure HIV and make it go away. Each injection cost 180 rupees. I had ten injections in the thigh but then I stopped because they were so painful. My injections cost about 1,800 rupees. My husband got thirty injections.

This comment, as well as my observations at T. A. Majeed's clinic (see Chapter 4), illustrates the ways in which medical practitioners from various systems of medicine throughout India have made claims to have developed cures for

HIV/AIDS. Majeed does so through Ayurvedic medicines, and Saraswati's other doctor was offering allopathic "cures."

Nonallopathic medicine has been found to help strengthen the immune system and improve well-being in people living with HIV/AIDS. For example, because Siddha treatments have been found to strengthen the immune system and thus aid the body in fighting opportunistic infections, the government provides these medicines for some opportunistic infections to HIV/AIDS patients at the Government Hospital of Thoracic Medicine in Tambaram. However, it is glaringly apparent that many individuals are taking advantage of the emergence of HIV/AIDS in India by selling so-called cures to people in desperate straits in the absence of affordable antiretroviral treatments. This is a particularly grave problem in the Indian context, where medical practitioners can operate largely unregulated. Given that Saraswati was denied prenatal care from the private hospital after her HIV-positive diagnosis, it is no surprise that she was willing to undergo this other treatment. No other doctor was advising her about the possible dangers to her health and the health of her baby from receiving these injections to "cure" her of HIV.

Saraswati went on to describe the events of the birth.

> Ten days before my due date, I went to that Government Hospital in Erode and checked in.[5] But suddenly, after three days in that hospital, when I showed the nurses my papers with my HIV-positive test results, one nurse said, "You people from Namakkal, you have no other work but to come to our hospital for all these kinds of things. We can't treat you!" She ripped up the "chit" with the test results and told me to go back to Namakkal. Then the doctor who had said that he would attend my delivery in that hospital came and scolded those nurses and said to me, "See, the staff here won't cooperate so it's better if you go to Namakkal." He gave me the name of a private doctor in Namakkal who would attend my delivery.

Perhaps the nurse ripped up the evidence of Saraswati's HIV test so that the hospital could claim to be referring her for some other reason and would thus be exempt from blame for discriminating against an HIV-positive patient.

Saraswati's birth story continued: "When I reached that private doctor in Namakkal, he said that he could care for me but he said that it might be hard to save me or my baby, and he asked us to have 20,000 rupees ready. The doctor said that since I was HIV-positive, I might die having a normal delivery so I would have to have a cesarean. He also said that a cesarean might help protect the baby." The explanations given for performing a cesarean section are confusing here.

Cesarean section is recommended to prevent HIV transmission from mother to child, although it was not performed routinely for that reason in the public hospitals in Tamil Nadu that had PPTCT programs because it was considered too costly to carry out for all HIV-positive mothers. But for this private practitioner, cost would not be an obstacle since he was charging Saraswati 20,000 rupees for this procedure. This was approximately three and a half months of her husband's total income at the time and, like the vast majority of Indians, she did not have access to any kind of health insurance to defray her medical costs. What is confusing is that Saraswati also said that the doctor claimed that the cesarean section was necessary to save her own life. It is not clear whether she misunderstood him, he incorrectly believed this, or there was some medical reason for this, or whether this was purely driven by a profit motive; or perhaps the doctor thought the cesarean posed less risk of HIV transmission to himself, given that it would allow for greater control over bodily fluids emitted.

Saraswati went on.

> Before the surgery, they started the "drip" [IV]. But then I needed to change into the hospital gown for the surgery and I could not change into it by myself since I was hooked up to the "drips." But the nurses refused to help me change so I had to wait until a "lady doctor" came, and she helped me change. And then, after the delivery, at 10:00 p.m. in the night, the "glucose drips" were running out and I needed a new "glucose bottle." But the nurses who were there refused to change the "bottle" for me. Two of the nurses there said that they had developed a high fever since they had touched me the day before and so none of them would change the "bottle." So I said, "Instead of letting it go dry, I will just pull the needle out of my hand myself." I started crying and my mother started wailing. Then the doctor heard this and came in, and the doctor changed the "bottle" himself. I was kept in a separate room in that hospital, and the nurses would stay outside the door and peep at me from outside.

This passage reflects a classic form of discrimination that occurred in many, although not all, medical settings. Similar experiences have been reported to me by other women. For example, Thameena, whose first delivery took place in a public hospital in 2005, complained of the poor treatment she received that made her feel as though she was being singled out and humiliated. Thameena described her experience.

> In the Government Hospital they keep us [HIV-positive people] separated and they talk badly about us when they come to give us an injection. They will only

give me an injection at the end, after giving everybody else their injections first. All the other patients would see this and give me insulting looks and talk about why they were giving me injections last. The doctor will not give me injections in the same way that he gave injections to others. For me only, he will wear gloves when he gives an injection. Not for the others. When I saw this, I felt very sad and hurt. After he gave me an injection, he washed his hands with alcohol, and that also made me feel very hurt.

Of course it is difficult to ascertain what in fact transpired during Thameena's birth. Why, for example, would a doctor or nurse have given her the injection last? Is it possible they are using the same needle for all patients? Is it possible they are not using gloves and sanitizing their hands with all patients? It may well be that this was her interpretation of what was going on and not in fact exactly what happened. Yet medical staff in some hospitals did complain about the lack of an adequate supply of syringes and gloves, suggesting that these may indeed be real material constraints that these medical personnel were working under. Regardless of what may have actually occurred, Thameena's anguish over feeling stigmatized in the medical setting was palpable.

In Saraswati's account it is interesting to note her different representations of the nurses and the doctors. It is clear that she thought it was the nurses who were the prime perpetrators of discriminatory practices, whereas the doctors—both male and female—were represented as much more caring and as stepping in to do the work of the nurses when the nurses refused. This is quite different from stereotypical representations of doctors and nurses in American hospital settings, where nurses are often said to be more nurturing and doctors more impersonal, aloof, and condescending.

My previous study of the biomedicalization of childbirth in Tamil Nadu revealed a similar pattern (Van Hollen 2003a). Birthing women were critical of the hospital nurses for scolding and denigrating women who expressed their pain in labor but spoke with more affection about the role of the doctors. My earlier analysis attributed this difference to differential performances of "professional dominance" (Freidson 1970). The medical staff, such as *ayahs*[6] and nurses, who came from a similar social milieu as the patients felt a greater need to demonstrate their position of superiority within the medical sphere to create social difference, whereas that social difference between the patients and doctors was more self-evident and therefore exhibited in more maternal ways by the predominantly female doctors (Van Hollen 2003a: 128–34). I suspect that this social difference may in part explain the apparent differences in the nurse-patient and doctor-patient relationships described by Saraswati. In addition, however, I think that in this context of treating patients with HIV, this difference may be a reflection of better education and training on the treatment and care of HIV/AIDS patients provided to doctors than to nurses and other supporting staff at that time, resulting in fewer fears about HIV transmission among the doctors than among the other medical personnel. It may also be related to the fact that, because of their social class, female nurses may have a difficult time discussing the potential for HIV transmission resulting from their work with their spouses, who are already ambivalent about their wives working in a profession that may involve touching men's bodies. Therefore they go out of their way to avoid any potential contact with HIV-infected patients.[7]

When I asked Saraswati if she or the baby received any treatment to prevent the transmission of HIV, she said that she did not think so, that she was never informed about anything like that, and that she did not remember having any tablets or injections for that during delivery. She did, however, remember the doctor's advice about caring for her newborn.

> After the baby was born, the doctor told me that I should wash my hands carefully every time before I touched my baby, that I should not breast-feed the baby, and that I should not lie near my baby since my breath should not touch the baby. When people saw me treating my baby this way, everyone came to know about my status. My son was very active, and the older women in the village would say, "Even when you haven't given mother's milk, your son is so active. Imagine how healthy and active he would be if you would breast-feed!" When these older women said that, my grandmother told them why I was not breastfeeding, and in that way the whole village came to know about my HIV status.

Although Saraswati's earlier comment suggests that the doctors were more knowledgeable about the modes of HIV transmission, here we see that this knowledge may have been uneven in 2000 because the doctor needlessly told Saraswati to avoid breathing close to her baby yet also advised against breast-feeding, which can be a mode of mother-to-child transmission. We also see in this section how HIV-positive women in Tamil Nadu may be criticized by their community for not breastfeeding their newborns because of a strong value placed on breastfeeding, and this public critique may lead to unintended disclosure of their HIV-positive status, often resulting in community-wide stigma.

Jayanthi Gives Birth: 2002

Two years after Saraswati delivered her child, Jayanthi gave birth knowing that she was HIV-positive. Jayanthi discovered her HIV status during the eighth month of her pregnancy with her second child. She had not been tested in her first pregnancy. I was introduced to Jayanthi at the sex-gender workshop in Namakkal, where I interviewed her. She was 26 years old at that time. Married at the age of 20, she became a widow at the age of 24, three days before the birth of her second child. After the death of her husband, Jayanthi, like Saraswati, left her in-laws' home and returned to live in her parents' home with her two children, both of whom were HIV-negative.

As with Saraswati, Jayanthi's account of the process of discovering her HIV-positive status reveals the kind of behind-the-scenes strategies of both family members and medical personnel. In her case her husband had fallen ill during her pregnancy, and Jayanthi's own father had taken her husband to the hospital for an HIV test, whereupon they discovered that her husband was HIV-positive. Her husband and father did not inform Jayanthi that they were going for the test or that he was HIV-positive, but they did inform the doctors at the hospital where Jayanthi was receiving her prenatal care. Jayanthi's husband and her father asked the doctor to inform Jayanthi of her husband's status through the prenatal counselor.

Similarly, I heard of some cases in which another family member was told by a doctor about a woman's HIV-positive diagnosis even before the woman herself was informed. For example, Suguna got her first HIV test at Apollo hospital, a prestigious private hospital in Chennai. She had opted to not get tested while her husband was dying of AIDS because she was worried that an HIV-positive diagnosis for her would put too much psychological strain on her husband and exacerbate his suffering. After the death of her husband, Suguna's father took her to Apollo for the test, and the results were first conveyed to her father, who then told her. Suguna explained that this was done because the doctors thought that women would not be able to handle such news alone; it would be too traumatic for them. We see from these two examples that doctors and other personnel working in the health service sector are often expected to play important roles as mediators for families, facilitating communication of this morally charged and emotionally difficult information within a family.

The United States mandates confidentiality of a patient's HIV status, reflecting a perception of HIV as a private, individualized disease, and this has become standard for international guidelines on HIV testing. Indeed, although patient confidentiality and informed consent are core components of biomedical practice in general, they are considered of paramount concern for medical care of HIV/AIDS patients because of the extreme stigma associated with AIDS, thereby contributing to the notion that "AIDS is unlike other diseases and must be handled with greater guarantees for individual privacy and autonomy" (Whyte et al. 2010: 85). This is referred to as AIDS exceptionalism. Among the communities in Tamil Nadu where I conducted my research, knowledge of someone's HIV status was perceived as a family affair—as something to be either disclosed or kept secret from particular relatives and sometimes from spouses—and medical personnel participated as brokers in the flow of this knowledge among kin. The Tambaram hospital used a computer program to track down family relations to get them tested. Thus community practice and state practices parallel one another but diverge from the global health policy that mandates patient confidentiality.

Researchers from other parts of the world have similarly revealed that global standards of HIV confidentiality are bent in practice as health care workers contend with "local moral worlds and specific clinical realities" (Whyte et al. 2010: 82). As Whyte and colleagues found during their research in Uganda, there is no such thing as patient anonymity in tight-knit rural communities where health care workers are friends or relatives of their patients. Thus, Whyte and colleagues argue, "The dense social networks that characterize rural life are based . . . not so much on confidentiality as on discretion" (Whyte et al. 2010: 82). The health care workers in Uganda find themselves breaching international codes of confidentiality, but they do so to be able to, in their minds, provide more personalized and thus better care for their patients. Through this example, Whyte and colleagues demonstrate the distinction that Arthur Kleinman (1995) makes between ethics and morality in the field of medical care.

> He [Kleinman] sees ethics as about abstract regulating principles established by experts about the good and right way for professionals to offer services to their clients. Morality is concerned with what is at stake in everyday experience in particular local worlds. . . . Moral decisions . . . are less about abstract values than practical dilemmas in the processes of social life. . . . However, as we have shown, ethics too are appropriated in specific moral worlds and thereby take on new significance in local interactions. (Whyte et al. 2010: 97)

Jayanthi continued recounting the events of her delivery.

After discovering that I was HIV-positive, while I was still pregnant my doctor gave me a tablet and told me to take the tablet as soon as I began to have my

pains. My pains came in the night, but I did not want to take that tablet because I was afraid that it would harm my baby. I didn't get proper information
about that. My husband had died three days before my labor began. I went to
the hospital in the night. It was a Taluk hospital [a public hospital for secondary care, also known as a District Headquarters hospital]. My mother and two
of my best friends came with me to the hospital.

We did not go to the same hospital that we went to for my checkups, so the
staff did not know that I had HIV. But the next day, one of my cousins came
and told the nurses at that hospital that I had HIV. She said, "Her husband
died because of HIV. Do not treat her or you might get the disease." They
asked me to leave. They asked me to go to the "GH" [Government Hospital for
tertiary care] in Namakkal. If I went to the Namakkal "GH," they might have
given medicine through the umbilical cord to the child. I knew they didn't
have that medicine here in this hospital. But I said that I would not leave now,
that I would not go to the Namakkal hospital until after the baby was born.
Then all of the "sisters" [nurses] went home and left me. I gave birth to my
baby like that, alone without any nurses there to help. I had terrible pain. I
didn't receive any treatment. Not a single drop of medicine. Not a single injection. After a little while, one "sister" came back. My mother gave her money.
Maybe she came back because of that.

There is no mention of any doctor present during her delivery, leading me to
assume that there was no doctor on night duty at that hospital, reflecting the
problem of understaffing in rural public hospitals in India that has been widely
documented. This account is reminiscent of the ethnographic work of Carolyn
Sargent and Joan Rawlins on hospital births in Kingston, Jamaica, where poor
women are stigmatized for being potential carriers of STDs and are therefore left
alone to deliver, unattended by any medical staff (Sargent and Rawlins 1992).

When I asked Jayanthi why she had not gone to the Government Hospital
in Namakkal when she knew that they had treatments to prevent the spread
of HIV there (she refers to this as "medicine through the umbilical cord to the
child"), had given her the tablets to take, and told her they would attend her
delivery, she explained that it was because she had a friend who was also HIV-
positive who had delivered her baby at that Government Hospital in Namakkal
just before her own baby was to be born. Her friend told her that no one at that
hospital helped her and that she had been forced to deliver her baby alone with
no medical staff assisting. Not wanting to have such an experience, Jayanthi
hoped that she could deliver at another hospital without them knowing about

her HIV status. In the end, her cousin came and blew her cover, so she had to suffer the same alienating experience as her friend in a hospital that had no preventive treatment available. Furthermore, her distrust of the medical system also led her to throw out the pills provided to prevent HIV transmission. It is not surprising that women like Jayanthi act pragmatically to fool the medical institutions if they think that this is the only way to receive treatment.

Without interfering cousins such as Jayanthi's it is also possible that such pragmatic efforts for survival could contribute to the spread of HIV in medical settings that are not set up to practice universal precautions for each and every normal delivery. Discriminatory practices at the hospitals lead to these kinds of strategies of secret resistance, which can fuel the spread of HIV and which also help explain why hospitals may not subscribe to informed consent and confidentiality for HIV testing. This creates a vicious cycle, detrimental to both HIV prevention and care. As Kavita Misra explains in a study of debates surrounding the discourses of confidentiality and rights within HIV/AIDS NGOs in India, this conundrum points to "larger philosophical and political debates on weighing collective versus individual good in the deployment of governance and in the construction of health as a site of governmentality" (Misra 2006: 55).

Saraswati's grandmother "outed" Saraswati's HIV status to the village in her attempt to defray the harsh criticisms about Saraswati's decision not to breast-feed. Jayanthi's cousin went out of her way to come to the hospital in the middle of the night to disclose Jayanthi's HIV status to the hospital staff, thereby making this known to the village community.[8] Saraswati's mother and father cooked up a scheme to force her husband to be tested to reveal his HIV status, and Jayanthi's father acted in concert with her husband to keep Jayanthi from knowing that her husband was being tested and, initially, from knowing her husband's HIV-positive status. These cases demonstrate that in Tamil Nadu the social experience of HIV/AIDS runs along the grooves of kinship and marriage relationships that serve at times to protect the dignity and health of these women and at other times to expose them to public indignities and prevent them from gaining access to the knowledge and health care needed to protect their health and the health of their future children. Clearly, as Carsten notes, inclusion through kinship is not as "intrinsically desirable" as anthropological analyses tend to assume (Carsten 2000: 28); it "can take both benevolent and destructive forms" (Carsten 2004: 9).

It is also important to note that, although in most cases the choice not to disclose one's HIV status to others stems from a desire to protect oneself from stigma and discrimination, at times it is a decision made in the interest of protecting others. Several women reported that they did not have the heart to tell their own parents, especially their mothers, that they were HIV-positive because they did not want to upset them. Some feel the same way about protecting their spouses. For example, Suguna did not even want to get tested for HIV after her husband tested HIV-positive and he was dying because she was worried that if he knew that she too had this disease, it would compound his suffering, thereby ruining his chances for recovery. She waited until just after his death to get tested. Rajeswari summed up this sentiment succinctly: "I feel sad in my heart. Let my sorrow be with me only." Yet she also understood how stressful it could be to keep something so profound secret.

> My husband and I are both HIV-positive, but no one in the family knows. I feel very sad about this. Whenever I am in the home, I am afraid, wondering: Who will come to know? How will they come to know? What will I do if they come to know? If they ask "Why are you taking so many tablets?" what will I say? What will I do if they come to know through that? What am I going to do? I am always very scared, thinking about these things.

Vijaya Gives Birth: 2004

HIV/AIDS can disrupt and wreak havoc on kinship and marital relationships at the same time that kinship norms provide a framework for the social responses to HIV/AIDS. HIV/AIDS is thus reproducing and transforming kinship and marriage in Tamil Nadu, just as new reproductive technologies have been reported to do elsewhere (Strathern 1995; Franklin and Ragoné 1998; Becker 2000; Inhorn and van Balen 2002). This is starkly apparent in the growing number of young AIDS widows (like Saraswati, Jayanthi, and Suguna) and the strategies that they and their families use to respond to these premature disruptions of family life. Vijaya also became an AIDS widow in 2000 when her first child was 4 years old. However, she would not come to know her own HIV status until four years later, in 2004, when she was in the ninth month of her second pregnancy after having gotten married again, this time to the older brother of her deceased husband (as discussed earlier).

Much has been written about the stigma of widowhood in the Indian context and about cultural proscriptions against widow remarriage (Agarwal 1994; Lamb 2000). The added stigma of being a widow did indeed exacerbate the already stigmatized position of being an HIV-positive woman, and both widowhood and an HIV-positive status often foreclosed the possibility of remarriage for women. This could be quite disastrous for women in a cultural context in which marriage alliances are arranged to provide economic and social support as much as emotional support. Veena Das (drawing from Pierre Bourdieu) demonstrated that in the aftermath of the violence of the partition of India and Pakistan, people were willing to engaged in modes of "practical kinship" to cope with the tragedies they had survived and perhaps even to forgive those who had perpetrated crimes in the crush of war and migration (Das 1995). I suggest that the same kind of practical kinship was operating in response to the tragedy of HIV/AIDS and the need to forgive in the face of moral accusations associated with this disease.

In Vijaya's case, rather than follow the cultural script forbidding widow remarriage—a pattern that was historically associated with primarily higher caste communities but that now cuts across many caste communities—her family, which belonged to the non-Brahmin *kovilpusari* caste, chose to follow another cultural possibility, that of levirate marriage, a possibility that coexists with the taboo against widow remarriage in Tamil Nadu (Agarwal 1994: 415–20). Others, however, are creating newer, unscripted kinship ties, like Renukha, who left her first husband (whom she later believed to be HIV-positive) and married her own sister's husband while her sister was still married to him. Each sister then had two children with the same husband, and they all lived together in one household. As discussed in Chapter 6, this was a highly unconventional marital arrangement.

I met Vijaya in one of the HUNS Positive Living Centers in Namakkal District in 2004. She was 34 years old and living with her mother-in-law, her second husband, and her two children. Her husband was engaged in construction wage labor, earning approximately 50 rupees per day (just over US$1) and supporting the family on his earnings alone.

Vijaya and her family knew that her first husband had died from AIDS. She herself had accompanied him to the Tambaram hospital. While she was at the hospital, she agreed to get an HIV test, but before collecting the results of that test, she journeyed back to Namakkal to look after her young child, whom she had left behind and who, she said, was crying for her mother to come home. Although she had understood then that she could have gotten HIV from her husband, neither she nor her parents realized that it would be possible for her to transmit it to her second husband or to a future child. "If I had known," she said, "I would have never agreed to remarry." She explained:

When my first husband died from AIDS, my family knew that it was because of AIDS, but they did not know that this could spread to the second husband.

My first husband used to drink a lot. So to overcome the "stigma," my family told other people that my husband died from a heart problem associated with alcoholism. My husband's brother was living away, and when he came back to Namakkal to take care of me and my child, the villagers said, "You should marry her." He didn't want to because he didn't want to get married at all. But finally he agreed. Then I told him about the fact that my first husband died from AIDS, and I told him that I should go back to Tambaram to get the result of the HIV test I had taken. But my second husband said, "Don't worry. You won't have it." So I never did go get the result.

Vijaya's experience of learning about her HIV status did not involve the same kind of duplicity that characterized the stories of Saraswati and Jayanthi. She learned that she was HIV-positive on her first prenatal checkup in a Taluk hospital in Namakkal District in the ninth month of her pregnancy. This was a hospital that had a PPTCT program in 2004. She received pretest counseling, gave informed consent for the testing, and received post-test counseling when she was found to be HIV-positive.

Unlike Saraswati, who deceived her husband into getting the HIV test, or Jayanthi, whose husband got tested without informing her and then told the medical staff about his status, Vijaya was open about her HIV status with her husband but was hesitant about having him get tested, even though the counselors at the PPTCT center strongly urged her to convince him to do so. In fact, she even pleaded with him not to get tested.

I told only my husband about the results of the HIV test. How could I hide it from my husband when he loves me? He was very supportive. He didn't even show his emotions initially. When I was crying, saying that I should not have gotten pregnant, he said, "Don't worry. The doctor said she can give you medicines to prevent the spread of this to the baby." At first I didn't want him to get tested because I thought if he was HIV-positive, I would feel badly. I cried, asking him not to get tested. He got tested after the baby was born. He tested HIV-negative. I would have felt bad if he was "positive" because I would know he had gotten this through me, that it would have spread from my first husband to my second husband through me. I understood from the PPTCT counselors that that was possible.

Vijaya said that she thought her husband was supportive of her HIV status because she was open with him about the issue right after they got married and because he recognized that it was, after all, because of his own brother that she had gotten HIV. His supportive attitude could perhaps also be due to a broader community-wide change in attitudes about HIV/AIDS between Saraswati's experience in 2000 and Vijaya's in 2004. Yet Vijaya was far from public with her status, suggesting that HIV/AIDS was still a highly stigmatized disease. Apart from the members of the HUNS network, Vijaya had not disclosed her HIV status to anyone other than her husband. Neither her in-laws nor her own parents had been informed. As she said, "Even my own mother does not know." Vijaya described the day of her child's birth.

> I went to the Taluk hospital when I started having labor pains. But the doctors and nurses would not see the delivery there. They referred me to "GH." People from HUNS helped me go to "GH." They got me admitted without telling the staff about my HIV status. It was only once I had been admitted into the hospital that we revealed my status.
>
> My baby is two months old. They have tested her four times, and the result has been HIV-negative. But they have asked me to reconfirm the test when she is eighteen months.

From Vijaya's account it is clear that even in 2004 women living with HIV in Namakkal District, one of India's districts with the highest HIV prevalence, still faced great obstacles in accessing basic maternity care at the time of delivery. The particular hospital that first refused to admit her when she was in labor was officially a PPTCT hospital. In fact, I visited that hospital on the very same day that I met Vijaya and was told about their PPTCT facilities. Yet the doctor with whom I spoke in that hospital did point out that the only HIV-positive women who presented in labor at that hospital thus far had been referred to the Government Hospital. Her explanation was that not all the medical personnel in that Taluk hospital were part of the PPTCT program, and those who were not trained in the PPTCT program would intervene and insist on referring the HIV-positive mothers. In a cynical aside she also said that those same doctors who insisted on referring patients to another public hospital sometimes referred HIV-positive patients to their private clinics, which they attended in the afternoons after completing their morning shift at the public hospital. This particular critique of the conflict of interest that arises for doctors who work in public hospitals in the mornings and at their private clinics in the afternoons and evenings is commonplace in India.

Just as Jayanthi attempted to access obstetric care while keeping her HIV status under the radar in 2002, this tactic was still being used in 2004, even in a Government Hospital with a PPTCT program. What is significantly different, however, is that Vijaya had the backing of the HUNS network to help her navigate the obstacles of the medical system. Among other advocacy activities, HUNS was providing access to legal aid for people living with HIV/AIDS who were facing all forms of discrimination, including discrimination in medical settings. The long queue of women who lined up to consult with the High Court lawyer at the workshop I attended in Namakkal was testimony to the importance of legal support for these women. Once admitted into the Government Hospital with the help of HUNS, there was no refusing Vijaya her treatment, and she and her newborn received nevirapine to help prevent the transmission of HIV to her child.

Despite the fact that others might view her experience as a circuitous path to obstetric care, riddled with obstacles, when I asked Vijaya how she felt about her birth experience, she replied, "I was completely satisfied with all the treatment and care I received from both the Taluk Hospital and GH." Similarly, Robbie Davis-Floyd found that most middle-class American women who hoped for a natural birth in a hospital setting but whose births, in fact, followed predictable patterns of medical intervention, resulting in cesarean sections, in the end reported overall satisfaction with the care they received. For the American women whom Davis-Floyd interviewed, their final sense of satisfaction was attributed to their belief that all the medical interventions were necessary for the safety of their babies, even though Davis-Floyd suggests that this was not always the case (Davis-Floyd 1992). Vijaya's satisfaction with her medical care must be placed within the historical context of Saraswati's and Jayanthi's birth stories. From this perspective we can appreciate the fact that Vijaya's birth was a victory for poor women living with HIV, but a victory that still required a struggle. As I reflect on accounts like Vijaya's, it sometimes seems as though women the world over are reduced to feeling grateful for whatever medical care they are dealt, just by virtue of the fact that it is provided and that their babies survive.

Kanakavalli Gives Birth: 2008

Kanakavalli lived in a village outside Namakkal, studied through the eighth standard, and at the age of 21 married her mother's brother's son, who was a lorry driver, and they set up a home together on their own. I met her nine years later, following a prenatal doctor's visit at the YRG Care center in Taramani, Chennai. She was 30 years old and six months pregnant with her first child. What had happened in those intervening nine years when most women from her village would have been raising small children at home?

As was expected, Kanakavalli did get pregnant soon after her marriage, but that pregnancy ended in a miscarriage. After recovering from that, she got pregnant again, only to suffer another miscarriage. After that, in 2002, two years after their wedding, Kanakavalli's husband fell ill with a continuous high fever. His father (Kanakavalli's maternal uncle) took him to a private doctor. She assumed that he must have had an HIV test, but her husband said he had not been tested. She kept pestering him, asking him if he had gotten the test and what the results were. As she explained to me, "AIDS is in our town. I knew two or three people who had died of AIDS. That's how I knew. That's why I kept asking." Ten days later her husband admitted that he had indeed been tested and that he was HIV-positive.

Kanakavalli was devastated but tried not to show her concern: "After he told me, I was crying all the time. But I was not crying in front of him because if I cry in front of him, he will become even more sick. I was weeping alone and then telling him, 'Don't worry; everything will be alright.'" But when Kanakavalli's HIV test also came back positive, her sympathy turned to anger. When her parents heard the news, they came and took Kanakavalli home with them. Her husband then went to live with his parents. She said that initially he called often, asking her to come live with him again, but she refused to even speak with him because "I was very angry that he did this to me." After five or six years passed, he began calling again. By then her anger had subsided, and she enjoyed talking with him regularly. Eventually they decided to move back in together, and within a few months she was pregnant again.

During one of her prenatal visits to a local Government Hospital, an outreach worker from YRG Care recruited her for their project. She had also joined a network during the years of separation from her husband, and she said that other members of the network had told her of the challenges they had faced while seeking obstetric care in the public and private hospitals around Namakkal and that they too had said YRG Care was preferable. So the offer of the YRG Care recruiter seemed too good to pass up, and she accepted. When I met her, she was in the sixth month of her pregnancy and she had come for her initial screening to participate in what she referred to as the "scheme" (using the English word). Most of the women I met in 2008 who were receiving prenatal care through YRG Care told me that they were receiving treatment through the scheme. They knew that this meant they were entitled to many more free services than they would have been had they gone to a public hospital, although that seemed to be the extent of their understanding of what it meant to participate in such a scheme. This is what Kanakavalli and other women participating in this particular scheme could expect from YRG:

1. Two prenatal visits (screening and one visit just before delivery). Patients coming from out of town were encouraged to seek regular prenatal care from a nearby hospital.
2. Cesarean delivery in a private hospital in the heart of Chennai where both HIV-positive and HIV-negative women would go for deliveries.[9]
3. Postnatal care visits one, two, and three weeks after delivery and then at longer intervals after delivery: five weeks, nine weeks, twelve weeks, twenty-four weeks, forty-nine weeks, and finally ninety-six weeks.
4. Formula for up to six months (plus bottles, a *paaladai*,[10] and a boiler pan in which to boil the bottles and *paaladai*).
5. One dose of nevirapine during labor, and for the baby a 2-milligram dose of nevirapine per kilogram of baby weight within seventy-two hours of birth.
6. Three different combinations of several other ARTs for the mother, which would be administered for seven days or twenty-one days after delivery, depending on which scheme group the mother was placed in.
7. All transportation costs to and from YRG Care, including the cost of bus fare for women who lived in distant villages, towns, and cities.
8. Accommodations for seven days for the delivery.[11]

All the women I interviewed who were participating in this program stated that they would not have been able to afford such comprehensive medical treatment if not for this scheme; private care would have been beyond their means, and all these treatments were not available through the government's PPTCT program. For example, if they had requested a cesarean section in a Government Hospital, they would have had to pay for it themselves because it was not routinely performed for HIV-positive women through the PPTCT program. The formula and bottles themselves were a major expense and too expensive for some of these women. Although the government had rolled out a program to provide ART in the middle of 2004, there were clearly problems with access. For example, Suguna, who was receiving ART as part of her prenatal care through YRG Care, explained to me that before becoming pregnant and receiving prenatal care at YRG Care, she and her husband were both purchasing ART at a 75% discounted rate through the Global Fund[12] program administered through YRG Care. Even with the discount, however, she said that the cost of these medicines for herself and her husband combined was a serious strain on them financially because they were paying 2,000 rupees monthly, and this had to come out of a monthly income of 6,000 rupees, which was significantly higher than the income of most of the women I met. When I said that my understanding was that starting in mid-2004 they could receive ARTs for free through select Government Hospitals, such as Tambaram and asked why they did not opt for that, Suguna replied that they would have to travel to Salem (a five and a half hour bus ride from Chennai, to which they had recently moved) to get the ARTs through the Government Hospital there. Even if they wanted to avail themselves of the free ARTs in Salem, they would first have to procure a ration card to make them eligible, and that, she said, was a long and complicated process and they might have to pay costly bribes to local officials to obtain the card. Was the government's ART program highly cumbersome and inefficient? Or did Suguna and her husband misunderstand how the program was being administered? Either way, clearly it was not working to serve their needs, and the same may well have been true for others.

Furthermore, based on the testimonies of many other women I met who had delivered babies through the YRG Care scheme that same year, Suguna and Kanakavalli could expect to receive something equally valuable to women: love and affection. Fatima's sentiment was echoed by many others. She explained:

> To tell you the truth, my husband could not have afforded to take care of me with the financial problems we are having. And even if I could have afforded to get treatment in a private hospital, I would not have received this level of care. When my husband was not feeling well, we went to the "GH." There, even for treating simple illnesses, they will charge twenty or thirty rupees. But here the treatment is all free. Moreover, they are taking care with love and affection. I don't know what would have become of me if I had had to get treated in any other hospital.

Shalini also had high praise for the care received from YRG Care compared to the Government Hospitals: "Here everything is nice. If I would have gone to the Government Hospital in Trichy [Tiruchirapalli] as soon as I conceived, they would not have taken much care. They get plenty of money but they do nothing for society. Whereas here, they are taking care of me with love. Here we get treatment to our hearts' content, though we reach here with difficulty by bus." Geetha went so far as to characterize the doctors at YRG Care as a divine gift from the gods: "We do believe in the doctors here. We feel that these doctors are the divine spirit, and they will help us by giving us good treatment and helping us to get rid of this disease. We believe the doctors here are sent by god."

It is no wonder, then, that women were coming to YRG Care from far-flung places all over Tamil Nadu and even from the neighboring state of Andhra Pradesh. In my sample of twenty women whom I met through YRG Care (all Tamil speakers because of my own ability to speak Tamil with them), I met women who were traveling from as far away as Theni, Nagapattinam, Madurai, Dharmapuri, Tiruchirapalli, and Namakkal. For Kanakavalli the bus ride from Namakkal took six hours. Another woman, who was coming from Theni, said the bus took eleven and a half hours. Had the bus fare not been made available, these women may not have been able to come. For some the distance from home was welcome because it provided them with increased privacy, which helped to ensure that knowledge of their HIV status would not spread through the community as a result of the increasing number of medical personnel who knew of their status. Yet, despite their gratitude for the bus fare and all the top-notch treatment and care they received, several women did say that the constant travel over long distances, not only late in the pregnancy but also frequently for the follow-up visits with infants in tow, caused tremendous strain on them physically.

. . .

Each of these four births took place after the government's PPTCT project had been initiated in Government Hospitals (either in its pilot phase or in its subsequent programmatic phase) and after treatment to prevent mother-to-child transmission of HIV had been made available in some private hospitals as well. Yet the mere fact that such treatments and programs exist tells us little about the lived experiences of pregnancy and childbirth for women living with HIV. My discussion of the births of Saraswati, Jayanthi, Vijaya, and Kanakavalli reveals that even though programs to prevent mother-to-child transmission were formally available, these four women all faced difficulties in obtaining obstetric care, primarily because of stigma and discrimination in medical settings but also because of what was perceived to be inadequate medical care itself.

The practice of medical care for mother-to-child HIV prevention programs is not universally implemented in the same way across the globe; it is shaped by local social organization and cultural understandings of HIV and birth. The local understandings and practices at times inform the state's interpretation of global health policy, as we can see in the state's choice of nomenclature of the PPTCT program and the state's more family-centered interpretation of patient confidentiality. When we examine the social uses and practice of medicine in Tamil Nadu, it is apparent that HIV testing and care, particularly in the context of reproduction, are not viewed as matters pertaining exclusively to the patient as an individual; rather, they are seen as events that involve broad networks of kinship and marriage. In Tamil Nadu an HIV diagnosis in the context of reproduction demands a careful and strategic but varied selection of alliances along kinship and marital lines that informs how knowledge flows and how care is, or is not, provided.

My study of women's HIV experiences also demonstrates how medical personnel in Tamil Nadu are drawn into these family alliances and how the practices of medical care for HIV/AIDS—including the absence of uniformly applied informed consent for HIV testing and confidentiality—are responses to local sociocultural contexts. Medical personnel may become coconspirators trying to keep an HIV diagnosis hidden from some family members or trying to expose HIV status to other family members. In turn, family members may inform medical personnel of someone's HIV status even when a patient is trying to keep that information away from the doctors and nurses. Sometimes the medical personnel's links to and participation in kinship and community networks were beneficial to the women in this study, and at other times these connections worked against their own interests. Above all, what these case studies reveal is that, whether women living with HIV are confronting stigma and discrimination in medical institutions or within their extended kin and community networks, their vulnerable situation itself demands that they engage in complex, pragmatic, and often creative strategies just to obtain basic obstetric services.

The combination of medical care and psychological support that women like Kanakavalli received at YRG Care is impressive and seems to suggest a positive development. On closer examination, however, it is clear that it does not mark an improvement per se; rather, it points to a solution for improvement. The package that these women were receiving was clearly superior to anything else that they could afford, thereby significantly reducing the risk of HIV transmission to their babies.[13] But at what cost? What does it say about the success of the government's PPTCT program that women living in poverty are crossing state borders and traveling more than eleven hours by bus to receive obstetric care?

Equally disconcerting is the fact that for many of the women there were strings attached to receiving this care, strings that seemed invisible to them. Namely, they were participating in a National Institutes of Health (NIH) sponsored clinical trial with pharmaceutical support provided by Abbott Laboratories, Boehringer Ingelheim Pharmaceuticals Inc., Gilead Sciences, and Glaxo Smith Kline (all headquartered in the United States and Europe) to evaluate antiretroviral strategies to reduce nevirapine resistance (the study is NIH Clinical Trial ACTG 5207). The trials were conducted independently of the Government of India but required government approval.[14] The National Institute of Allergy and Infectious Diseases reported in its *2007–2008 Biennial Report on Women's Health Research* that this clinical trial was being carried out in parts of Africa, India, Haiti, and Thailand[15]—all areas of the world where single-dose nevirapine treatments are more widespread than in North America and Europe. During this same time period, YRG Care was also involved in another NIH-sponsored clinical trial for babies of these mothers as well as a clinical trial for discordant couples who were expecting a baby.

Another project for pregnant women was funded by USAID through Population Services International and implemented by YRG Care. This was the Connect project and was a service project rather than a clinical trial. The Connect project also offered women elective cesarean sections and free formula. In addition to the single dose of nevirapine, additional antiretroviral medicines were given to pregnant women enrolled in this program, and these ARTs were subsidized by the Global Fund.[16] These women were given only a one-month supply of ART at a time. This was to ensure that they would come for regular monthly checkups. Furthermore, I was told that rationing was also done to prevent women from giving their free medications to their HIV-positive husbands, which was apparently a common practice.[17] The women I interviewed who were enrolled in this program thought that this was a burden because, unlike the NIH clinical trial, transportation costs were not included in the Connect project.

When I interviewed women who were coming for their prenatal or postnatal care or women who were at YRG Care recovering from their deliveries, it was apparent that all were aware that they were getting benefits through YRG Care that were not available elsewhere, but most did not know whether they were participating in a clinical trial or in a service project. They did, however, know whether or not their transportation expenses were being covered, and this became the primary way for me to discern whether they were participating in a clinical trial or a service project. Those who did know they were participating in a clinical trial said that they had given consent, but they did not know which clinical trial they were participating in and they did not seem to be concerned about their role in such trials. The bottom line for these women was that they knew what services they were receiving and that these services far outshined what was otherwise available to women in their economic bracket.

I have no doubt that the women who were participating in the clinical trials were informed about the trial and gave their informed consent. YRG Care is careful to follow strict international guidelines pertaining to the ethics of research and informed consent, and women reported giving consent for the care they were receiving at YRG Care. However, the broader significance of the role they were playing in the global research and production of drugs by and for multinational pharmaceutical companies did not seem to register with them. These were not women who were choosing between a full package of PMTCT care and the same thing with new trial drugs. They were choosing between being able to afford to safely provide replacement feeding and not being able to, knowing that breastfeeding could increase the risks that their child could be HIV-positive; or between being able to have a cesarean section and not being able to, knowing that a cesarean section could prevent transmission of HIV from mother to child. These are the things these women think about when they give consent. They become vessels for Western pharmaceutical companies' research in the process, and global inequalities are thus reinscribed through their bodies.

In the early days of the epidemic, AIDS activists tied to the gay rights movement in North America, Europe, and Australia demonstrated what Nguyen described as a "strong therapeutic militancy" when they demanded to be included in clinical trials for HIV/AIDS treatment as a form of politics (Nguyen 2010: 91). Nguyen considers these demands to reflect a kind of therapeutic citizenship that "[grows] out of a sense of duty so that others may benefit from treatment eventually found to be effective" (Nguyen 2010: 92). When clinical trials for AIDS treatments later moved outside North America, Europe, and Australia to less affluent parts of the world, they became mired in controversy and were sometimes denounced as racist; for example, some patients were given placebos or were kept on certain therapies when other therapies had already been found to be more effective (Nguyen 2010: 92–93). My own concern with the women participating in the clinical trials through YRG Care is not that some of them were provided with better ART treatment than other participants in the same trial. Rather, it is that these women were making their bodies bioavailable not out of a sense of duty for the greater good, about which they could have felt some pride, but in order to receive the basic components of the full package of PMTCT care to prevent HIV transmission to their children, which otherwise would not have been available to them. As Adriana Petryna writes in her penetrating analysis of the post-1980s outsourcing of clinical trials for U.S.-based companies, "The increasing 'choice' of citizens in transitioning economies to become experimental subjects parallels their poverty status and often reveals the limits of local standards of care and the failure of states to protect citizens" (Petryna 2009: 31). Women should not have to make such circumscribed "choices."

According to Nguyen, this "choice" also represents a kind of therapeutic citizenship. In this case it is because of the exceptionalism of the global response to AIDS, combined with the absence of adequate governmental medical care for HIV-positive people in India, that HIV-positive people in India, such as the women I interviewed at YRG Care, become enmeshed in complex webs of rights and obligations to

> a consortium of NGOs, foreign donor governments, Northern universities,[18] hospitals, research institutions, churches, pharmaceutical firms, and even the American military. It is they who now administer life-saving treatment for millions living with HIV in Africa and, indeed, in other parts of the world, through tangled organizational webs that ensure distribution of money, drugs, and resources. . . . They directly govern the lives of populations with HIV and, in fact, exercise the power of life or death over them. (Nguyen 2010: 187)

The Indian state and the state of Tamil Nadu are by no means absent players, as seems to be the case in Nguyen's study of Côte d'Ivoire. Therefore I would include these state institutions in the larger consortium that Nguyen captured so well and described as exercising "the power of life or death" over HIV-positive people living in poverty around the globe.

8 Breast or Bottle?
HIV-Positive Women's Responses to
Global Health Policy on Infant Feeding

AS I HAVE DEMONSTRATED IN THIS BOOK, responses to HIV/AIDS in India bring cultural values and social relations into sharp focus, as they emerge like photographic images in troubled waters of a darkroom. At the same time, responses to this disease lead to social and cultural metamorphoses more akin to the creative manipulation of reality with digital photography. In this chapter I explore how public health efforts to prevent the transmission of HIV from mother to child through breast milk and responses to these efforts simultaneously reflect and transform core cultural values and socioeconomic relations in Tamil Nadu.

Without any interventions, worldwide HIV transmission rates can vary from 15% to 30% without breastfeeding and can be as high as 40% with breastfeeding up to twenty-four months (WHO 2002). Studies suggest that the risk of HIV infection through exclusive breastfeeding itself for up to six months is approximately 4% (WHO 2007: 2). According to the SWEN Study Team's 2008 report in the *Lancet*, "Breastfeeding continues to pose a significant risk of HIV transmission to infants born to HIV-infected mothers, accounting for about 150,000 infant infections per year, mainly in low-income settings" (SWEN 2008: 300).[1]

However, risks of malnutrition, dehydration, or infection from improper use of replacement feeding may exceed 4%, and the risk of HIV transmission with mixed breastfeeding and alternative feeding (whether formula, milk, or other liquids and solids) is higher than the risk with exclusive breastfeeding (WHO 2007: 3). The potential for such risks is high among poor communities, particularly in the global south, where lack of access to clean drinking water or fuel to boil water and bottles for sanitation may preclude access to safe replacement feeding. Furthermore, cultural taboos against bottle feeding may compel some women to mix bottle feeding with breastfeeding. In such cases policies that advocate exclusive replacement feeding may increase rather than decrease health risks to infants of some HIV-infected mothers.[2]

As a result, following the lead of international organizations such as WHO and UNICEF, NACO and TNSACS also chose to move away from an earlier policy of uniformly advocating replacement feeding for all HIV-positive mothers. Instead, they adopted a more nuanced approach in which counselors in the PPTCT program were charged with the task of evaluating whether or not the following criteria were in place to guarantee the success of replacement feeding: affordability, feasibility, acceptability, sustainability, and safety. These five factors are collectively known as AFASS. If all AFASS criteria were deemed to be met, a counselor could recommend replacement feeding if a mother requested the counselor's advice. As a rule, however, the new guidelines recommended that counselors provide mothers with the pros and cons of both feeding methods and then allow the mother to make an informed choice.[3] Unlike some other countries, the Indian government does not have a program to provide replacement feedings or bottles free of cost to HIV-positive mothers.

Drawing primarily from my interviews with those thirty-two women who knew about their HIV-positive status during their pregnancies and births, in this chapter I seek to reveal how low-income HIV-positive women make decisions about infant feeding and how they respond to the shifting terrain of public health recommendations. By doing so, I hope to demonstrate just how complicated, if not impossible, it is to determine the AFASS criteria for individual women in Tamil Nadu, given the complex and sometimes contradictory interplay between cultural and economic determinants in this decision-making process.

This chapter contributes to a growing body of social science literature on HIV and infant feeding that explores the cultural and economic determinants of infant feeding options for HIV-positive women around the world. Most of the earlier studies on this topic have been based on research in sub-Saharan and West African countries (e.g., de Paoli et al. 2002; Desclaux 2004; Doherty et al. 2007; Kerr et al. 2008; Blystad and Moland 2009; Hofmann et al. 2009; Traoré et al. 2009). Others are large-scale comparative studies across several countries (e.g., Cook and Dickens 2002; Desclaux and Alfieri 2009). In this vein, my study is significant because it provides in-depth ethnographic insights into the previously undocumented circumstances, perceptions, and decision-making processes surrounding infant feeding by poor women living with HIV in India. In their 2004 article "Breastfeeding and Infant Feeding Practices Research in India: A Critical Review," published in *AIDS and Maternity in India* (Cohen and

Solomon 2004), Lakshmi Lingam and Siddhi Mankad suggest that in studies on breastfeeding in India "the presentation of quantitative data is given precedence over its qualitative analysis" (Lingam and Mankad 2004: 205), and they point to the need for a "socio-anthropological perspective" (206) to this research in the Indian context. Furthermore, they state that there were no qualitative Indian studies on the relationship between HIV and infant feeding at that time (203). My in-depth ethnographic analysis on this topic serves to fill these gaps.

Like my study, several of the mentioned qualitative studies demonstrate how global health initiatives become localized when implemented on the ground. In particular, these studies often foreground the "local cultures of breastfeeding" (Desclaux and Alfieri 2009: 822) and examine the symbolic value given to breastfeeding and other forms of infant feeding in various communities. Studies conducted in sub-Saharan and West African countries point to the central role that breastfeeding plays in the cultural construction of motherhood; the investigators argue that, given this high cultural value associated with breastfeeding along with the problems of entrenched poverty, exclusive breastfeeding of infants of HIV-positive mothers will have greater success than replacement feeding (Hofmann et al. 2009). One of the reasons that women in these studies mention for not wanting to use replacement feeding is a concern that this will be interpreted as a sign of their HIV-positive status and will therefore lead to disclosure of their status, which they are trying to keep secret (sometimes even from their spouses), and they fear that this disclosure will lead to stigma and discrimination (Desclaux and Alfieri 2009: 825; Traoré 2009). My study also demonstrates a high cultural value placed on breastfeeding for mothers in India. Nevertheless, like most of the women in the three-country study comparing Burkina Faso, Cambodia, and Cameroon (Desclaux and Alfieri 2009: 824), most of the women in my study also said that if they could afford replacement feeding, they would choose that option, despite the concerns about being criticized for not breastfeeding. These women, in consultation with counselors and medical practitioners, developed creative means to defray such criticisms. Furthermore, the concern that replacement feeding would be interpreted by others as an indication of being HIV-positive was not expressed by the women in my study. This is because, compared with some sub-Saharan and West African countries, HIV-prevalence rates in India are quite low and most people in India are not aware of knowing anyone with this disease (Namakkal was the exception to this rule in my study). Moreover, although most of the women in my study were careful not to disclose their HIV status to many others inside or outside their kin groups, in no case did I meet an HIV-positive woman who said that her spouse was not aware of her seropositive status, even when the spouse was HIV-negative.

My study also supports the arguments made by others (Desclaux and Alfieri 2009: 825) that women not only must weigh deep-seated cultural values and economic realities in their decision-making process but also must negotiate what appear to be mixed messages from two different vertical public health campaigns, one being UNICEF's Baby Friendly campaign, which advocates the nutritional benefits of breastfeeding, and the other being the HIV/AIDS prevention campaigns, which in the past recommended replacement feedings and now recommend either replacement feeding or exclusive breastfeeding, depending on each woman's circumstances. To add to this confusion, and like other investigators (Desclaux and Alfieri 2009), my research suggests that the nature and content of counseling is uneven across hospitals and even among counselors in the same hospital; in theory counselors are supposed to provide women with informed choices, but in practice they tend to be directive, recommending one method of feeding or another.

Other studies have tended to use ethnographic evidence to make a case for specific policy changes, such as more forceful advocacy for breastfeeding in "resource poor" countries, particularly in cultural contexts where breastfeeding is the norm and is associated with good mothering (Coutsoudis et al. 2008). Other examples of specific policies are recommendations to pay particular attention to certain kinds of information when counseling (such as whether or not the woman has access to piped water or certain fuels and/or whether or not she has disclosed her HIV status) and to use those specific indicators to direct counseling (Doherty et al. 2007). Another example is recommendations that suggest including grandmothers or spouses in decision making in order to have more success with adhering to either replacement feeding or exclusive breastfeeding (Kerr et al. 2008; Traoré et al. 2009).

Making specific policy recommendations regarding the benefits of breastfeeding or replacement feeding for most of the women in resource-poor settings or even in poor communities in India is outside the purview of my expertise. However, in addition to the ethnographic specificity in the South Indian context, my research diverges from these earlier studies in several important ways. First, I provide specific case studies of HIV-positive women who have bottle-fed one baby but breast-fed another, and I examine their reasons for doing so in each circumstance. More important, I demonstrate the complex logic that women use as they attempt to make sense of shifting policy recommendations on infant feeding over time and provide insight into women's own interpretations of the relationship between the different feeding methods they used and the health outcomes of their children.

Finally, my study differs because it does not view culture as a static factor that influences decision making. Rather, I demonstrate how cultural values themselves are being transformed as HIV-positive women make sense of their lives and make decisions about their bodies and the bodies and lives of their children. Astrid Blystad and Karen Moland's study in Ethiopia and Tanzania also points to a cultural transformation of women's perceptions of motherhood and the body. However, their study depicts a negative transformation from viewing milk as a symbol of nurture and love to a symbol of death, thereby, they argue, inhibiting the possibility of activism in the context of PMTCT programs (Blystad and Moland 2009). My research also demonstrates the confusing, contradictory symbols of mother's milk in the PPTCT program. However, my study hints at the possibility for transformations of subjectivity that foster activism within the context of the PPTCT program. Specifically, I found that local notions of women's power (*sakti*) were evoked in the process of translating biomedical concepts about immunity (both in conversations of the loss of immunity resulting from HIV/AIDS and in conversations about the immunological benefits of breastfeeding). These concepts were further becoming fused with feminist and human rights discourses of positive living found among women involved in the networks. This fusion enabled women to challenge cultural ideas about the centrality of breastfeeding in the construction of motherhood, thereby making replacement feeding not only more acceptable but also potentially a sign of their power as HIV-positive mothers and of their resistance to the stigma and discrimination they faced because of their HIV-positive status. In short, my study demonstrates how some poor HIV-positive women are actively negotiating and refashioning the discourse of global health agendas and of international rights movements in local idioms to serve their own interests.

Assessing AFASS Criteria in Counseling

Despite the new guidelines regarding informed choice and the use of the AFASS criteria in counseling, some of the UNICEF representatives I met lamented that, in practice, counseling is rarely so in-depth as to allow a counselor to either assess the AFASS criteria of the mother or to provide full and balanced options. In practice, they explained, counselors tend to steer the mothers one way or another. This was certainly what I found in my interviews and observations. A counselor working in one Government Hospital with a PPTCT program told me that "we tell them not to breast-feed; to only give bottled milk." A counselor in yet another Government Hospital said, "It is best if they give mother's milk [*taay paal*] since that provides the baby with immune power [*ethirppu sakti*], so we tell the mothers that."

Ethirppu means "opposition," "protest," or "resistance" (*Dictionary of Contemporary Tamil* 1992), and *sakti* can be translated as "power." So *ethirppu sakti* can be literally translated as "resistance power," and it is the term used by health care practitioners to translate the biomedical concept of immunity or immune power into Tamil. The power connoted in the term *sakti* is gendered. In Hindu cosmology *sakti* is understood as a kind of female regenerative power associated with women's reproductive abilities and with the divinity of the goddess or Devi (Wadley 1980; Van Hollen 2003a, 2003b). According to Hindu conceptions of personhood, although both men and women are said to have *sakti*, women are generally thought to have more *sakti* than men because of women's reproductive capacities as mothers. Toward the end of this chapter I explore the significance and creative uses of this term for the HIV-positive women I met.

In some instances the same counselor would advise some mothers to breast-feed and others to give replacement feeding, which seemed to follow the flexible AFASS counseling approach. For example, one day I met two HIV-positive mothers who had recently delivered their babies through the PPTCT program in one of the government maternity hospitals in Chennai. The first woman, Saroja, who had delivered her baby the day before I met her, told me, "The people in the hospital told me to breast-feed for five months." But the second woman, Amaldevi, who had delivered her baby two days before Saroja in the same hospital, explained, "Since breastfeeding may cause HIV to pass to baby, the 'counselors' said that I should not breast-feed. Formula [*paal podi*] is expensive, but there is no other option." Both of these women stated unequivocally that they were given clear instructions from the counselor at this hospital, not that they were given the options and told to decide themselves.

I was curious to understand how the counselors had assessed the AFASS criteria of these two women. Reflecting on this, I reviewed the notes from my own interviews with them. Both were from villages on the outskirts of Chennai. Saroja had never attended school, whereas Amaldevi had completed the ninth standard, so I thought perhaps that was an important AFASS factor. Amaldevi had agreed to undergo sterilization following her delivery, whereas Saroja did not want to go through with this surgery but was determined to never get pregnant again. Perhaps the counselors correlated both higher education and sterilization with a higher AFASS rating? Yet Saroja reported a slightly higher household income at 4,000 rupees per month, compared to Amaldevi's

3,500 rupees per month. Saroja's husband sold ready-made clothing, whereas Amaldevi's husband worked the night shift at a printing press. Saroja earned extra income doing "coolie" work, and Amaldevi was a housewife. Furthermore, Saroja was much older, age 35, and in her second marriage, compared to Amaldevi, who was only 22 and having her second child. One might think that increased age would increase the AFASS rating, but perhaps being in a second marriage was thought to decrease one's AFASS score. Saroja's first husband died of AIDS, and she believed she got the virus from him and she berated his bad character. Amaldevi, on the other hand, was convinced that her husband had received HIV from a blood transfusion he received five years before their marriage and told me that "neither my husband nor I have done anything wrong." I wondered, Was it possible that unconsciously AFASS assessments followed the all too well traveled paths of viewing some HIV-positive people as innocent and therefore more qualified for AFASS replacement feeding, whereas others were considered immoral and were therefore scored lower on the AFASS scale? In short, I was baffled as to how counselors might assess the AFASS criteria of these two women in such a way as to make opposing recommendations.

The next time I came to the hospital, I asked the counselor in charge about these two cases. He explained that it all came down to one factor, even though, according to WHO guidelines, all five AFASS criteria must be met in order to recommend replacement feeding. Amaldevi was receiving care and support through a local NGO. The counselor thought this was essential for the sustainability of replacement feeding. Saroja was not affiliated with any such organization, and therefore her family would not be able to overcome the social stigma that she would face from community members if she did not breast-feed. But then he added (in English), "It's really their choice." This supports arguments made by others that the criteria counselors use to make their assessments are often limited. For example, Desclaux and Alfieri (2009) found that in Cameroon "the assessment by health workers of mothers' means was based on an informal assessment using a few features such as the woman's appearance, origin, social status, and occupation, without objective criteria explored in a systematic way" (824).

HIV-Positive Women's Decisions and Perceptions About Infant Feeding

I wondered about the future impact of this kind of assessment on the lives of Amaldevi and Saroja and their newborn children. What might they think down the road about the "choice" of method for infant feeding they were making? I looked to the experiences of other HIV-positive women who had used different methods of infant feeding to get a sense of how they assessed their choices in retrospect. Most interesting were those cases in which the same mother had breast-fed one child and given replacement feeding to another. Why had they done so? How did they themselves evaluate these different feeding practices and their outcomes? How did the AFASS factors come into play in their own decision making and self-evaluations?

Devi, Karpagam, and Renukha were all HIV-positive mothers who had not breast-fed their first child but had breast-fed their second child. Yet the reasons for the differential feeding methods varied in these three cases, the HIV outcomes were not uniformly patterned, and the mothers' opinions about the risks and benefits of breastfeeding and replacement feeding were not consistent. Each case demonstrates cultural and/or economic logics at play, yet not in a patterned way that would justify uniform counseling or the kind of directed counseling that was being practiced. In short, these three cases are not intended to be representative of all the women in my study but are presented to demonstrate variability. Following these three case studies, I discuss some core cultural and economic issues that did cut across the lives of the women in my study.

Devi

Devi was 34 years old when I met her. She lived with her husband and their two young children—a 4-year-old daughter and a 1½-year-old son—in a tiny thatched squatter house built up against another building in a narrow alley in the heart of Chennai. It was during my conversation with Devi in the Gandhi Mandapam Park that she revealed to me her assumption that her conversion to Christianity was a prerequisite for receiving care and treatment from World Vision.

Originally from Salem District, Devi, who had never attended school, entered into a love marriage with her first husband, but she left him because of his "bad habits" (*mosamaana pazhakangal*), especially pickpocketing. After that she and her brother came to Chennai looking for work, and, through a connection with a woman from her community in Salem, she got a job carrying bricks and sand at a construction site. That woman then convinced Devi to come with her to a suburb of Mumbai called Mulnund, promising to find her a better job there. Instead, the woman sold Devi into prostitution to a *hijra* who ran a brothel. Although Devi was concerned about STDs during her years in Mumbai, she had no knowledge whatsoever of HIV/AIDS.

> While I was engaged in prostitution, I did not know anything about HIV and no one warned me to be careful. If we asked the "customers" to use condoms,

they would go out and complain and our boss would beat us. I used to demand that a condom be used because I was scared I would get sores. I did not know about HIV. Other women who were with me there told me that I would get sores.

I do not know if the men who came to me in Mumbai knew about AIDS. I myself came to know about HIV only after coming back here to Chennai. People who have sex with prostitutes are twenty-one years old and up. Both married and unmarried men come. But they never talked about AIDS.

Three years later, after Devi had unsuccessfully tried to escape from the brothel several times, the brothel was raided by the Tamil Nadu state police, who were in search of Tamil women who had been sold into the Mumbai sex trade. Devi's boss gave her a train ticket to flee back to Chennai. Unlike many of the women who were shunned by their families after being returned to them on the Mukti Express after this brothel bust, Devi was fortunate that her brother took her in, even though he knew that she had been employed as a sex worker. She stayed with him for two years before she got a job as a domestic servant and went to live on her own in a hostel. It was at that time that she met her second husband and they began living together.

Devi's new husband had not been married before, and she did not inform him about either her first marriage or her involvement in the sex industry. In 1999, when she was five months pregnant, she went to a government maternity hospital for her first prenatal checkup. It was then that she was first tested for HIV. But, rather than return to the hospital to get the results of the test, as she had been instructed to do, following Tamil cultural norms, Devi left for her native village in Salem to have a home delivery in her parents' home with a local midwife (*marruttuvacci*), and she remained there for several months. When the counselors from the hospital discovered her HIV status and Devi had not come to collect the results, they tried in vain to track her down in Chennai using the Chennai address she had provided. But because Devi lived in a squatter hutment, the address was imprecise and they could not locate anyone who knew of her.

Devi said that when her daughter was born in the village, she tried to give her mother's milk but her daughter didn't like it (*pidikillai*), and after a short while, she didn't have any milk to give. So using a *paaladai*, she fed her baby with Aavin cow's milk. Aavin is formally known as the Tamilnadu Co-operative Milk Producers' Federation Ltd. Aavin milk is widely consumed throughout the state and is considered high-quality milk at reasonable cost. Devi had no idea at this point that she was HIV-positive or that HIV could spread to a baby through breast milk. The choice of replacement feeding in her case was independent of her knowledge of her HIV status.

It was not until Devi was in the seventh month of her next pregnancy in 2002 that she returned to the same hospital in Chennai for a prenatal checkup and learned that she was HIV-positive. The counselors had her name and status on record, so they were immediately able to make the connection that she was the same woman they had tried to track down a few years ago. Now they were able to give her post-test counseling, and she decided to have her second delivery at this hospital; she also agreed to undergo sterilization immediately following the birth. Devi brought both her husband and her daughter in for testing, and both were found to be HIV-negative.

During her delivery—a vaginal delivery—Devi and her newborn each received a dose of nevirapine to prevent HIV transmission. According to Devi, the counselors explicitly told her that she should not breast-feed the baby. Devi's husband, however, was opposed to this advice and insisted that she breast-feed the baby for nine months before introducing cow's milk. He felt strongly that this would be best for the baby. Devi explained that her husband had not been happy that she had not breast-fed their first baby, but his opinion did not weigh so heavily from afar. After the birth of her son, however, she was living with her husband, and he insisted that she breast-feed this baby. Therefore, even though this went against the advice of the counselors at the hospital, she breast-fed her baby. When her son tested HIV-positive a year and a half later, Devi felt certain that it was due to her breastfeeding and she laid blame squarely on her husband: "My son got HIV only due to my breastfeeding. My husband thought that mother's milk was best for the baby and he forced me. He said it was not acceptable for a mother to feed her baby with a bottle." Because numerous factors need to be considered in mother-to-child transmission of HIV, biomedical practitioners would argue that Devi's definitive conclusions are unfounded.

Devi's anger toward her husband over this issue must also be viewed within the context of their broader marital problems. She said that the fact that they were a discordant couple with her being positive and her husband being negative led to endless quarrels between them, especially because she had never disclosed her history as a sex worker to her husband. She also complained vociferously about her husband's inability to find regular work, stating that although he claimed to be opposed to bottle feeding for the sake of the baby, she thought it was in fact because he was not willing to work hard enough to make the money needed to buy the milk.

When I met Devi, her son's CD4 count had dipped as low as 70 and he was receiving ART for free from World Vision. When I asked her what her hopes were for the future, she replied, "I want to educate both my children well. I want to put my girl in an English medium LKG [lower kindergarten]. I am trying to get help for this since I have no jewels to pawn in order to get money." Having entered into two love marriages, Devi had never received any jewels as part of a dowry from her family.

Devi's story points to several social and cultural issues of relevance to the successful implementation of counseling regarding infant feeding. First, we see that, although she tested HIV-positive in a Government Hospital during her first pregnancy, she never returned for the results and instead went back to her natal village for the delivery and postpartum period. This is a common practice in Tamil Nadu (particularly for a woman's first birth) and differs from the social practice of birth in most North Indian communities (P. Jeffery et al. 1989; Van Hollen 2003a). Counselors working in Government Hospitals that serve poor communities in Tamil Nadu often deal with patients who may come to the hospital for one checkup but then move to their natal home for subsequent care at home or at another hospital, and it is often extremely difficult for counselors to follow up with them. These patients come from poor communities and therefore may not have a telephone number through which they can be contacted (especially in a confidential matter), and they may also live in squatter colonies and therefore have imprecise addresses, making contact again challenging. If patients do not return to the hospital, counselors cannot give them test results and counseling or help them adhere to one feeding method or another.

Further, through Devi's story we can see that even when women do receive counseling and care from the hospital, as Devi did with her second birth, they may not be able to adhere to the counselors' recommendations. Devi's story gives us a clear example of the extent to which husbands can indeed influence the reproductive health decisions of women. Studies conducted in other countries have argued that support from the infant's father for a particular feeding method is critical and that the father often has the final say in a patriarchal family context (Desclaux and Alfieri 2009: 825; Traoré 2009). Yet, because women in Tamil Nadu often return to their natal homes for their first births (and sometimes subsequent births) and may be absent from their spouses for months after the baby is born, it would also be helpful to include the women's parents in counseling regarding infant care if the women have disclosed their HIV status to their parents. My research suggests that when women did not disclose their status to their own parents, that decision was usually motivated by an interest in protecting their parents, especially their mothers, from emotional pain more than by a concern about being stigmatized and discriminated against by their parents.

Devi's story evokes both a cultural and economic reason for her husband's preference for breastfeeding. On the one hand, she states, "He said it was not acceptable for a mother to feed her baby with a bottle." It is likely that this opinion was influenced by both long-standing cultural norms as well as pro-breastfeeding public health campaigns, which have been active in Tamil Nadu in recent decades. Yet Devi doubts the sincerity of her husband's statements, and instead she frames his preference in economic terms. She suggests that her husband pretends to have noble reasons for insisting that she breast-feed when in fact the real reason is that he is too lazy to work to earn money to pay for replacement feeding. The decision-making process surrounding infant feeding in this example is clearly exacerbated by a marital conflict concerning the discordant HIV status of this couple. My reason for elaborating on these points is not to ascertain the veracity of Devi's statements or to know what truly motivated her husband to insist on breastfeeding. Rather, my point is to demonstrate the complexity of social relationships within which infant feeding practices are negotiated and determined. It is unlikely that counselors in a hospital who are trying to assess the AFASS criteria of replacement feeding through brief pre- or postnatal questionnaire-based interviews would be able to either predict or influence a situation such as Devi's.

Karpagam

Karpagam's life parallels Devi's in many ways. Karpagam was born in the town of Marakanam, south of Chennai near Pondicherry. Never having attended school, she was taken to Vellore by a man from Marakanam on the pretext of getting her settled in a job as a domestic servant. Upon her arrival in Vellore, she was promptly sold into commercial sex work. She was 15 years old at the time. She believed that she contracted HIV in Vellore, because, even though she took birth control pills to avoid getting pregnant, she had no knowledge about condoms and HIV/AIDS at that time. While in the Vellore sex trade, Karpagam was arrested three times; on the third arrest she was taken to the Vigilance Home in Mylapore, Chennai, where arrested sex workers were kept in custody of the state. It was while she was in the Vigilance Home that she came to know that she was HIV-positive, and it was during that time that she met her husband, who was also HIV-positive. He worked for an NGO that was involved in providing food to women at the home. Karpagam and her husband were open about their previous sexual history. As she said, "He had been a fisherman in Bombay. At that time he had 'sex' with many women and thus became HIV-positive. So he married me even though he knew that I too had had 'sex' with other men."

After Karpagam and her husband were married, she was released from the Vigilance Home to live with her husband. She began attending PWN+ support group meetings, and her husband attended the TNP+ support group. Karpagam said that it was due primarily to the confidence she and her husband gained through attending these meetings that they chose to have two children, and her husband's parents supported their decision. Her first child was born in a government maternity hospital in Chennai before the official PPTCT program was in place, and she described this delivery as a humiliating experience.

For the first delivery in the hospital they behaved insultingly. No one attended for half an hour after the birth. The *ayah* cut the umbilical cord. They did not allow me even to visit the bathroom. Also I was put in the ward for people with chicken pox. I did not breast-feed the first child because they said not to since he may get HIV. I breast-fed only for one month. Then I gave cow's milk [*pasum paal*]. They kept me in the hospital for one month in order to interview me for research.

Her second son was born two years later in another government maternity hospital in Chennai. There, she said, the medical staff was more supportive and treated her well during her delivery. Once again, they recommended replacement feeding for the baby, but at that time, she explained, she had no money to buy either formula or cow's milk because her husband's AIDS-related illness had rendered him bedridden and unable to work. So she breast-fed this child for the first year. In the end, her first child was HIV-negative and her second was HIV-positive, and she attributed this to the two different feeding methods. Her second son had been taking ART for one year when I met her, and she herself had begun ART seven months before our meeting. World Vision provided both of them with their medication free of cost because there was no free ART available through the government at that time.

Karpagam's story demonstrates that even when the same woman is given the same advice about infant feeding for two different births, her life circumstances can change suddenly so as to dictate her decision making. In this case Karpagam's husband became too ill to work just at the moment when she had to decide about feeding her second baby, thus making replacement feeding financially impossible. Furthermore, people's ideas about what constitutes exclusive bottle feeding or exclusive breastfeeding must be scrutinized. Here Karpagam begins by stating that she did not breast-feed the first child because of the risk of HIV transmission. Yet in the next sentence she says she breast-fed for one month—the time when there is the greatest potential for HIV transmission (SWEN 2008: 301)—and she introduced cow's milk after one month, which is known to pose a greater health risk to infants than properly sterilized formula but which is substantially cheaper. The fact is that in India even people who say they are engaging in exclusive breastfeeding often mix breastfeeding with other supplements, most notably gripe water (a remedy given to infants to treat colic), sugar water, and sometimes brandy to calm a baby down. In addition, an herbal medicine known as *pillai maruntu* (typically made with ginger, asafetida, and roasted garlic) is often given to young infants in Tamil Nadu to ensure regular bowel movements (Van Hollen 2003a: 198).

My study relied primarily on interviews, and there is little doubt that the gap between what people say they will do or have done and what they actually do in practice with respect to infant feeding is sizable. This makes the benefits of specific counseling recommendations difficult to evaluate, particularly because counselors and health care practitioners attached to the major Government Hospitals with PPTCT centers are not engaged in home visits to monitor feeding.

Renukha

Like Devi, Renukha also came from a village in Salem District and she had never been to school. As discussed earlier, Renukha had previously been married to another man in Salem but had left her first husband and had unofficially married her older sister's husband. Renukha and her new husband had two sons, ages 4 and 2, when I met them.

Like Devi and Karpagam, Renukha had given replacement feeding to her first child and then breast-fed the second. In her case she had known her HIV-positive status during both deliveries, but the counselors had given opposing advice to her following each delivery in the same hospital, one in 2000 and the other in 2002. As she explained:

> For the first child, the doctors and counselors in the Government Hospital told me not to breast-feed. So I bought Lactogen [formula made by Nestlé]. I diluted it with water. It was "special" milk that was very thick. We were advised to give that, but we couldn't afford so much so we decided to add more water to it so that we could give it for more days. I thought that would be good because it was

so thick to begin with. For the first three months I fed this to my baby with a spoon or a *paaladai*. It cost twenty-seven rupees daily to give the Lactogen!

This meant that during those first three months, Renukha's family spent 810 rupees per month on formula alone. This represents 22% of the average total monthly household income reported for all seventy of the HIV-positive women in my study who were not being fully supported by charitable organizations. Renukha continued:

> After three or four months I started feeding Aavin milk with a "tumbler" [a stainless steel cup]. Buying milk was difficult because it was costly. I didn't have to worry about people questioning why I was not giving mother's milk because I was working as a servant and my employer had given me a place to stay. They gave me milk in the morning and the evening and once at night. My husband worked in a tea shop and he was able to get some milk from them as well. But still it was costly. We needed one and a half liters of milk each day. I rarely came out of that house so no one knew that I was feeding my baby Aavin milk and not mother's milk. Even the people I worked for did not know; they thought the milk that they gave me was for me to drink. They did not know that I was HIV-positive; if they had known, they would have thrown me out. Then the woman in the house saw me giving my baby cow's milk and she asked me why I was doing that. I told her it was because I didn't have any mother's milk.
>
> Like that, for the first child the doctors told me not to breast-feed, but for the second child, they told me that I should breast-feed. Both deliveries were in the same hospital, but they told me different things about milk.

When I asked, "Why do you think there was that difference? Why did they tell you not to breast-feed the first baby and then tell you that you should breast-feed the second one?" Renukha replied:

> When I was pregnant with the first child, they gave me tablets so that the HIV would not go to the baby. So I think those tablets protected the baby enough so that it did not need mother's milk, so then it was safe to give cow's milk and that would also help so that the baby would not get HIV from the mother's milk.
>
> But when I was pregnant with the second child, they didn't give me those tablets. They only gave one injection when the baby was born. So the baby did not get *ethirppu sakti* from all those tablets, I think. So that is why I had to give the baby mother's milk for the first three months so that it could get *ethirppu sakti* from the mother's milk. I even gave colostrum [*cimpaal*] because they

said that would give *ethirppu sakti*. And after that, after three months, they said that I should start giving cow's milk.

Renukha's first baby was born in 2000 and the second was born in 2002. Between the birth of the first child and the birth of the second child, there was a shift from the pilot phase of the PPTCT project, during which time zidovudine was administered in the form of several pills during the pregnancy, to the actual implementation of the official PPTCT program, in which nevirapine was administered as one shot to the mother and one dose of syrup to the baby at the time of birth. At the same time, there had also been a shift from recommendations to not breast-feed toward a tendency to recommend exclusive breastfeeding. In her attempt to make sense of the changing procedures and protocols, Renukha blurred these two distinct phenomena in a highly innovative and logical way by equating the quantity of pills ingested with *ethirppu sakti* in contrast to the single injection. I was impressed by the conclusion she had come to in order to make sense of these shifting tectonics of policy and medical practice.

When I asked about the health of both of her children, Renukha said that fortunately both were HIV-negative. But, she added, the first son was sickly, frail, always tired, and constantly catching colds [*sali*]. In short, she said the first son was *oru maadiri* (a bit strange; not quite right), whereas the second son was healthy and active, and she attributed this to the different methods of feeding. Indeed, observing the boys as they played, I had been struck by their similar height, even though they were two years apart in age. "Just today," Renukha said, "I had to go buy another 'tonic' [medicine] for my first son." She was bitter about the fact that her first son had not benefited from the *ethirppu sakti* of her own milk. As she put it, "I may be losing all of my *ethirppu sakti*, but I should at least give *ethirppu sakti* to my child. Isn't it so? That's why I gave mother's milk to my second child."

Affordability

A common concern expressed across all these interviews was that of affordability of replacement feeding, whether in the form of powdered formula (usually Lactogen) or cow's milk (such as Aavin milk). Indeed, by reviewing the comments made by Devi, Karpagam, and Renukha, we can appreciate why it is that affordability is the first AFASS criteria listed. Earlier I noted Amaldevi's statement that "formula is expensive, but there is no other option." Devi suspected that the real reason her husband was opposed to replacement feeding was the cost. Karpagam explained that, although the counselors recommended replacement feeding for her second child, just as they had for the first, she simply could not afford it and so had breast-fed instead. Renukha described her struggles with trying to cover the cost of replacement feeding as she diluted the formula powder to make it go further and then switched to milk after three months, benefiting from the generosity of her employers, who gave her some milk, and from the unique circumstance of having a husband working as a tea master. Yet she still complained of the financial strain caused by feeding her baby while she was giving formula those first three months.

Vijaya (from Namakkal District, whose birthing story was described earlier) also spoke of the burdensome cost of replacement feedings. She held her 2-month-old baby on her lap, feeding her from a bottle, as she explained:

> I chose not to breast-feed my baby. The doctor explained about breastfeeding and bottle feeding and then said, "It's your choice." I chose formula and cow's milk. . . . I give cow's milk daily. It costs fifteen rupees daily for one liter. I also give Lactogen one time each day. I spend 170 rupees each month on Lactogen. It is too costly to only give Lactogen so I switch back and forth: cow's milk sometimes and Lactogen sometimes. When neighbors ask me why I am not breastfeeding, I say that my body is weak and that I have no milk. So they don't ask anymore.
>
> My baby is two months old. They have tested her four times and the result has been HIV-negative. But they have asked me to reconfirm the test when she is eighteen months old.

This statement means that Vijaya was paying 620 rupees per month on both kinds of replacement feedings combined. When infants are given mixed feedings like this, switching back and forth between different kinds of replacement feeding methods, it poses increased health risks to an infant's digestive system and is discouraged by UNICEF.[4]

Maliga also recounted the financial challenges of replacement feeding.

> I bottle-fed my baby from the beginning. I gave Lactogen for four months. Then I started giving Aavin milk. Now my son is an Aavin baby. Both our families knew that I should not breast-feed. When others asked me about this, I told them that I had a sugar problem [i.e., diabetes] and that I was weak. I needed 300 rupees monthly for Aavin milk and much more for the Lactogen. Being "middle class," that was difficult. After changing to Aavin milk it was not so hard.

When she said "my baby is an Aavin baby," she picked him up from the cot where he was lying and gave him a loud kiss on his cheek. When I asked her managed to afford the formula and the milk, she explained, "My father-in-law gave 8,000 rupees for my delivery. He pawned my jewels and did not reclaim them. That is how he could give 8,000 rupees for me so that also helped with the Lactogen and the milk." Maliga believes that because she is middle class, giving replacement feeding is a financial strain for her, the implication being that it would not be a problem for wealthier families. In fact, compared to most of the women I met, Maliga was highly educated, with a bachelor's degree in commerce, and was financially quite comfortable, with a husband in a salaried job earning 5,000 rupees per month working for the police, and she herself was earning 3,000 rupees per month working for a network. Their total monthly household income was 8,000 rupees compared with the average total monthly household income of 3,726 rupees for all the HIV-positive women I interviewed who were not fully dependent on charity. Furthermore, Maliga had entered into an arranged marriage, so her parents had provided her in-laws with wedding jewels as part of her dowry, which could be used to cover these expenses.

If buying replacement feeding was a struggle for middle-class Maliga, imagine how difficult it must have been for most of the women I met who were living in poverty, like Punitha, who explained:

> I did not breast-feed the baby. I was upset about that. I bought four bottles, sterilized them, and fed the baby. I gave cow's milk from the beginning. We gave Aavin. I could not afford to buy formula. The money was not there. I would buy one liter of milk a day. It cost me 400 rupees for each month. After two years I gave milk from a "tumbler." By then I was giving one and a half liters each day. My daughter started walking when she was nine months old.

To get a sense of how difficult this must have been for Punitha to buy milk for her newborn, consider her description of how she managed during her pregnancy with this child: "When I was pregnant the second time, I went without food for four days even though I was also working at that time in an onion 'godown' [warehouse]. On most days I would take my day's wages and buy broken rice to make rice porridge for all of us. That's all that we would eat. The remaining money was for house rent. My husband did not work and I had pawned all my jewels."

Indeed, most of the women in my study did struggle financially to provide replacement feeding. Yet their accounts clearly suggest that they were rarely able to provide formula exclusively for six months, which is what is recommended by international guidelines for women who choose the replacement feeding option. However, the women who were receiving care from YRG Care were in a unique position. They were receiving the full package of PMTCT care free of cost, including a full six-month supply of formula as well as bottles, a *paaladai*, and a pan in which to boil the bottles and *paaladai* for sterilization. All the women I met through YRG Care had high praise for the services they were provided by the organization. They were aware that they would not be receiving these concessions through the Government Hospitals. This was cited as one of the reasons for coming to YRG Care, despite the long distances they had to travel.

Cultural Perspectives on Breast Milk

The repeated comments about various excuses that these women deployed to defray criticism of neighbors and others about their choice not to breast-feed point to a powerful cultural norm in favor of breastfeeding in Tamil Nadu. They also reflect the strength of maternal and child public health campaigns to promote breastfeeding in an effort to counteract what is thought to be a modern turn toward formula feedings. Not breastfeeding is therefore perceived as not performing one's culturally scripted role as a mother and also as not following the advice of the state's maternal-child health policies and thus not being a good citizen. In Namakkal District, where HIV prevalence rates were quite high, not breastfeeding was increasingly being interpreted as an indication of one's HIV-positive status. But this was unique to Namakkal at the time and did not appear to be a concern elsewhere in Tamil Nadu.

It is not simply that breastfeeding is the cultural norm in the sense that it is the most common practice, but, according to Margaret Trawick in her ethnography *Notes on Love in a Tamil Family*, in the Tamil cultural context, "Mother's milk was a special substance because it was mixed with the feelings of the mother and transmitted them to the child. In particular, mother's milk contained the mother's love" (Trawick 1992: 94). Trawick also explains that in Tamil culture a mother's love for her child, known as *taay paacam*, is "the strongest of all loves and the most highly valued" (93). Thus we see that breast milk is viewed as a substance that transmits the strongest and most highly valued form of love of which humans are capable.

In his analysis of premodern Tamil literature, George Hart points to the elevated cultural value of women's breasts as a symbol of their fertility and sexuality. He argues that in ancient Tamil poetry "woman" as a category is highly sacred and a woman's breasts are viewed as the "seat" of her sacred power (Hart 1973: 240). Hart sees in these poems a connection between the sacred power of the mother's breasts and the heroism of her sons. For example, in one poem a mother threatens to cut off her breasts if her son is a coward, and in another poem, when a mother recognizes "the valor of her dead son, her breasts give milk again, showing that her joy was so profound that the seat of her sacred power, long since impotent, is suddenly charged with power again" (Hart 1973: 240). Finally, in the best known Tamil epic, the *Cilappatikaram*, which is thought to have been written in the first century C.E., the heroine, Kannaki, "after her husband has been executed unjustly, tears off her right breast and with it causes the city of Madurai to be consumed by fire" (Hart 1973: 243), further underscoring the symbolic power of a woman's breast and the milk that flows from it in Tamil culture.

Furthermore, breastfeeding is one of the most potent symbols of Tamil cultural identity. In Sumathi Ramaswamy's analysis of the deification of the Tamil language as the mother goddess—Tamil Tay—in Tamil nationalist identity formation, she points out that one of the ways in which Tamil speakers develop a feeling of kinship with one another is through the construction of the goddess Tamil Tay as the mother of all Tamil speakers; they have all shared her womb and they have all been nourished and loved by her breast milk. Tamil language, and thus Tamil identity, is also seen as being transmitted through the breast milk of all Tamil-speaking mothers. Like the interpretations of ancient Tamil poetry discussed by Hart, Ramaswamy also argues that the emphasis is placed on the filial bonds between mother and son and the brotherhood kin ties among brothers who have shared the same mother's breast milk. As Ramaswamy writes, "Indeed, in the discourses of Tamil's devotees, there is a ready slippage between *tamil; Tamilttāy; tāyppāl,* 'mother's milk'; *tāy,* 'mother'; and *tāymoli,* 'mother tongue,' all of which over time come to be synonymous with each other" (Ramaswamy 1997: 17). There is a fusion here where the Tamil language is the goddess who breast-feeds her children (all Tamil speakers) and the notion that Tamil language and, thus Tamil identity, is transmitted through the breast milk of all Tamil-speaking mothers.

Thus in the political context of historical periods of perceived competition between Tamil and Indian identities, Ramaswamy (1997: 67–68) quotes the Tamil poet Bharatidasan, who wrote in 1958:

"O glorious Tamilian! What is the name of your nation?"
When I ask thus, he sheepishly says "India," O mother!
How will this child ever improve if he confuses the evergreen
Tamil nation with India, O mother!

Will he ever change, the one who does not recognize his mother as mother,
and declares the evil that destroys his motherland as mother, O mother!
Sitting in [his] mother's lap and nursing on the breast-milk of Tamil, how
can this child not know [his] mother's name, O mother!
Tamil *is* [his] mother tongue, and Tamilnadu is his motherland.
Does not the Tamilian realize this?

In addition, in 1956, during legislative debates about replacing English with
Tamil as the official language in Madras, one member of the Legislative Assembly in favor of promoting Tamil wrote, "Today our mother tongue reclines
royally on the throne of government. For a child, its mother's milk is far more
necessary than bottled milk. Even if the children who grow up on bottled milk
survive, there are excellent substances [*cattu*] in their mother's milk. Children
who drink their mother's milk have fine dispositions as well" (Ramaswamy
1997: 107). *Cattu*, the word used to describe the substances of breast milk here,
is a polyvalent word meaning "truth," "virtue," "goodness," and "moral excellence" (Ramaswamy 1997: 107). This metaphorical equation of Tamil : breast
milk :: English : bottle milk, thus aligns bottle feeding with the colonizing
"other," the antithesis of truth, virtue, goodness, and moral excellence.

It is only with an understanding of these symbolic meanings of breastfeeding and bottle feeding in the Tamil cultural context that we can truly appreciate
why HIV-positive women who do not breast-feed are shamed into justifying
their actions.

Excuses for Not Breastfeeding

At times, community criticism of HIV-positive women for not breastfeeding became so intense that these women or members of their family felt compelled to
divulge the truth about the role of HIV in their decision not to breast-feed, and
this in turn sometimes had a devastating, negative effect on the women because
HIV/AIDS is highly stigmatized. For example, recall Saraswati's postpartum
experience in Namakkal District. Her grandmother could no longer stand the
criticism of the other elder women in the village who chastised Saraswati for
not breastfeeding. Finally, the grandmother broke down and divulged the truth
about Saraswati's HIV status.

To avoid public stigma, women have learned to manufacture creative excuses to avoid the critiques and also to avoid disclosure of their HIV status and
the stigma and discrimination that may ensue. For example, Punitha explained,
"When neighbors asked me why I was not breastfeeding, I told them that it was

because I had jaundice. When I went to the Corporation hospital to ease the milk accumulation in my breasts, I used to buy my own syringes. I told them to use my syringe because I had jaundice. After the injection, I would discard the needle myself." Punitha's mother said, "When people asked why she was not breastfeeding, I told them she had cancer. When people asked why we were getting various forms of help, I told them it was because she had had cancer surgery." Vijaya simply stated, "When neighbors ask me why I am not breast-feeding, I say that my body is weak and that I have no milk. So they don't ask anymore."

In fact, I found that doctors and counselors themselves helped women to develop similar explanations for not breastfeeding. Lack of milk, lack of strength, jaundice, diabetes, cancer, asthma, chest pains, blood clots, or even having a common cold were considered effective conversation stoppers that women came up with and that doctors and counselors recommended. Women told me that the doctors themselves would sometimes even give these explanations to other family or community members to preempt any questioning when patients did not want anyone other than their spouses to know about their HIV status. Research from Cameroon and Burkina Faso also shows that HIV-positive women manufacture excuses, such as "bad milk" or breast cancer, to justify replacement feeding. In those cases, however, women typically felt compelled to begin breastfeeding initially for a few days or a few weeks in order to publicly demonstrate their interest in breastfeeding before using one of these excuses to stop (Desclaux and Alfieri 2009: 826).

Stopping the Flow

Women who chose not to breast-feed used a variety of traditional and allo-pathic medical methods to stop the flow of milk. As mentioned by Punitha, women received injections from allopathic doctors to dry up their milk.[5] A doctor in one hospital explained to me [in English]: "If a positive woman wants to bottle-feed but she is worried about the social pressure, we have medicines to solve this problem. We can give the woman an injection to dry up her milk so no questions will be asked about why she is not breastfeeding. You see, there is a medical solution to respond to all these social situations!" Maliga's doctor provided her with pills to serve the same purpose: "Because I was not going to breast-feed, I was given tablets and warm water fomentation to stop the milk. I did not put jasmine on my breasts or anything like that to stop the milk." Several other women did report rubbing the buds of jasmine on their breasts to stop the flow of milk. This was a method I had heard about during my previous research on childbirth in Tamil Nadu, and doctors confirmed that jasmine flowers, which are abundant in Tamil Nadu and are typically worn in women's hair, had indeed been proven to stop breast milk production. For Saraswati, no injections, pills, or jasmine seemed to do the trick, but she experimented and finally found something to help her: "I tried many things to stop my milk. First I took tablets. It did not stop. An injection did not work. Then they gave me some kind of powder to eat. I ate the powder and it still did not stop. Then we tried jasmine flowers and roses; that didn't work. Finally, they covered my breasts with cabbage leaves and that stopped the milk."

"My Baby's an Aavin Baby"

Although most of the women I met who were trying to provide replacement feeding used medical excuses to counteract public scrutiny, some, like Maliga, were able to enthusiastically embrace a middle-class identity associated with bottle feeding. Despite the strong cultural norm in favor of breastfeeding, it is nevertheless also the case that practice is never a mirror reflection of normative cultural values, and in fact many mothers in Tamil Nadu do not breast-feed their babies for a variety of reasons. Elsewhere, I have written that the Tamil Nadu state government and the Government of India have adopted UNICEF's Baby Friendly Initiative in maternity hospitals to promote breastfeeding and to deter all non-HIV-positive mothers from using formulas or cow's milk (Van Hollen 2002, 2003a).[6] The Baby Friendly Initiative aims to undercut the move to adopt bottle feeding as a sign of the "modern." Although I support the Baby Friendly agenda, I have also seen it overzealously promoted in Tamil Nadu, to the point of blaming women who bottle-feed, without changing the structures of work that might compel working mothers to adopt bottle feeding to be able to seek employment. For example, I remember witnessing one instance in which a woman who was receiving training to become a multipurpose health worker was forced to leave the training when she admitted that she had left her baby at home to be bottle-fed in her absence so that she could get the training and one day gain employment to help support her child.

The Baby Friendly Initiative also seeks to counteract long-standing taboos in Tamil Nadu (and elsewhere in India) against feeding newborns colostrum. This explains why Renukha made a point of saying, "I even gave colostrum." Many women in India consider colostrum to be "polluted" because of a belief that when menstruation stops during pregnancy, the blood that would normally flow each month accumulates in the breast and is transformed into colostrum, only to flow from the breast for the first few days of the newborn's life. Thus, because menstrual blood is viewed as highly ritually polluted, colostrum—as transformed menstrual blood—is also considered polluted. For breastfeeding advocates, however, colostrum, along with the subsequent breast milk, is crucial for the well-being of infants because both are high in antibodies, which boost the immune system. The taboo against colostrum has been difficult to overcome (Van Hollen 2003a).

Despite the high cultural value placed on breastfeeding in literary and nationalist political rhetoric, combating the power of advertising of multinational corporations that market infant formula has been a formidable task. Since the 1970s much has been written about the power of companies (such as Nestlé, which manufactures the popular brand of formula sold in India known as Lactogen) to win over consumer converts around the globe, in part by equating bottle feeding with modern living, freedom for women, and high social status. Scholars working on this topic have also documented the potentially life-threatening consequences of this for infants in resource-poor communities around the world (Raphael 1979; Van Esterik 1989, 2002).

Aavin uses similar tactics to win over the hearts and minds of Tamil mothers to promote milk consumption. One only has to look on the Aavin website to see that the sole image on the homepage is of a chubby white toddler drinking from a glass, with what appear to be Jersey cows in the background, reminding us of the ways in which "whiteness" often gets used as a symbol of the modern in the Indian context.[7] The use of the glass here is significant because it is not common to find glassware among poor families in India, who would use the more indestructible stainless steel tumblers. In addition, not only do cows in India look very different from Jersey cows, but also buffalo milk is commonly mixed in with what is called *pasum paal* in India. Given such advertising, it is not surprising to see Maliga proudly and affectionately kissing her baby as she declared him to be "an Aavin baby," as if this were a known category indicative of good middle-class parenting skills. Although Maliga represents a small minority of the HIV-positive women I met who did not seem ashamed of bottle feeding because of a degree of middle-class status attached to it, others were emboldened to move beyond the shame of bottle feeding not because of its association with modernity or social class but as a stance against the discrimination of HIV-positive mothers. In the next section I examine this emerging phenomenon.

From Cultural Acceptability to "Resistance *Sakti*"

Elsewhere, I have written about the ways in which women in Tamil Nadu perceive modernity and new biomedical childbirth technologies as transforming their *sakti*, or female regenerative power (Van Hollen 2003a, 2003b). Once again, in this research on HIV and breastfeeding, I found the concept of *sakti* constantly rising to the surface of women's discourse. Because Tamil speakers comprehend the modern allopathic concept of immunity through the use of the Tamil phrase *ethirppu sakti*, there is clearly a sense that HIV/AIDS depletes *sakti*. On the other hand, once again in translating allopathic "immune power" into Tamil, people also say that breast milk (and colostrum) increases *ethirppu sakti* in babies.

Self-sacrifice (*tyaagam*) is one of the most powerful attributes of the gendered construction of womanhood in Tamil culture, most notably of motherhood. Nowhere have I witnessed this more than in my discussions with HIV-positive mothers. When asked the open-ended question, "What are your hopes and goals for the future?" at the end of most of my interviews, across the board the first thing each woman said was that she was not worried about herself but thought only about the need to secure the future of her children, especially because she thought she would not live long enough to guide her children into adulthood. It is this ethic of self-sacrifice that rings out when we hear Renukha say, in explaining her decision to breast-feed her second child, "I may be losing all of my *ethirppu sakti*, but I should at least give *ethirppu sakti* to my child. Isn't it so?"

Yet it is also clear that women are willing to forgo breastfeeding as a great sacrifice to protect the health and lives of their babies. Punitha, a member of PWN+, told me that to not breast-feed was a great sacrifice but that this sacrifice itself can also add to a woman's *sakti*. She explained that, to engage in positive living and be a mother, she would need to have the extra *sakti* necessary to endure both the economic hardships and the social stigma of replacement feeding. Therefore an HIV-positive woman who could publicly overcome the stigma of replacement feeding without shame would have more *sakti*, more power. She told me that, although in the past she and her mother had fabricated excuses about why she was not breast-feeding, after she became more centrally involved with PWN+, her perspective on this changed and she no longer felt ashamed about being open about her HIV status or about the fact that that was why she was not breast-feeding. She had even agreed to speak out on television programs about HIV-positive motherhood.

Based on their research in Ethiopia and Tanzania, in which most of the low-income women in their study were desperately trying to adhere to an exclusive breastfeeding regime, Blystad and Moland argue that "the PMTCT programme and the structural conditions surrounding pregnancy and breastfeeding do not constitute a basis that is suited for HIV related activism" (Blystad and Moland 2009: 107). My study, however, suggests that those women who are affiliated with the positive people's activist networks in India and who are struggling to bottle-feed their infants are in fact attempting to mobilize elements of the PPTCT program as a basis for activism.

Organizations such as PWN+, which advocate positive living for HIV-positive women as part of a global discourse of human rights and women's rights, link this global discourse of rights and empowerment to the local concept of *sakti* to explain how HIV-positive women in Tamil Nadu, who face multiple forms of discrimination, can find the strength to stand up to cultural norms that threaten their ability to live positive lives with this disease. As Angamma from the HUNS network in Namakkal put it:

> This disease has depleted the *ethirppu sakti* in my body, but at the same time, I feel that I have gained another kind of "resistance *sakti*" in my life by joining this "network." Being in the "network" is a very soothing experience. I get affection there. I made many friends. I felt wanted. I never used to be forthcoming with people. Now I have self-confidence, I conduct meetings and have discussions. I am able to be open about my HIV status. I did a TV program on HIV. This was seen in the village. When people asked if I was in the show, I was spontaneously able to ask, "Oh, did you see me on TV? I'm so glad!"

This feeling of self-transformation as a result of participating in one of the positive people's activist networks has been noted in other parts of the world as well (Robins 2006; Nguyen et al. 2007) and was echoed by many women I met. What is interesting in Angamma's statement is the way in which she glides from the Tamil use of the phrase *ethirppu sakti* when speaking of the body to a partial translation, using the half-English half-Tamil "resistance *sakti*," to refer to the notion of empowerment through collective activism; by speaking this way, she implies that these phrases are in a sense equivalents, that resistance *sakti* has become a replacement for the loss of *ethirppu sakti*. Perhaps even more significantly, we can glean a sense that this replacement has led to an improvement in Angamma's life. HIV-positive women like Punitha who become active players in these networks strive to experience replacement feeding within this broader framework of replacing *ethirppu sakti* with resistance *sakti* while simultaneously transferring both of these kinds of *sakti* to their children.

The code switching witnessed here is of a different register from that described by Stacy Pigg in her analysis of language and translation among HIV/

AIDS health educators in Nepal (Pigg 2001). In Pigg's example development workers struggle to translate biomedical terms into local idioms (such as *ethirppu sakti*) to promote what is considered a system of knowledge lacking in the local population. At the same time, they cling to the English terminology of "sex" in response to a perceived lack not of knowledge but of comfort and ease in discussing sexuality because of "cultural" obstacles. The use of the English word resistance in "resistance *sakti*" could also be read as reflecting a perceived lack of a homegrown perception of activism. I would suggest, however, that use of the bilingual term "resistance *sakti*" not by an NGO educator but by a member of an activist organization should be interpreted as an example of a conscious, or unconscious, play with code switching itself. It is a sign of participating in a transnational rights discourse in which Indian women recognize the ways that cliché, New Age uses of the concept of *sakti* are pragmatically mobilized to gain legitimacy in the eyes of international development donors and programmers bent on "localizing." Crafting a phrase that combines this local element with the term resistance as a women's discourse may be considered doubly attractive to international donors, who assume that Indian women have much to resist but lack the agency to do so. Perhaps I am reading too much into what may be an isolated turn of phrase coined by Angamma. But Angamma herself credits her participation in a rights-discourse-based organization with transforming her life, so I do not think it is too far-fetched to interpret her phrase in this light. In any event, Angamma's comment to me reflects a genuine sense that to participate in this movement and to think with this concept of resistance *sakti* has indeed transformed her subjectivity and helped her to live positively. Women like Punitha have found ways to publicly embrace bottle feeding as an act of resistance against both discrimination against HIV-positive people and narrow normative values that consider breastfeeding essential for good mothering.

. . .

It is repeatedly said that international public health organizations and national- and state-level organizations must take local social and cultural contexts into consideration when developing their programs. Indeed the shift by such organizations as WHO, UNICEF, NACO, and TNSACS from a policy of recommending exclusive bottle feeding for all HIV-positive mothers to a more nuanced approach of informed choice and consideration of AFASS criteria reflects the ways in which international organizations and local governments have recognized the need to come to terms with complex local realities. In principle, this new approach is laudable. It is clear, however, that it was not being fully implemented in the way it was intended. In practice, counselors and medical personnel seemed to be instructing mothers either to breast-feed or to give replacement feeding rather than enabling mothers to make decisions for themselves. More important, however, my research points to the overwhelming complexity of assessing the AFASS factors for any given woman in Tamil Nadu, throwing into question whether such an assessment can even be adequately made.

Furthermore, it is both valid and easy to criticize the AFASS approach and the apparent shift more in favor of breastfeeding than replacement feeding in resource-poor communities along the lines of Paul Farmer's vehement critique of the argument of the "limited good" (Farmer 1999). Clearly, affordability is a key factor taken into consideration in the AFASS approach. It is a determining factor in the choice made by some of the women I met to breast-feed. But Farmer and others remind us that we should not be complacent in the face of such seemingly "realistic" approaches to public health policy. Simply put, we should not accept this reality. According to this critique, we should not be content to say that because women cannot afford to provide replacement feeding in a safe fashion, breastfeeding provides a lesser health risk. Rather, we should redistribute economic and educational resources such that every HIV-positive mother, no matter where she lives in the world, has the means to provide replacement feeding safely to prevent the transmission of HIV to her baby and thus help stem the global spread of this disease. These are hard-fought political struggles and ones we should all be engaged in. As mentioned earlier, this critique is warranted in the Indian context when we consider that only 0.7% of India's GDP went toward health care in 2004. It also seems warranted when we consider that the international funds to provide a full supply of formula feedings and bottles seem to quickly materialize when women submit their bodies to clinical trials.

Yet people's quotidian lives go on while these political battles are being fought. Although we know that this is a created and not an inevitable reality, it is nonetheless the one in which the women in this study live. Even though Farmer admirably rails against the sustainability rhetoric of international development organizations, people like Karpagam bluntly tell me that "we had no money to buy either formula or cow's milk, so I gave mother's milk for the first year." Further, women like Renukha dedicate on average 22% of their total monthly household income just to give their babies formula, only to feel afterward that the health of their children who were bottle-fed was compromised as a result. In this regard, if counseling is to be meaningful at all, it does indeed need to take the economic factor into consideration as much as possible. How to effectively evaluate this from a brief, decontextualized interaction in a hospital is exceedingly difficult, as my ethnographic examples demonstrate.

In addition to the difficulty of assessing the economic factors in counseling, my research also vividly demonstrates that the cultural meanings of breast milk are highly charged. Mother's milk and the act of breastfeeding are highly valued in the Tamil cultural context, and they are promoted forcefully through the government's Baby Friendly Initiative. We also see how creative and flexible mothers can, must, and are willing to be in order to accommodate these values. The fact that mothers who give replacement feedings are compelled to devise all manner of medical excuses to ward off their critics speaks to this entrenched cultural norm. Ethnographic and historical research sheds further light on how breast milk and breastfeeding are viewed in this cultural context. Only by understanding that breast milk is considered both the highest symbol of human love and also the essence of Tamil cultural identity, of truth, and moral excellence can we recognize what kind of mixed message is being conveyed to women when they are told not to breast-feed out of love for their children. We can begin to see that recommending replacement feeding may necessitate a transformation of women's understanding of themselves as women or a transformation of other people's perception of them as women, as members of positive networks are recognizing.

In short, when we contemplate the factor of cultural acceptability within the AFASS framework, we see how extraordinarily complex things can get. On the one hand, the profound cultural value and active public health campaigns in favor of breastfeeding make replacement feeding seem unacceptable for some. For most, however, it is something to be creatively navigated through acts of public deception. For some the use of replacement feeding offers an opportunity to strive for a modern, middle-class identity. And for others the challenge to the cultural norm that considers breastfeeding essential for good mothering can become highly valued among women activists, who are mobilizing against the particular gendered nature of discrimination against HIV-positive women and mothers. Ginsburg and Rapp argue that reproduction must be analyzed not only as a site for the reification of sociocultural forms but also as a site for sociocultural transformation (Ginsburg and Rapp 1995). Because HIV/AIDS prevention has come to occupy a central role in public reproductive health care and policy in India, reproduction has indeed increasingly become a site for such cultural contestation and transformation, as evidenced by mothers involved in the human rights–based positive people's networks. I have demonstrated in this chapter how all these responses to the vexing question of infant feeding for HIV-positive women coexist and jostle against each other in one part of the world.

9 Creating a Storm

Activists' Hopes and Mothers' Fears

IN CHAPTER 8 I DEMONSTRATED THAT HIV-POSITIVE WOMEN in Tamil Nadu were beginning to overcome their stigmatized identity. Although most still thought that they had to keep their HIV status hidden like a shameful secret, some women were beginning to step out into the limelight in their efforts to combat the stigma and discrimination that women living with HIV/AIDS in India face. And they were doing so with the emotional, legal, political, and economic support of the networks and other civil society organizations, such as YRG Care. By speaking out, they experienced a transformation in their subjectivity that went beyond the mere fact of overcoming AIDS-related stigma to a sense that their lives were more meaningful than they had been before learning of their HIV status.

That sense of purpose gave them the strength to combat social conventions in other domains of their lives. Two such arenas were widow remarriage and legal inheritance rights for widows. In this final chapter I explore the processes by which women living with HIV/AIDS were beginning to forge new marriage alliances and to demand their legal rights to property after their first husbands died from AIDS-related illnesses. Charting such courses was by no means simple, as these stories attest, and the steps these women were taking were neither radical nor transformative in and of themselves. These stories do, however, demonstrate how women pragmatically negotiate the sociocultural structures within which they must operate. In so doing, these women open up space for changes in those structures—changes that have the potential to diminish stigma and discrimination for people living with HIV/AIDS and the potential to help achieve greater gender equity more broadly, benefiting women in general. In these ways, responses to HIV/AIDS can be seen once again as not only reproducing sociocultural norms but also creating the space for the possibility to transform them as well. Yet, although these women may have been instrumental in facilitating social change and although their participation in rights-based activism may have infused them with a sense of hope, that optimism was heavily guarded, tempered always by a foreboding sense of anxiety about what the future would hold for their children.

Before discussing the pragmatics of remarriage and inheritance rights, it is important to first describe the depths of despair that some women felt as a result of their HIV status. Only after this description can we then appreciate the nature and reach of the discourse of optimism and of collective activism engendered within the contexts of the meetings organized by the networks for HIV-positive women. I then examine how the discourse of rights that drives these networks and the feeling of social solidarity or "biosociality" (Rabinow 1999) generated through participation in these groups get mobilized and articulate with the other structures of women's lives as they engage in decisions about remarriage and inheritance rights.

"I Will Have Peace Only After I Come Out of This HIV"

Some of the women I met could not shake the sense of absolute despair they felt about their HIV-positive status. It was as though their HIV-positive status had become their identity. It tainted everything they did, and they were constantly reminded of it. This was true for Thameena, who was HIV-positive but whose husband was HIV-negative. She said that, although HIV can spread through several different means, people only think about the sexual transmission and they think badly of her as a result. She complained that even in the Tambaram hospital, she thought the counselors were judgmental about her sexuality.

> When we go to the hospital, the question they ask is also like that only [i.e., about sexual history]. There are other sources [of transmission] too, but they do not ask about that. In Tambaram too the counselor will ask the first question like that only: "With whom have you had your sexual contact?" Why not ask about the other sources? In every hospital they ask like that only. . . . When educated people are asking such questions, what can we expect from the people in the villages?
>
> When I go to Tambaram, or here [YRG Care], wherever I go, I always have the feeling that I have HIV. I have come here only for that. This thought will be with me until I come out of this HIV. I will have peace only after I come out of this HIV.

Given her feelings that "I will have peace only after I come out of this HIV," combined with the fact that there is no cure for HIV/AIDS, it is not surprising that Thameena is one of the HIV-positive people I met who told me that she had contemplated suicide. Her HIV status had been discovered during her pregnancy, and she had chosen not to abort the child and said that that was what kept her alive.

Susan Estroff once wrote that diseases become categorized into "I am" and "I have" diseases. "I am" diseases are those that tend to claim the identity of those people suffering from a particular disease such that they cannot view themselves apart from the disease, whereas "I have" diseases do not have such power to abduct identities wholesale. Estroff explains the reasons for these different categories of illness: "It appears that compared to 'I have' conditions, 'I am' illnesses are more mysterious and more stigmatized, entail more disruptive, disapproved expression, are more likely to be centered in the brain or to involve cognitive function. They are also more offensive to the moral convention regarding the individual—for example, drinking to excess (alcoholism), driving a car recklessly (paraplegia, quadriplegia)" (Estroff 1993: 257). Estroff's research at the time was focused on schizophrenia, which accounts in part for her emphasis on illnesses that affect cognitive function. Although HIV/AIDS does not necessarily entail impaired cognitive function, it certainly is "mysterious" because there is no cure for it and because it can remain unexpressed in the body for a long time. Above all, it is a disease that is highly stigmatized and viewed as being "offensive to moral conventions." The moral attributions associated with HIV/AIDS combined with the absence of a cure can result in this disease fusing with the identity of the person who suffers from it, as indicated by calling someone "HIV-positive" (as in "I am HIV-positive"). When the disease is as intensely stigmatized as HIV/AIDS is in India, the identity can become quite literally unbearable to live with. It can, as Goffman wrote, reduce "life chances" (Goffman 1963: 5).

Typically when a disease fuses with the identity of the person suffering from the disease, it is detrimental to the psychological well-being of that individual. As Thameena said, "I will have peace only after I come out of this HIV." This suggests that as long as she is HIV-positive, she lives within the disease; she inhabits the disease; the disease has not just fused with her self, it has enveloped it. Networks for people living with HIV/AIDS that espouse the discourse of positive living help counsel people to transform this from an "I am" disease into an "I have" disease, to reclaim HIV-positive individuals' sense of self and rights to living normal lives, like anybody else. As Punitha said, "I told the doctor that I could live a happy life myself even with the HIV virus, and I told him that I knew how to raise a baby whether the baby was HIV-positive or HIV-negative." Unlike Thameena, who views herself as living "in" HIV and who longs to come "out" of it, Punitha views herself as living "with" the virus and not letting it interfere with her life's aspirations. Activist organizations have worked to shift the discourse from saying that people *are* HIV-positive to using the expression "people living with HIV/AIDS." For Punitha, HIV/AIDS is not her self.

Some women involved in the networks that strive to reclaim the dignity and human rights of HIV-positive people took this to another level. They not only expressed their acceptance of living with this disease but also, at some level, almost celebrated it for the positive changes it had brought to their lives as a result of getting involved in the networks. As Angamma said, joining the network as a result of her HIV-positive status led to a positive transformation in her life and provided her with "resistance *sakti.*" This sentiment was echoed by other women as well; they told me that in the past their lives had been constrained and confined to their roles as daughters and wives and mothers, but the networks opened up new avenues for them and enabled them to express themselves in public, even when what they were expressing was precisely the fact that they were living with HIV/AIDS. Backed by the networks, they felt that their HIV positivity allowed them to have a public identity that had been denied to them in the past because of gender-, class-, and caste-based forms of discrimination. This was evident in the monthly support group meetings I attended at PWN+, but it was even more pronounced at the gatherings of more specialized and more public events, such as the PWN+ Five-Year Vision Workshop held over the course of two days at a hotel in Chennai in February 2004.

Creating a Storm

The Vision Workshop brought together members of all the PWN+ networks, which at that time included Tamil Nadu, Kerala, Karnataka, Andhra Pradesh, and Maharashtra. The facilitator for the workshop was a member of INP+ from Chennai. A representative from UNIFEM came from Delhi for the event. I was there to observe and document the workshop for PWN+'s records. Because of the linguistic diversity of India, the women coming from the five different states spoke five different languages. English was the most common denominator, and most of the meeting was therefore conducted in English. However, most of the participants did not speak English, so a substantial amount of time was reserved for translating comments into each of the five languages.

The meeting began with motivational gimmicks to break the ice—to help participants feel comfortable not only in a room full of strangers but also in a room full of women living with HIV/AIDS. We began by going around the circle telling a story about something funny that had happened to each of us. All these stories were unrelated to HIV/AIDS, except for one woman's anecdote. She recounted a story about being at a monthly support group meeting when a woman who was coming to the meeting for the first time came to the door timidly and said that she was all right but that she had "just a little bit of AIDS," whereupon the woman from the group who met her at the door said, "You have only a little bit of AIDS, but come inside and you will see a lot of AIDS in there!" The women present at the Vision Workshop erupted into laughter upon hearing this story. The ice receded rapidly from there on out.

The workshop had several components, including a PowerPoint presentation by the PWN+ president on "Involvement of WLHA [Women Living with HIV/AIDS]: Experiences of PWN+"; an open discussion about various issues or concerns that women wanted to talk about; role-playing session about the importance of PWN+; a presentation on "Women's Vulnerability and Gender Dimensions of HIV/AIDS" by the representative of UNIFEM, who provided an overview of the importance of the United Nations CEDAW and its relevance for women living with HIV/AIDS; state-based small-group brainstorming sessions about the vision for PWN+ five years from then, in which each group created a poster representing their vision; state-based small-group discussions in which each state had to come up with a one- or two-sentence mission statement for PWN+ and a list of things that PWN+ should focus on in the coming year; a full group discussion in which participants were asked to say who was represented by PWN+ and create a poster including all of those represented groups; and a large group discussion about how to achieve the goal of PWN+ involvement at the national level. In short, much ground was covered.

The state-based brainstorming sessions about the vision for PWN+ five years down the road and the posters created during the sessions were exemplary of how far women imagined they could stretch themselves beyond the confines of their familial obligations through their participation in this network. Take, for example, the poster created by the women from Tamil Nadu. Most of the items listed on their poster were relatively pragmatic, achievable goals. Here is how they were presented to me by one member of the group as she read the list and translated it from Tamil into English:

- We will have our own building.
- PWN+ was initiated by a few people. But in the coming years we will have more workers and more support.
- PWN+ will be an information center aimed at building confidence.

- We will have a job center to identify skills of WLHA and provide contacts for them to seek employment. Job referral center.
- We will have a care center.
- We will have a short-term stay home/shelter. It will be a place where WLHA can come for 10–15 days for rest, support, and help with family conflicts.
- In five years we will provide educational support for children and we will have a hostel for positive children and children of positive people in all states.
- We will provide support for women to adopt positive children or children of positive parents who cannot care for them due to death or illness.
- We will have a crêche (day care) for children.
- PWN+ has the responsibility to provide women with information about how to take care of themselves (e.g., nutrition and medication). Positive people themselves should be the ones to provide advice about how to take ARTs since doctors don't provide proper advice.
- Every village should be aware of HIV/AIDS. Now everyone has heard about it, but they don't understand fully.
- There should be a PWN+ shelter for women who are totally abandoned.

In addition, their poster expressed a much more ambitious goal.

- There should be a representative from PWN+ in Parliament. In five years time, we will have a Chief Minister!

Next to this they drew a picture of a flag with the international HIV/AIDS image of the red ribbon in the center. When they were presenting their poster to the whole group, they pointed to the flag and said, "That will be the political symbol for our political party."[1] They even envisioned reaching beyond the national arena to the global community.

- It will be not only at the national level but at the international level.

They also envisioned a legacy that would live on forever, well past the five year mark.

- Even if you die, three letters will live forever: PWN.

Next to this line they had drawn a picture of a man with a white hat and dark glasses. This was a picture of the immensely popular former chief minister of Tamil Nadu and founder of the AIADMK political party, M. G. Ramachandran (known by most as MGR). Like many of Tamil Nadu's most prominent politicians, MGR had gotten his start as an actor in the Tamil cinema.

The women at the PWN+ workshop from the Tamil Nadu group said that when they wrote, "Even if you die, three letters will live forever: PWN," they were alluding to a song from one of MGR's films called "En Kadamai" (My Duty). They explained: "The song says, 'In three words my soul will be there after I have passed away. Even after that, everyone will talk about that: duty [kadamai], dignity [kannyam], and discipline [kattupaadu].' Like that, PWN stands for three words [i.e., Positive Women's Network] and also represents duty, dignity, and discipline."

At the bottom of their poster they had drawn several pictures. On the bottom left side, there was a picture of two kolams (geometric designs, made of rice flour, with which women decorate their front doorsteps each morning). One of the kolams had four peacocks arranged in a square, and the other looked like interlocking parallelograms. The women explained, "Like kolams, we are all small dots; together we make the whole picture." On the bottom right side of the poster they had drawn a flower, a peacock, an elephant, and a tree, and they gave their reasons for these drawings:

A rose is soft and delicate.

A peacock is very active.

An elephant is strong.

Leaves from the mango tree are auspicious.

PWN+ has the qualities of all of these combined.

The workshop ended after two days, with another motivational ritual. We all stood in a circle, and the moderator from INP+ led us all in a game she called Creating a Storm. First one person would rub her hands together to create a soft swooshing noise, and one by one each of the other women would join in, moving around the circle. When it got back to the first person, she switched to snapping her fingers, and that went around the circle. Next it was clapping hands. And then we were loudly stomping our feet. At the end of that, we reversed our motions and clapped, then snapped, and finally rubbed our hands softly again and stopped in silence. The moderator explained the symbolic meaning of this: "If we all work together, we can create a storm [stomping our feet], and then we can make people listen and can make change in the world. Having accomplished this, we can find peace [the return to gently rubbing hands and silence]." Gimmicky though it was, this stunt (which comes from a transnational motivational speaking repertoire) seemed to embody the experience of the two-day workshop. By the end, women who had not known each other at the beginning of the meeting were holding hands—a typical gesture of friendship among women in Tamil Nadu—and exchanging telephone numbers as the meeting shifted into casual conversations and we broke for a tasty buffet lunch provided by the hotel, a space and experience that would have previously been beyond the financial grasp of most PWN+ members.

Ripple Effects from the Storm

Would this activist optimism transcend beyond the walls of this meeting room? Did the work of these networks in fact lead to change? In addition to understanding how HIV/AIDS "radiates social conditions," as Farmer and Kleinman state (2001: 353–56), can we also see how this disease might lead to social change? If so, in what ways? In this book I have demonstrated that, although HIV/AIDS in the context of reproductive health brings sociocultural structures into focus and those structures affect how low-income women in Tamil Nadu can and cannot act before and after they receive an HIV-positive diagnosis during pregnancy, most women do not simply submit to the despair they may feel upon receiving the initial diagnosis. They do not resign themselves to a negative fate but rather actively engage with the social and cultural circumstances that affect their lives as they come to terms with their identities as women living with HIV/AIDS.

They do this at every stage as they engage with the reproductive health care apparatus: when deciding about HIV testing, when deciding whether or not to continue with a pregnancy, through the process of childbirth, and while making decisions about infant feeding. Although their choices are constrained, they actively negotiate their options as best as they can as they pursue a better future for themselves and particularly for their children. In the process social and cultural norms are reproduced, but they are also challenged, opening up the possibility for social change that could begin to overcome both gender inequality and the problem of stigma and discrimination for HIV-positive people in India.

While the changes imagined in the PWN+ Vision Workshop ranged from the pragmatic to the fantastic, signs of transformation were evident during my research. One such sign was the growing trend for women who knew they were HIV-positive to still choose to marry. This was particularly remarkable among young AIDS widows in a cultural context in which widow remarriage was frowned upon, particularly when those widows were also mothers of young children. A second sign could be found in the growing movement for HIV-positive widows to demand property rights in a cultural context in which women were often discouraged from claiming such rights.

HIV-Positive Marriages

The fact that men and women who knew they were HIV-positive were entering into marriages together and were sometimes doing so with the knowledge and even the support of their family members was an indication of a certain level of acceptance of people living with HIV/AIDS and of a move to overcome the stigma and discrimination associated with being HIV-positive, in particular, with being an HIV-positive woman. Of the seventy HIV-positive women I interviewed, five of them had entered into a new marriage after learning of their positive HIV status.

The story of Karpagam (discussed earlier) provides a vivid example of the extent to which marriage after an HIV-positive diagnosis can provide women with support in the present and open up new possibilities for hope for the future. For Karpagam this was her first marriage, and it allowed her to transition away from her previous life first in the sex trade and then under police custody in the Vigilance Home. She and her husband entered into the marriage each knowing that the other was HIV-positive. It is not that marriage is a panacea that leads women out of life's struggles. In fact, for most of the women I met, it was marriage that put them at risk for HIV in the first place. Marriage alone did not solve all of Karpagam's problems. As we saw in Chapter 8, she was not able to afford replacement feeding for her second child because of her husband's AIDS-related illness, and she thought this was why her second child was HIV-positive. Nevertheless, after their marriage they felt that their future was promising enough to opt to have two children, and it was clear from speaking with Karpagam that she felt validated as a woman by becoming a mother, something that is not surprising in a cultural context that views motherhood as the central aspect of a woman's identity. HIV-positive women are often denied this basic right to marriage (and thus to the future possibility of motherhood) once their HIV status becomes known, because of the intensity of the stigma associated with HIV/AIDS and the negative assumptions about their sexuality. In that sense, then, Karpagam was luckier than many others.

The four other women I met who had married after learning of their HIV-positive status were all widows of husbands who had died of AIDS; they were entering into their second marriages. This put the remarriage rate among the widows in my sample at 12%. This is a relatively high percentage in a cultural context in which widow remarriage is considered taboo, particularly for women with children. The taboo against widow remarriage was historically more pronounced among high-caste communities. However, ironically, the Widow Remarriage Act implemented by the British in 1856, which ostensibly was intended to give widows more rights to remarriage, had the effect of "reducing widows' rights among the lower castes, which had always condoned widow remarriage. The new act brought with it legal restrictions regarding the disposal of the widow's property and children on her remarriage: these were to remain within her deceased husband's patrilineage. Many widowed women, now facing a choice between marrying again and keeping their children and property, refrained from remarriage" (Lamb 2000: 215). Given that women in my study were widowed at a young age and given the cultural value placed on marriage, especially for women, it is not surprising that this group of women would want to challenge the taboo against widow remarriage and it is not surprising that their families and friends would support them in this decision. Nevertheless, it is important to recognize that these women had to swim against two powerful currents—namely, the stigma of HIV/AIDS and the taboo against widow remarriage—to get what they wanted.

Many found their second husbands through network meetings, and in most cases their new husbands were also HIV-positive. YRG Care was also actively involved in helping to arrange marriages between HIV-positive men and women who were patients at YRG Care. Kaliamman's first husband died three years after their marriage. Although she had only learned about her HIV status at the time of her pregnancy with their first child, she learned that her husband had known he was HIV-positive before the marriage, and he told her father that he had been taking pills for HIV for ten years. After his death, like most HIV-positive widows I met, Kaliamman was sent away from her in-laws' house and back to her parents' house. She lived with her parents for two years before remarrying. Kaliamman met her second husband through a network, and, with the help and encouragement of a friend, she started up a relationship with him on the phone. She thought he would take good care of her. Kaliamman recounted the story of her mother chasing her first mother-in-law down the street, berating her for having arranged for their HIV-positive son to marry her daughter without disclosing information about his status. Kaliamman herself had railed against her own parents for arranging that first marriage to an HIV-positive husband. A few years later, knowing the seropositive status of Kaliamman and her soon-to-be second husband, her family was enthusiastic about the relationship, offering up a good dowry and arranging for him to get training for a new job. She was in the seventh month of her pregnancy when I met her. She and her husband were receiving good medical care through YRG Care, and their future seemed bright.

In June 2005 the AIDS-INDIA e-mail discussion list reported that in the city of Ahmadabad, located in the North Indian state of Gujarat, HIV-negative women were responding to matrimonial advertisements of HIV-positive men, whose HIV status was publicized. The report said that many of these women were young widows or divorcées with children who needed the financial and psychological support that a husband could provide, and it seemed to suggest the extent to which these women lacked power if they were willing to knowingly enter into a marriage with an HIV-positive man. Yet I met two women—Vasuthi and Sumitradevi—who were both AIDS widows, and both said they had married HIV-negative men who knew that their wives-to-be were HIV-positive. Here we are witnessing something different. Although in both cases it could be argued that women are remarrying in part because of their lack of economic and social independence, when HIV-negative men choose to marry HIV-positive women, this indicates a new level of social acceptance of HIV-positive people and particularly of HIV-positive women, who usually face even more stigma as a result of their seropositive status than men, particularly within the domain of the family.

In Vasuthi's case her second husband worked for an NGO involved in an HIV/AIDS project in Salem District. Vasuthi said that his training for that job made him aware of the myths and realities of HIV transmission and gave him an understanding of the problems of stigma and discrimination. He was working to end such discrimination and practiced what he preached through his marriage. Vasuthi knew something about HIV/AIDS discrimination. Recall that a doctor in the hospital where she had been working tricked her into getting an HIV test and immediately terminated her job upon discovering her HIV-positive status. Her first husband, who had tested positive one month earlier but who had never told her about the test, died in between the time she had the blood test and the time she received the test results. She had been married for only three months. Overnight Vasuthi became an unemployed AIDS widow. Because she had nurse's training, however, she was able to get another job as a health worker for a network. She was enthusiastic about her work with the network. As she said, "I have learned a lot in this job. I knew very little before. I have made many friends. I am happy. I feel I can help at least a few others, not financially but in other ways. I counsel others and have even prevented suicides." Furthermore, it was because of her job with the network that Vasuthi met her second husband. They had recently married at the time of our interview. As for children, they were planning to adopt children after two years of marriage.

Sumitradevi's second marriage was a bit more tenuous because it was to a man who was already married. Sumitradevi's first husband had fallen severely ill in 1995, when their two children were young. At that time he tested positive for HIV, as did Sumitradevi, but their two children were HIV-negative. Her husband died one year later, and, after supporting her two children on her own for three years, Sumitradevi married her maternal uncle, who was already married and had two children and was taking her as a second wife. According to Sumitradevi, she was not marrying him for financial support. As she said: "I do not expect to have his earnings. If I do that, there will be conflict. What I earn is enough for me. He comes once in a while." Nor apparently was the marriage based primarily on a sexual relationship.

> I have had a hysterectomy. Once, in a quarrel with my first husband, I took poison. I drank insecticide. My uterus was damaged.[2] In 1999 I had the surgery. My second husband recommended that I get that operation. Since my uterus has been removed, I don't feel any desire. I lost weight after my first marriage. But now I am better. My second husband gave me lots of advice. He understands me better now than at the beginning. When I was eligible for marriage the first time, he was not able to marry me. Since he couldn't marry me then, he has married me now, even though he knew I am living with HIV.

As discussed earlier, in Dravidian kinship systems cross-cousin marriages and maternal uncle–niece marriages are considered preferred marriage alliances normatively speaking, and in my research I found that many of the women I met did have their first marriages arranged with such a partner. Anthropologists have demonstrated that within communities with this kind of kinship system, a particularly close relationship emerges between such partners because of their kinship positions, even if a marriage is not in fact arranged between them. Furthermore, kinship terminology is specific with respect to relatives from the matriline versus the patriline such that a woman would use one kinship term for her mother's brother (*maaman*) and another kinship term for her father's brother (*appaa*), whereas in English both would be called by the same term, *uncle*. As a result of the normative marriage patterns and the kinship terminology, it is not unusual for a Tamil woman to grow up with particularly strong feelings for whomever she calls *maaman* (Trawick 1992). It seems that this may have been the case with Sumitradevi and her *maaman* and that even though a marriage was not arranged for them with their first marriages, once she was widowed, the affection borne from their kin relationship surfaced again.

Nevertheless, despite Dravidian kinship patterns, it was considered remarkable that an HIV-negative man would choose to marry an HIV-positive woman who not only was a widow but also had two young children to raise, albeit both HIV-negative. Perhaps in this case the fact that she did have children would lead a woman's maternal uncle to feel a certain kind of obligation to support her and her children. Still, this alliance was so outside the norm that some questioned the veracity of Sumitradevi's story, especially because her second husband did not come forward in public to acknowledge the marriage. As Sumitradevi said, "When the Health Secretary heard my story, she was in disbelief that an HIV-negative man would marry an HIV-positive woman, and she wanted to meet my second husband to see for herself. But he did not go. He did not marry me for fame or to impress anyone. Wherever I ask for help, people ask to meet him and he refuses. So some people do not believe me. I think that is because they are jealous."

Although these second marriages of HIV-positive widows seem to point toward acceptance, nevertheless they also often reveal conflicts. For example, although Suguna's parents and her new in-laws were highly supportive of a second marriage, when Suguna became pregnant after the marriage, this changed the equation, as mentioned earlier. I met Suguna when she was in the seventh month of her pregnancy and coming from Pondicherry to YRG Care for her prenatal care. Suguna had married her maternal uncle when she was 17 years old. Their first child died of AIDS at 9 months of age, and her husband died of AIDS shortly thereafter, only two years after they had been married. She had not known anything about her husband's HIV status or its effect on her child until after her husband died, when her husband's doctor told her the cause of his death and the probable cause of the baby's death and advised her to get tested. Because her family had more money than those of most of the women I met, her father took her to the prestigious private Apollo Hospital in Chennai for the test. There the doctors first informed her father of her status, and he, in turn, conveyed the positive diagnosis to her.

Initially Suguna took Siddha medicines in the form of a *lekiyam*.[3] Her father had seen an advertisement for cures for HIV/AIDS and had traveled to Madurai to buy the medicine for her. But that did not seem to help, and a few years later she began traveling to YRG Care in Chennai to receive treatment. While she was coming for her treatments, she met another HIV-positive man who was also coming to YRG Care for treatments, and they developed a friendship. She said that she never had any intention to get married again because,

I felt as though my life was wasted so why should I waste another person's life? And not only that, but I felt that if another person's family was not able to afford treatments for him, then I would have to bear the cost of the treatment.

And suppose both of us got sick, who would be there to help us? Because of these thoughts, I never considered marrying him. But my family and my friends told me, "You should have a partner for your future. If you need any help, he can help you; if he needs any help, you are there for him. You must have one person to help avoid all the problems."

Her parents took the initiative and spoke with the man's parents over the phone. Suguna said, "After that, the marriage was arranged, and I went to live in his house with his parents." All parties seemed to be pleased with the arrangement. She was 27 years old when she remarried.

When the marriage was arranged, Suguna and her husband did not want to have any children of their own. After the marriage, however, they became more aware of the treatment options through YRG Care, and they decided that they would like to have a child "for our future support" and because they were confident that, with the YRG Care services available, their child would be HIV-negative. The desire to have children—particularly sons—so that those children will be able to care for their aging or elderly parents is typical in the Indian sociocultural context. But this kind of logic was less prevalent among many HIV-positive people I met; they were not confident that they would even live long enough to raise their children, let alone long enough for their grown children to care for them. Wanting to have a child speaks to the level of optimism Suguna and her husband felt about their future, an optimism made possible through the good-quality medical care they were able to receive. This quality of care was not available to many other women I met; they had to rely primarily on public hospitals, and access to ART was either not available or not easily obtained. Most HIV-positive parents I met feared for the future of their children because they feared they would not be able to raise them to adulthood. In that light, it is not surprising that Suguna's new parents-in-law were displeased with the news of her pregnancy. Fearing that the burden of caring for the child would fall on their shoulders, Suguna's in-laws forced Suguna and her husband to move out and set up a separate nuclear household, and the relationship between the couple and her in-laws was strained when I met her.

Conflicts might also arise if the new marriages are facilitated through the networks or other support organizations, such as YRG Care, but are not fully supported by the families. The story of Pushpa is one such example. I met Pushpa at YRG Care where she was coming for her prenatal care with her second child. She was in the last month of her pregnancy. Pushpa was from a village near Thanjavur. She said that she was either 13 or 14 when she entered into an arranged marriage with her maternal uncle, who was then 25 years old. After their first child was born, her husband began to suffer from tuberculosis and was therefore tested for HIV. When his test came back positive, both Pushpa and their son were tested, and both were also found to be HIV-positive. Her husband died six months later, leaving Pushpa widowed with a 2-year-old HIV-positive son. Once alone, the other men in the village began to flirt with her and harass her, and even her father-in-law (who was also her grandfather), with whom she had been living since the time of her marriage, began to sexually harass her. Pushpa said that her father-in-law/grandfather had a reputation for having a bad character and for engaging in many extramarital affairs. Because of this, she fled and went to live with her mother and brother. But her father-in-law/grandfather came and took her and her son back to live with him. She found her way into a network in Thanjavur, and the support she found through this group benefited her: "The people who come there will not be sad. They will all be happy and 'jolly.' They will not hide anything in their heart. Only after going there was I able to become relaxed. I forgot everything and came to feel normal. I had the feeling of being one among them, like them, and only after that could I feel relaxed." It was through the network that she met and married her second husband, who was a biryani cook and also an HIV-positive man. She and her son and her new husband were all three living separately when her grandfather (her former father-in-law) came and took her son away against her will. She told me that her grandparents were angry that she had remarried and that was why they had taken away her child. She was worried that they would not know how to take proper care of her son, to get his CD4 count done regularly and give him proper antiretroviral treatments when the time came for him to need them. Both of her grandparents worked outside the home, and Pushpa was also concerned that this would mean that they would be leaving her son at home all by himself. She wanted to wage a legal case to reclaim custody of her son. Pushpa did not get much sympathy from the female elders in her village or the *panchayat,* who would say to her, "Why are you complaining when they are taking care of your son? And anyway, you have remarried someone else now." The networks were trying to help her at least gain visitation rights to see her son.

Pushpa and her husband had not planned to have children, and when she got pregnant, she wanted to have an abortion, but she said that her husband, who had never been married before and had no children of his own, insisted that they have the baby. Because she knew by then that she could get the full package of PMTCT care through YRG Care, she was reassured that the baby would be HIV-negative, and she agreed to have the baby. When I asked Pushpa what her hopes were for the future, she replied:

> I have many wishes. My son has been away from me for the past so many years. I wish to have him with me. I pray to God that the child that is going to be born will be HIV-negative. He should live well. Like that I have lots of wishes. The first child is HIV-positive and we both are HIV-positive; at least this child should be born HIV-negative. That is my wish. We are a normal family. Until the end I wish we both should be normal. That is enough for me.

When I asked her what she meant by normal, she explained, "Financially and health-wise, if we are like this continuously, that is enough."

Despite the rift with her grandparents, it seemed that remarrying and having children after becoming an HIV-positive widow had afforded Pushpa the luxury of normalcy that had seemed so illusive when her first husband had died and her father-in-law/grandfather had first sexually harassed her and then taken away her only son. This renewed sense of normalcy was possible because she had joined one of the networks for HIV-positive people. With the social and psychological support of the network, Pushpa and her second husband had the courage to go against social convention to marry, despite the fact that she was a widowed mother. In this case, however, it seemed that her decision to marry as a widow had cost her a life with her first son. The cultural context in which choosing to remarry as a widow is frowned upon makes it extremely difficult for a woman to get custody rights or to claim the right to a share of her deceased husband's property, although this too was something that women involved in the networks were trying to change.

HIV-Positive Widows Seek Inheritance Rights

A substantial portion of time at the PWN+ Vision Workshop in Chennai was set aside for a presentation on the merits of CEDAW by a visiting representative from UNIFEM, and the same was true for the Legal Literacy Workshop I attended in Namakkal. However, when I met with Geeta Ramaseshan—the lawyer in the High Court in Chennai who had volunteered her services to the networks—she told me that, although CEDAW provides a useful framework for understanding gender-based discrimination and garnering funds for NGOs and networks, it does not have much practical relevance for individual women's lives. On the other hand, she thought that the legal process could benefit women living with HIV/AIDS in their efforts to combat discrimination. She was involved in providing free legal aid to women living with HIV/AIDS on cases involving inheritance rights for HIV-positive widows and their children, and she was providing legal aid for both men and women living with HIV/AIDS who were facing discrimination on the job as a result of their HIV-positive status. She was also available to provide legal aid for cases of discrimination against people living with HIV/AIDS in medical settings, although she said those cases were extremely difficult to win because it was easy for medical personnel to use some other medical explanation as an excuse for why a patient was referred to another hospital. Most of the pro bono work she was doing was for HIV-positive widows, who were attempting to gain rights to their husbands' property after the husbands' deaths.

The property rights for most Hindus in India today are governed by the Hindu Succession Act of 1956. As Bina Agarwal explains, this act was intended to create gender equality in inheritance rights. Put simply, "Under the Act, in the case of a Hindu male dying intestate, all his separate or self-acquired property, in the first instance, devolves equally upon his sons, daughters, widow, and mother. In addition (and simultaneously with the mentioned four categories of heirs), if there is a pre-deceased son, his children and widow get the share he would have received if alive" (Agarwal 1994: 212). Several provisions within the law are dependent on earlier forms of customary laws, for example, with respect to joint family property. Some of these provisions limit gender equity, but these do not typically pertain to communities in Tamil Nadu (Agarwal 1994: 214).

Despite the goal of achieving gender equity through law, Agarwal notes that "the divergence in many regions of South Asia between contemporary inheritance laws and social practices governing marriage and residence makes for a considerable tension, leading either to women forfeiting their claims or to social and legal conflict" (Agarwal 1994: 101). Daughters are the least likely to enjoy the legal benefits of inheritance because of social norms. Widows' inheritance seems to be somewhat more socially acceptable, but widows too face social barriers when they try to claim their right to their husbands' inheritance, and most do not pursue legal means as a result. As Agarwal explains:

As *widows*, women's claims enjoy somewhat greater social legitimacy than their claims as daughters. In India, for example, the perception that a widow has a right to a share in the deceased husband's land appears to be fairly widespread. In practice, however, the fragmentary available evidence suggests that many of those who are eligible to inherit do not, and those who do inherit do so mostly on severely restricted terms. In a rural Hindu household in India, for instance, the extent and nature of rights that a widow enjoys in her husband's land are contingent in practice on a variety of factors, such as whether or not she remains single and chaste; whether she has sons and her sons (if any) are minors or adults; whether the deceased husband has partitioned from the joint family estate before his death; and so on. To begin with, as under traditional Hindu law, a widow usually loses her right if she remarries, is unchaste, or leaves her husband's village on his death. If she has only daughters or is childless, she often gets only maintenance. . . . A woman with minor sons is usually allowed use of the husband's estate as a trustee on behalf of her sons till they grow to adulthood, after which she is expected to live with one of them. (Agarwal 1994: 254–55)

The discrepancy between law and practice was apparent in many of the stories I heard from AIDS widows in Tamil Nadu. What was striking, however, was that because many of the women I met had come into contact with the networks, they were also becoming increasingly savvy about their legal rights and, with the help of lawyers like Ramaseshan, they were beginning to actively pursue those rights. TNSACS also established a Legal Cell through which people living with HIV/AIDS could file legal complaints and receive free legal aid. K. Dheenabandhu, the project director for TNSACS in 2004, encouraged HIV-positive women to collect all their complaints of discrimination through PWN+ so that PWN+ could present them together to the Legal Cell at TNSACS. In addition, the HIV/AIDS Unit of the Lawyers Collective worked at the national level to protect and promote the rights of HIV-positive people throughout India through legal reforms, legal aid, and advocacy.

The HIV/AIDS pandemic has led to a demographic change, with rising numbers of young widows in the reproductive-age group. These women face the double stigma of being HIV-positive and widows, and they are denied rights on both accounts. However, because of their growing numbers and because of the organized activism of the networks, they are beginning to push back. This activism on the legal front to claim their inheritance rights has the potential to not only help overcome the stigma and discrimination of HIV-positive people but also to turn the tide for women in general to successfully claim their inheritance rights as widows and even as women more broadly.

The attempts of the widows I met to claim inheritance rights, not only for themselves but also for their children, were mired in controversy, and none had been fully resolved to the women's satisfaction at the time of my interviews. However, the fact that they were willing to pursue these claims in the first place demonstrates a degree of what could be characterized as highly guarded optimism and once again represents ambivalence coupled with pragmatism.

Recall the story of Leelavathi, whose mother-in-law and brother-in-law conspired to prevent her and her HIV-negative children from gaining inheritance rights to her husband's property upon his death (see Chapter 5). Although her father-in-law was supportive of her claims and was willing to sign a statement indicating that he owed her the amount of the property she should inherit, he seemed impotent in the face of his wife and son, and so Leelavathi was turning to Ramaseshan to help file a suit to obtain the rightful shares for herself and her children.

Saraswati was also turning to Ramaseshan for help, and this gave Saraswati renewed optimism when she was beginning to lose all hope. As she explained, she asked her in-laws for cash compensation in lieu of property when her husband died. Even the *panchayat* supported her and said it should be given, but the in-laws refused. Saraswati said that when she went to the police station about the matter, they did nothing. When she went to her in-laws' house with members from a women's self-help organization, the in-laws still refused and said she could sue them if she wanted to. And so Saraswati went to the courts to seek help: "I went to court for many days. Each time the case was postponed. Now I have stopped going to court. If the money is to come, let it come. I am fed up." But the next day, when I met her again, she had just met with Ramaseshan, who had agreed to help her with her legal case; her optimism was renewed.

Some women had the benefit of learning about their legal rights and how to pursue them with the help of the networks even before their husbands died. This was the case for Maheswari, whose husband was dying. She had one son in a hostel and was pregnant with another child when I met her. She explained to me that if a husband dies and there are children, the property should go to the wife and the in-laws will have to give it: "I know this because I went to a meeting three days ago organized by the 'network.' Big judges and police officers all came and spoke about that. They promised us that in case we need help getting the property, they are willing to help too." I had attended a public hearing organized by PWN+ in February 2004 at which several members of the network gave testimonials to high-level public officials about various forms of discrimination they faced. Among those present was the prominent retired justice J. Kanagaraj, who also pledged to help guide women living with HIV/AIDS to legal services to which they are entitled under the Legal Services Authority Act of 1987. For women with little or no education and living in poverty in both rural and urban communities in Tamil Nadu, the access they could gain to such figures through the networks was unprecedented in their lives, and it gave them hope for the first time that they may in fact be able to use the legal system to their advantage. This clearly demonstrates another facet of what Vinh-Kim Nguyen calls therapeutic citizenship.

Women often commented that "good in-laws" would give widows a share of the property and would also give widows shares of the property to hold for their children until they turned 18 and became legal adults. They said that in-laws with a good conscience would be willing to do this particularly because they would recognize that their daughter-in-law had been infected with HIV through their son and therefore would feel responsible for her well-being. Many also pointed out that if the marriage had been arranged, the in-laws would be more likely to feel responsible for giving the widow a share of the property. If a woman's family had provided a dowry at the time of marriage, at least this could be considered something that the widow was entitled to upon the death of her husband. Nine times out of ten, however, women reported to me that they had had to sell whatever jewels may have come with their dowry to pay for the hefty HIV/AIDS-related medical expenses for their husbands and sometimes for themselves and their children. Furthermore, most of the women I met thought that in practice their in-laws did not usually fall into the category of good in-laws. As discussed earlier, often the in-laws would accuse the widows of having infected their husbands with HIV and use that as an excuse for denying them a share of the family property (if they had any). In such cases, the women I met felt empowered by knowing what their legal rights were and, more important, by having access to people at high levels within the legal system who were committed to helping them obtain their rights.

Although women living with HIV/AIDS expressed guarded optimism as they began to imagine new futures through remarriage and began to actively engage in carving out a space for themselves within the legal system to gain access to property to which they were legally entitled, their feelings about the future prospects for their children were much more ambivalent. When I asked women about their hopes for the future, their responses were unanimous: They thought only of the future of their children, and they were worried. Their struggles to gain inheritance rights and even their plans to remarry were often couched in terms of providing financial and social security for their children in the long term. Even if they were choosing to give birth to children in the context of a second marriage, knowing they were HIV-positive, and even if they were giving birth through the PPTCT program and could feel relatively assured that their children would be HIV-negative, still they expressed extreme anxiety about their children. The precariousness of their own lives, especially in the absence of guaranteed ART and also resulting from the financial disruptions caused by HIV/AIDS, meant that the future of their children hung in the balance. In the final section of this chapter I discuss common concerns that HIV-positive mothers had about their children and the sometimes painful steps they were taking to guarantee that their children would be cared for in the long term.

"I Exist Only for the Children"

For most of the women living with HIV that I met, their primary aspiration was to live long enough to see their children survive and live full lives, even if they themselves must die prematurely. Many women said they wanted to live at least until their children were 10 years old. Ten seemed to be the age at which people thought their child was mature enough to cope in the world, and given the conditions of poverty in which they lived, many of the women could hardly expect their children to receive formal education beyond that age anyway, if their own life experiences were any indicator of the future for their children.

Others wanted to live long enough to see their children through puberty or marriage, especially their daughters. The legal age of marriage in India is 18 (when one is legally an adult), and although in practice many are married below the legal age, nevertheless the actual age of marriage has been increasing over the past decades. According to UNICEF, in 2001 the average age at marriage for women in India was 18.3 and for men it was 22.6.[4] Parents from poor families in Tamil Nadu who think that they cannot afford to contemplate advanced educations for their daughters often still begin to lay the groundwork for their daughters' marriages once they have gone through puberty. In fact, among *dalit* communities there is often a public ritual to announce a girl's puberty, which marks the beginning of a complex process of arranging a marriage. Parents who have successfully arranged marriages for their children—especially for the daughters for whom a dowry is expected (despite laws prohibiting dowry)—often believe that they have accomplished their primary obligation in life as adults. There is a sense that if they were to die, they would at least go with the assurance that they had done what they could to ensure a secure family life for their own children.

For other women, seeing their children reach the age of 5 was reassuring enough because early childhood illnesses often claimed the lives of young children. Once a child lives to age 5, the most acute fears of childhood mortality begin to subside. In fact, global health organizations, such as WHO, use the

"Under Five Mortality Rate" as a key indicator of children's health and of development in general.

Here are some comments that are representative of all the HIV-positive women I interviewed as they reflected on the relationship between their children's ages and their own sense of how long they themselves hoped to live:

I asked the counselors how long I can live. I don't want to live long, but I want to live for five years, at least until this child in my womb has grown up and can survive. They said with medicines I can live longer.
—Geetha, from Kovalam, a 24-year-old married woman
who was pregnant with her second child

I am planning to bring my child up to ten years and give whatever I have to my child and then I can go. After that, my child will be educated and can start to take care of himself.
—Shalini, from Perambalur District, a 30-year-old married,
pregnant woman whose first child died at the age of 4 days

I wish to live at least until my youngest daughter reaches ten years, at least until all my children are educated. After that it doesn't matter. I do not want my children to know that I am HIV-positive because I am afraid that they will face discrimination if others know.
—Fatima, from the village of Palikudi near Nagapattinam, a 31-year-old
married mother of five children, the youngest of whom was 5 days old

God cannot change what is written on my forehead [i.e., my fate], but I still pray to God pleading, "At least until the time my second daughter attains puberty, don't take me away." My husband has been very supportive. When I cry, he consoles me and tells me there will be medicines to cure this one day soon. Will people find a cure soon? What do you think?
—Vijaya, from Namakkal, a 34-year-old mother of two in
her second marriage after becoming an AIDS widow

I exist only for the children. The school does not know that our first daughter is HIV-positive, and we have not yet told our daughter that she is HIV-positive. My hope is that someone will find a cure before my daughter turns fifteen and matures. I want to live at least long enough to see her mature.
—Prema, from Pondicherry, a 24-year-old married woman
with a 5-year-old HIV-positive daughter and a 9-month-
old daughter whose HIV status was still unknown

I don't have anything else except this child in my womb. My child is all to me. My husband and I will not tell our child that we have HIV until the child is married because we do not want our child to be sad or worry about the future. After that, I will be free to go. I want this child to study in an English medium school.

—Minradha, from Chennai, a 25-year-old married woman in the eighth month of her pregnancy (her first pregnancy ended in a miscarriage; the baby born in her second pregnancy died at 5 months of age)

Some of the women I met had either already put their children in a hostel or put them up for adoption, or they were hoping to do so. For these women a hostel or adoption was their only hope for their children's future because they did not believe that they would in fact live long enough to raise them to a safe age. Even if they did actually survive, they believed that they would have no means to support their children and provide them with nutritious food and an education; they thought that they and/or their spouses would be too ill to work or that they would be widowed and unable to find a job to support their children because they lacked education and/or because their HIV-positive status had become known to their employers and had been grounds to dismiss them from the job.

Karpagam placed her eldest HIV-negative son in a hostel for his education while keeping her younger HIV-positive child at home, where she could nurture him. Although she felt assured that her first son was well cared for, her contact with him was severely restricted and she missed him terribly. As she explained:

World Vision arranged this for us and they cover all the costs. He has been there for four years now, ever since he was five years old. We don't have to pay for it. They provide food, clothing, everything. We see him once a year on his birthday. We go to see him and come back on the same day. We are not allowed to visit often. The hostel will not give him leave to come home. That is the rule at the hostel. They do this because they say that the child's education will be negatively affected if we visit too often. We can talk to them on the phone. We have agreed in writing that he will be there for ten years. If we wish, he can continue there after that. The hostel knows that we are HIV-positive, but we don't know if there are other children in that hostel whose parents are also HIV-positive or not.

Maheswari and her husband were relieved to be able to place their son in a hostel. She and her husband and their first son were all HIV-positive. The son was 4 years old and Maheswari was pregnant again when I met her. She explained to me that they were extremely poor and struggled to be able to eat one meal a day. As she put it, "If we have money, we will buy rice and make rice porridge. Otherwise we will starve only." Her husband was bedridden at the Tambaram hospital and had no income. After her husband entered the hospital, she went to work as a servant, earning 200 rupees per month. But her employers learned of her HIV status and stopped paying her, so she was looking for sporadic wage labor work. Previously, when her son was sick, a charitable organization had given rice and *dhal* to her whole family for three months. Then they also started to give her son ART. As his health improved from the ART, she explained, the charitable organization cut back on the free food provided to the family, after which point they could not afford to feed their son, even though he was receiving ART for free. Given all these factors, she was tremendously relieved when the same organization helped her to get her son situated in a hostel, even if it meant that she would spend little time with him.

I met Chellamma in the postpartum ward—a comfortable, private room—at YRG Care where she was caring for her 22-day-old daughter. Usually women did not stay in the postpartum ward for such a long time after a baby's birth, but Chellamma's case was different. Chellamma was a 25-year-old married woman from a village in Theni District in southwestern Tamil Nadu, and this was her third daughter. She told me that YRG Care was helping to make arrangements for her daughter to be adopted by a family from a foreign country; she thought it was a family from the United States. She had expected the family to visit the baby the day I met her, and the staff at YRG Care had brought new clothes for the baby to make sure she looked presentable for the potential adoptive parents. But no one had come and the YRG Care staff was not sure how much longer they could let Chellamma stay before they would have to send her back to her village, which was a long distance from Chennai. Chellamma explained why she was putting this child up for adoption: "This is my third girl child. My husband is dying from AIDS. He cannot work to earn money. We cannot afford to raise three girls. Our children should not undergo this type of trouble like us."

It is not merely coincidence that, as discussed earlier, Pushpa's parents-in-law/grandparents were fighting hard to hold onto custody rights of Pushpa's only son after she was widowed (and then remarried), even though her son was HIV-positive, whereas Chellamma was seeking adoption for her third daughter, even though she most likely would be HIV-negative because she had received maternity care through YRG Care. Although Tamil Nadu is considered to have greater gender equity than many other parts of India, as with India as a whole, Tamil Nadu has long faced a problem of what is sometimes referred to as son preference. This has sometimes manifested itself in disturbing ways through the practice of female infanticide and through sex-selective abortion with new prenatal technologies, especially ultrasound. The north-central regions of Tamil Nadu, such as Namakkal and Salem Districts, which have been the hardest hit by the HIV/AIDS epidemic, have also been identified as regions in which female infanticide rates are high. The Tamil Nadu government has been proactive in its attempts to develop policies to deal with this problem and incentives to prevent it, just as they have with HIV/AIDS prevention. To hear Chellamma say "We cannot afford to raise three girls" is thus hardly unusual. I have heard mothers voice this concern repeatedly, long before HIV/AIDS was a factor. But HIV/AIDS exacerbates this problem profoundly when people living in poverty have little or no access to treatments and when stigma and discrimination drive HIV-positive people away from jobs, medical care, and family support systems. In such situations it is no wonder that the possibility of placing one's daughter in a hostel or placing her in a supportive adoptive family can give HIV-positive mothers peace of mind. It was therefore not surprising that when I visited CHES—a home for children affected by HIV/AIDS—in Chennai in January 2003, the founder and director of the organization, Dr. P. Manorama, told me that they had taken in more orphan girls than boys.

. . .

In this final chapter I have shown that some women expressed newfound—though guarded—optimism with respect to remarriage and inheritance rights. I have suggested that their efforts might contribute to transforming gender norms in these arenas more broadly, but I have also demonstrated that the overarching concern of all the women I interviewed was the future well-being of their children, about which they expressed extreme anxiety. Such are some of the unintended consequences of a public health program aimed at preventing HIV transmission from mother to child.

The PPTCT program has been effective in stemming the tide of the transmission of HIV from mother to child in India, as in other parts of the world, but it has often done so at an enormous social and psychological cost to HIV-positive mothers, as has been demonstrated throughout this book. The research presented in this book reinforces the observations made by such medical anthropologists as Farmer and Kleinman, who state that illnesses "absorb and radiate the personalities and social conditions of those who experience symptoms and treatments" (Farmer and Kleinman 2001: 353–56) and who argue that the study of responses to AIDS in particular reveals much about social relations and cultural values.

My study of the impact of the PPTCT program in South India reveals, first, the ways in which global and national inequalities play out when counselors feel compelled to increase the number of pregnant women getting tested for HIV because of pressures from the government and ultimately international donor institutions interested in seeing quantitative indicators to demonstrate the success of their interventions. In the process, low-income, undereducated (or uneducated) women are not provided with full and accurate information with which to make an informed decision about their reproductive health care. Furthermore, even while being compelled to accept prenatal HIV testing and to go forward with birth if found to be HIV-positive, low-income women in this part of the world are not provided with the full package of prevention of mother-to-child transmission care. This care includes cesarean sections and free replacement feeding and provides substantially greater protection against HIV transmission. The low-income women who did receive the full package care were those who received services through an NGO and who often had to make their bodies available to the clinical trials of multinational pharmaceutical companies in order to obtain such comprehensive care.

My research also demonstrates how unequal gender relations are reinforced through such public health programs, because women are being singled out for HIV testing during their pregnancies and this is leading to women's HIV status becoming known to families usually before their husbands are even tested (or at least before a husband's test becomes known to others). In patriarchal, patrilineal, and patrilocal contexts in which newly married women have less power and authority than their male spouses, the discovery of their HIV status often places them in an extremely precarious position within the family of their in-laws, further exacerbating gender inequalities. Because many of these women become AIDS widows at a young age, the intense stigma attached to their HIV-positive status compounds the social stigma they face as widows and typically precludes the possibility of remarriage. Furthermore, it is not uncommon for a woman's in-laws to blame her for being sexually promiscuous and spreading HIV to their son and for them to use this as excuse to expel her from their home and family and to deny her inheritance rights once she becomes widowed.

The stigma of an HIV-positive status in India was particularly intense during my research in the beginning of 2004, before the government established a program to provide ART free of cost. Essentially, the PPTCT program amounted to an international and government-driven program to increase HIV testing among pregnant women to prevent new cases of HIV, but it offered no treatment to the women themselves and provided little protection from the stigma-related forms of discrimination they would face in their families and even, ironically, when seeking maternal health care. The discrimination they faced in medical settings was exacerbated by the lack of resources to provide universal precautions in many hospitals catering to the poor.

Since 2004, the Indian pharmaceutical industry has been able to produce generic first-line drugs at substantially reduced cost. As a result, NACO has been able to phase in an ART program with initial support from WHO. Dr. S. Rajasekaran, the deputy superintendent of the Tambaram hospital in May 2004, told me in a meeting right before the ART program was being phased in that the gender distribution of people on ART through this program at Tambaram was 50% men, 48% women, and 2% eunuchs. The fact that 48% of the patients enrolled in this new program were women was significant because it represented a higher percentage than the overall percentage of HIV-positive women and pointed to the fact that they were giving priority to women. In fact, Dr. Rajasekaran explained that they were giving particular priority to widows and women with children.[5]

My research in 2008 suggests that, although some people living with HIV/AIDS were able to benefit from the government's ART program, still others would have liked to have access to free ART but either did not know about it or were not able to make use of it because of the distance they had to travel or because of bureaucratic obstacles, such as the need to obtain a government ration card that would entitle them to the free treatments. In some cases people were in fact traveling great distances, even crossing state borders from Andhra Pradesh and Kerala, to come to Chennai to get ART from the government Tambaram hospital or YRG Care. Greater effort clearly needs to be placed on making sure that these medicines are reaching people in need. Barring this, the widespread HIV testing of low-income pregnant women can do as much social damage as it does public health good.

With support from activist networks for people living with HIV/AIDS (such as PWN+) and NGOs (such as YRG Care), some women are beginning to push back against the boundaries of society's gender conventions and against HIV/AIDS-related stigma and discrimination; they are entering into new marriages despite their status as HIV-positive widows (even choosing to have children in the second marriages) and are making demands for their legal rights to their share of their husband's property once they become AIDS widows. These efforts have not always been seamless, but they are indicative of socially and economically marginalized women's pragmatic struggles to overcome not only the severe stigma associated with HIV/AIDS in India but also, more broadly, gender inequalities that have exacerbated that stigma for women living with HIV/AIDS.

Epilogue
Memory Boxes

NETWORKS AND NGOS THAT PROVIDED PSYCHOSOCIAL SUPPORT for women living with
HIV/AIDS were aware that the greatest concern for most of these women was
the future well-being of their children, because HIV-positive women felt an
intense sense of insecurity about their children's financial and emotional futures, whether their children were HIV-positive or HIV-negative. The strong
consensus among the women I met was that it was best for parents not to disclose their HIV status to their own children until their children were grown.
This was reflected by Minradha, who said, "My husband and I will not tell our
child that we have HIV until the child is married because we do not want our
child to be sad or worry about the future." There was also a consensus among
the women I interviewed that if their children were HIV-positive, they should
not inform them about this until the latest possible time. Many thought that 16
would be the appropriate age at which to disclose this information to a child,
although how they intended to keep a child from knowing his or her own status
for that long if they were taking ART is hard to imagine. Avoiding disclosure
was viewed as a way of protecting children from worrying about the future and
from feeling responsible for the fact that they and/or their parents were HIV-
positive. Parents also feared that if their children knew about either their own
HIV-positive status or that of their parents and they happened to inadvertently
mention this to their friends, teachers, or other family members, the children
themselves would run the risk of experiencing stigma and discrimination. By
law, parents were not required to report their child's HIV status to school administrators, and, given the media reports during the time of my research of
schools in Kerala that had expelled children because of their HIV-positive status, there was a strong incentive to keep this information secret.

Keeping such secrets from anyone can be a tremendous psychological strain, as Rajeswari noted: "Whenever I am in the home, I am afraid, wondering: Who will come to know? How will they come to know? What will I do if they come to know? If they ask, 'Why are you taking so many tablets?' what will I say? What will I do if they come to know through that? What am I going to do? I am always very scared, thinking about these things." Keeping this information secret from one's own children added to women's sense of guilt, even if it was done to protect them.

YRG Care developed a creative approach to try to alleviate some of this psychological stress through the creation of what they called memory boxes. At one of their support group meetings HIV-positive mothers were provided with the materials to decorate small shoebox-size boxes with pink and purple tissue paper, newspaper clippings, colored markers, and stickers of hearts and Winnie the Pooh. Mothers were then encouraged to write a letter to each of their children. In the letter they were asked to write whatever they most wanted their children to know. They were supposed to write about things that they felt they could not say directly to the children but that they wished they could tell them or that they wanted their children to know in the future, including disclosing their HIV status. Then they put the letters in the memory box. The mothers did not want to bring these boxes home because they would arouse too much curiosity and there was no place to hide such things in small, crowded homes. So they asked YRG Care to keep them safe for them until they felt ready to give them to their children. The mothers instructed YRG Care to give the memory boxes to their children at an appropriate age in case they died before they could present the boxes to the children in person.

I saw the boxes all lined up inside a locked cabinet at YRG Care. The mothers had written in English or Tamil, "To: Child's Name. Love: Mummy/*Amma*. The researcher in me wanted to ask to see the letters inside the boxes, but another part of me knew this would be a violation of privacy. I found myself getting choked up, staring at those pink and purple boxes, imagining that most intimate moment when a child would open one of them to read the letter inside. And I wondered how HIV/AIDS would affect that child's life as she or he grew up and how it would affect the lives of that child's children.

Reference Matter

Notes

Prologue

1. This name is a pseudonym. To protect the confidentiality of the HIV-positive women participating in this research as well as the other women interviewed during their prenatal visits, I gave each woman a code number and did not include their real names on the tape-recorded interviews or in the notes. In my writing I have chosen to use pseudonyms for all the women interviewed and have avoided providing details about them that would expose their identities. Given the nature of stigma and discrimination associated with an HIV-positive status in India, maintaining confidentiality was of paramount concern. For interviews conducted with professional people involved in HIV/AIDS prevention and care, I asked whether they would like me to use their real names and whether I could identify their professional positions; the vast majority gave consent for this. Thus, unless otherwise indicated, the names of those professionals interviewed are real names.

2. The *panchayat* is a local government body traditionally composed of five members.

3. The exchange rate during the time of my research in 2004 was 44 Indian rupees to US$1.

Chapter 1

1. http://www.unaids.org/en/CountryResponses/Countries/india.asp, accessed November 2, 2009.

2. According to the 2001 census, the population was 1,028,737,436.

3. For example, in 2006 it was estimated that India had 5.7 million HIV-positive people. This figure put India in the number one spot as the country with the most people living with HIV/AIDS (UNAIDS 2006) until prevalence rates in the country were recalibrated in 2006. The recalculation, using a different demographic method, resulted in dramatically reduced prevalence rates and reduced estimates of the numbers of HIV-positive people for India as a whole and for individual states. In 2007 the government's National AIDS Control Organization (NACO) published a report that stated that 25–30% of the people living with HIV/AIDS were aware of their status (NACO 2007b), and another NACO report from the same year indicated only 13% awareness (NACO 2007a).

4. In precolonial India girls from the Devadasi community could be dedicated to marriage with a god, and these girls would dance in the service of the gods and the king in Hindu temples. Under colonialism this practice was deemed immoral, and it was outlawed. Subsequently many *devadasi*s have entered into prostitution to make a living.

5. This was an advertisement produced by the San Francisco AIDS Foundation in 1992.

6. As stated in the film *A Closer Walk* (Bilheimer 2003).

7. Interviews with these women lasted approximately one hour each. Women were given their choice regarding the location of the interviews. Many of the interviews were longer when I met women in their homes, network offices, or parks. In some cases I interviewed the same woman up to three times. Some interviews with women who were coming to YRG Care for prenatal or postpartum checkups were a bit shorter because I had to accommodate the doctors' schedules.

8. YRG Care is a nonprofit organization based in Chennai that is involved in education, care and support, and research and training in the field of HIV/AIDS.

9. At these support group meetings I had the opportunity to introduce myself and explain my research interests to the women living with HIV who were attending the meetings. During the breaks, I asked women if they would like to participate in the research and if they would be interested and willing to be interviewed for my project. If they said yes, I asked them where and when we could meet for an interview. When I met them for the interview, I explained the project to them again and obtained their informed consent to participate before beginning the interview.

10. Interviews with these pregnant women lasted approximately half an hour each.

11. My research was approved by the Institutional Review Boards at Syracuse University and YRG Care. All the interviews with HIV-positive women and with the women receiving prenatal care in the public hospitals were conducted in Tamil, with the exception of one interview, which was conducted in English. With consent, all the interviews were tape-recorded, and either one of my research assistants or I also took notes during the interviews. Following the interviews, my research assistants helped to transcribe and translate the tape-recorded dialogue. Participation in all the interviews was voluntary, and I did not offer monetary compensation in return for the interviews. I did, however, explain that I would make contributions to the organizations with which the participants were affiliated, and I made contributions to PWN+, HUNS, SPMD, and YRG Care. I told participants that I hoped that by writing about their experiences, it might make policy makers and medical practitioners and the public more aware of their plight and might thereby lead to changes that could improve the lives of women living with HIV/AIDS in India more generally. In a few cases women opted to meet in public places and therefore had to take extra time out of their busy days to meet with me. In those cases I also offered to buy them lunch or provided a picnic and covered the cost of their transportation to and from the meeting place.

12. The highest household income reported was 14,400 rupees/month, and the lowest was 250 rupees/month.

13. Some of the women interviewed, however, had much higher levels of education: four had B.A. degrees; three had received an M.A., and one of these three had both an M.A. and an M.S. degree.

14. The youngest was 20 and the oldest was 50.

15. As Libman and Stein write, "The CD4 cell count correlates highly with the progression of HIV disease and is the main surrogate marker for immunological function" (Libman and Stein 2003: 48). CD4 counts of HIV-positive individuals will typically decrease over time as the immune system becomes compromised. At the time of my research, once a person's CD4 count dipped below 200, it was recommended that they begin antiretroviral treatment, if available.

Chapter 2

Some sections of this chapter have been previously published in Van Hollen (2011c).

1. "Indian Premier Urges Major Push on AIDS," *New York Times*, July 27, 2003: 6.

2. Some of the information presented here about the dates and core components of Phases I, II, and III of the NACO program comes from NACO's *Annual Report 2008–09* (NACO 2009).

3. Gerrit Beger, "'Red Ribbon Express' Rides the Rails to Raise Youth AIDS Awareness in India," http://www.unicef.org/infobycountry/india_42022.html (accessed November 5, 2009).

4. http://www.cnn.com/2009/WORLD/asiapcf/11/12/india.gender.voting/index.html (accessed November 18, 2009).

5. The first case was detected by Dr. Suniti Solomon of YRG Care.

6. Tamil Nadu has some pockets of higher HIV prevalence, such as Namakkal, where TNSACS reported in 2003 that prevalence rates were greater than 2% (TNSACS 2004a) and others suggested that it was as high as 6.5% in 2002 (K. Jain 2002).

7. Information provided here about the formation of the networks in India is based on my interviews with Rama Pandian, President of TNP+, on March 15, 2004; and with K. K. Abraham, President of INP+, on December 20, 2002. Information on the development of the networks can also be found in K. Jain (2002: 223–40).

8. The other two centers were the JJ Group of Hospitals in Mumbai and the Regional Institute of Medical Sciences in Manipur (Dr. P. Paramesh, Superintendent, Government Hospital of Thoracic Medicine, Tambaram Hospital, personal communication, May 31, 2004).

9. Interview with Rama Pandian, President of TNP+, December 20, 2002, Chennai.

10. The HIV sentinel surveillance is a "collection of epidemiological information . . . regarding the distribution and spread of HIV infection to be relevant to planning, implementation and monitoring of HIV/AIDS prevention and control programs" (TNSACS 2004b: n.p.).

11. This figure is based on the presentation "The Gates Foundation's Experience," given by Ashok Alexander, of the Bill and Melinda Gates Foundation, India, at the 2004 Conference on "Strategy for the Second Wave: Learning from India's Experience with HIV/AIDS," organized by the Center for Strategic and International Studies, Washington, D.C., September 9, 2004.

12. This figure is from an article posted on the AIDS-INDIA e-mail list on March 1, 2005. The subject of this posting was "Second Phase of Anti-Retroviral Programme Begins: Tamilnadu, India." The article posted on the e-mail list was copied from an article published in *The Hindu*, February 28, 2005. According to a 2005 briefing paper by the Center for Reproductive Rights, among women who do not breast-feed, the risk of transmission without any other interventions is 15–30% (Center for Reproductive Rights 2005: 3).

13. Dr. V. L. Srilata, UNICEF, personal communication, March 4, 2004, Chennai. Eight of these PPTCT centers were in private hospitals, and the others were in public hospitals.

14. As of 2012, in the state of Tamil Nadu there were 786 PPTCT centers in government facilities and 77 centers in private hospitals as part of a public-private initiative. See the TNSACS website for the PPTCT program: http://www.tansacs.in/PPTCT.html (accessed May 22, 2012).

Chapter 3

1. Unless otherwise indicated, all quotes from interviews are translated from Tamil. English words used in the original interview will appear in quotation marks.

2. Another NACO report from 2007 indicated awareness rates as high as 25–30% (NACO 2007b: 1), and in 2009 NACO reported a 50% awareness (NACO 2009).

3. The window period is the time between when one is exposed to HIV and when it shows up in a positive test for HIV antibodies. Most people will test positive 2–8 weeks after exposure, but for some it may take longer. Because of the window period, it is possible to receive a false-negative test.

4. During March and April 2006 there was a discussion on the AIDS/India e-mail discussion list about the usefulness of the distinctive Indian emphasis on "parent" rather than "mother."

5. The salt referred to here is actually albumin, a protein that is normally present in blood and leaks out of the kidneys and into the urine in women with preeclampsia. This condition is also associated with hypertension, and salt restriction is seen as one way of controlling this component of preeclampsia. However, recent studies have shown no significant benefit of restricting salt, and there is concern that restricting salt might indirectly affect overall nutrition because saltless food

is unpalatable. References to albumin as salt is common in a variety of clinical settings in India, especially when talking to less educated patients who are unlikely to understand what a protein is. The usefulness of the metaphor is that it creates an (untrue) explanatory framework that can explain the need for salt restriction (Dr. Lalit Narayan, personal communication, April 11, 2012).

6. Counselors reported this to me and the program director, Shyamala Natarajan, also stated this when I interviewed her at SIAAP in Chennai on March 4, 2004.

7. Interview with Shyamala Natarajan, SIAAP program director, March 4, 2004.

Chapter 4

1. Some Mudaliar caste subgroups are considered Forward Castes by the Tamil Nadu government, whereas others are considered Other Backward Castes (OBCs). Given her lower class status, it is likely that this woman belonged to one of the OBC Mudaliar groups, although I cannot say for certain.

2. In Chapter 5 I elaborate on Susan Seizer's discussion of the term murai and the way it is used to denote both propriety and Tamil culture more broadly. Following her work, I have chosen to translate this one Tamil word using two different English words to best capture what I believe is the intent of the speaker.

Chapter 5

A version of this chapter was published in Van Hollen (2010).

1. This figure was calculated on the basis of the rural-urban distribution figures provided on the NACO website Facts & Figures: "HIV Estimates—2004," http://www.nacoonline.org/facts_hivestimates04.htm (accessed July 7, 2005) (NACO 2005).

2. Interview with Dr. Suniti Solomon, YRG Care, Chennai, March 9, 2004.

3. Jonathan Mann, statement at an informal briefing on AIDS to the 42nd session of the United Nations General Assembly, New York, October 20, 1987.

4. The length of time it takes for HIV to develop into AIDS depends on biological and socioeconomic factors, including poverty, which can jeopardize health and weaken people's immune systems, making them more vulnerable to AIDS.

5. A study conducted on HIV and AIDS support groups in Thailand reports a similar phenomenon in which women outnumber men in the support groups (Lyttleton 2004).

6. The term hostel is commonly used in India to refer to many different kinds of boarding residences, not simply those for orphans.

Chapter 6

A version of this chapter was previously published in Van Hollen (2007).

1. I use the term enable here in the positive sense of providing the opportunity, power, or capacity to act.

2. HIV diagnosis late in a pregnancy was also found to be an issue in studies in Thailand (de Bruyn 2002: 19) and the United States (Kirshenbaum et al. 2004).

3. Interview with Dr. V. L. Srilata, UNICEF, Chennai, March 4, 2004.

4. Interview with Dr. Suniti Solomon, YRG Care, Chennai, March 9, 2004.

5. VDRL stands for Venereal Disease Research Laboratory and refers to an antibody test. Many patients in India who are HIV-positive are also VDRL-positive.

6. The Tamil term veeriyam, meaning "potency" or "strength," is usually used in reference to medicines and seeds.

7. http://www.wvi.org/wvi/childsponsorship/faqsponsorship.htm (accessed April 19, 2005).

8. "Frequently Asked Questions" section of the World Vision website, http://www.wvi.org/wvi/childsponsorship/faqsponsorship.htm (accessed April 19, 2005).

9. Sometimes the women I interviewed would simply use the English word "character" (as in, "He had a 'character'") to imply that someone had a bad character.

Chapter 7

A version of this chapter was previously published in Van Hollen (2011a).

1. My study has not yet explored how HIV/AIDS is affecting the practices of midwives (known as *marutuvaacis* in Tamil Nadu and *dais* more generally throughout India). Such a study is of critical importance.

2. The CDC defines universal precautions as "a set of precautions designed to prevent transmission of human immunodeficiency virus (HIV), hepatitis B virus (HBV), and other bloodborne pathogens when providing first aid or health care. Under universal precautions, blood and certain body fluids of all patients are considered potentially infectious for HIV, HBV and other bloodborne pathogens" (http://www.cdc.gov/ncidod/dhqp/bp_universal_precautions.html, accessed June 3, 2010).

3. I once observed another lab technician in a government maternity hospital doing HIV blood tests without any gloves. When I asked him about this, his response was that he never uses gloves because it is difficult to feel the vein while wearing gloves, and he is experienced enough to take necessary precautions without wearing gloves.

4. Dr. Lalit Narayan, personal communication, April 11, 2012.

5. It is not uncommon for women from rural areas who have to travel far for their obstetric care to come to the hospital several days in advance of their due date and stay in the prenatal ward until they deliver.

6. In this context an *ayah* refers to a woman who is at the lowest level of the medical staff in the maternity wards. *Ayahs* prepare women for deliveries, assist doctors and nurses during deliveries, and clean and move mothers and babies following the delivery.

7. Dr. Lalit Narayan, personal communication, April 11, 2012.

8. Unfortunately I did not discover what motivated this cousin to reveal Jayanthi's status to the medical personnel, so I cannot say whether it was an act of revenge, an act of citizenship, or something else.

9. The hospital where the women from YRG Care went for their deliveries was partly funded by a trust that provided care for high-risk mothers with a range of medical concerns. This helped to bring down the cost from that charged for deliveries of HIV-positive mothers at most private hospitals. The total cost for delivery and all postpartum care for HIV-positive women at this hospital was 25,000 rupees. YRG Care covered this cost for those women coming through their projects. Dr. R. Shoba, personal communication, June 17, 2008.

10. A *paaladai* is a small metal vessel shaped like a tear drop that is used to feed infants liquids and herbal medicines.

11. Information about the treatment and care provided under this scheme was provided by the YRG Care staff member in charge of the clinical trials (personal communication, June 11, 2008).

12. The Global Fund to Fight AIDS, Tuberculosis, and Malaria is usually referred to simply as the Global Fund.

13. A doctor working on this project at YRG Care told me that with the combined interventions given through this scheme, they could reduce HIV transmission to 1%, whereas the government's PPTCT project with only single-dose nevirapine (without cesarean section and with breastfeeding) can reduce transmission to only approximately 11%. Personal communication, June 13, 2008.

14. Information about the clinical trial was provided by the YRG Care staff member in charge of organizing the trial (personal communication, June 11, 2008).

15. National Institute of Allergy and Infectious Disease (n.d.: 9). This report did not indicate where in Africa the study was taking place. In Africa, India, and Haiti this clinical trial was ACTG 5207; in Thailand it was PACTG 1032.

16. All non-ART medicines for this project were donated by two Indian pharmaceutical companies: Aurobindo and E. M. Cure. ARTs for the Connect project were available to women for free either through the Government Hospitals or through the Global Fund, which was administered through YRG Care. These ARTs were produced by the Indian pharmaceutical companies Cipla and Ranbaxy. HIV-positive patients at YRG Care who were not in the Connect project could also receive ARTs through the Global Fund program either free of cost or at a discounted rate, depending on their financial and medical needs. Those who paid higher prices helped to subsidize those who received the medicines for free, thereby making this a self-sustaining program. The Global Fund provided funds to NACO, which in turn provided funds to YRG Care. YRG Care began administering the Global Fund program in February 2005. YRG Care received the medications for free but charged some patients for these medications so that they could cover the costs of administering the medications to all their patients. These costs included ascertaining CD4 counts and paying doctors' consultation fees. On average, the cost of these ARTs without any subsidy was 2,500 rupees per month (this was for the lamivudine-efavirenz combination, which was the most common). Some ART regimens could cost as much as 7,000 rupees without subsidies. YRG Care was the one center in Tamil Nadu selected to administer this program. This information was provided by the YRG Care staff member in charge of the Global Fund program (personal communication, June 17, 2008).

17. YRG Care staff member in charge of the Global Fund program, personal communication, June 17, 2008.

18. YRG Care has direct links to a long list of some of the most prestigious universities in the United States.

Chapter 8

A version of this chapter was previously published in Van Hollen (2011b).

1. SWEN stands for Six Week Extended-Dose Nevirapine. The SWEN Study Team has an extensive list of members. The contact person listed for the SWEN team and its report is Prof. Robert C. Bollinger at the Johns Hopkins Center for Clinical Global Health Education.

2. Doctors at the Institute of Obstetrics and Gynecology in Egmore, Chennai, suggested that at their institute babies born to HIV-positive mothers who were breast-fed exclusively had lower morbidity and mortality rates than those who were bottle-fed. Dr. A. Sundarvalli, personal communication, March 12, 2004.

3. It is important to note that in 1996 UNAIDS and the UN High Commissioner for Human Rights jointly produced international guidelines on human rights for people living with HIV/AIDS. These guidelines stipulate that when a woman has access to the safe, nutritional use of replacement feedings, the infant has the right to that alternative; in addition, if a woman in this situation does not provide her infant with replacement feeding, she "may be subject to intervention by a child welfare agency on the ground that she is endangering her child." These same guidelines, however, recognize that when a woman does not have access to the safe, nutritional use of replacement feeding, breastfeeding may be more advantageous to the health of the infant, and such a woman would not be subject to intervention from a child welfare agency (Cook and Dickens 2002: 61).

4. This is distinct from the increased risk of HIV transmission from alternating between breastfeeding and replacement feeding, which was mentioned earlier.

5. According to Dr. Lalit Narayan, this is a controversial method of suppressing lactation be-

cause it probably refers to injecting high doses of estrogen or a related compound, which may cause life-threatening blood clots (personal communication, April 11, 2012).

6. See http://www.babyfriendly.org.uk/ for general information on UNICEF's Baby Friendly Initiative. Also see http://www.unicef.org/india/health_3000.htm for the UNICEF Baby Friendly Initiative in India. Both accessed on February 2, 2010.

7. See http://www.aavinmilk.com/ (accessed August 31, 2007).

Chapter 9

1. In India each political party has a symbol associated with it, and these symbols are central to political campaigns. For example, in Tamil Nadu, a state with vibrant populist politics, the symbols of the political parties can be seen painted on the walls of public spaces of cities and villages alike.

2. According to Dr. Lalit Narayan (personal communication, April 11, 2012), from a biomedical standpoint it is not likely that insecticide would damage the uterus, although it could have severe neurological effects.

3. A *lekiyam* is a form of medicine made from a sweet base (with white or brown sugar, or jaggery) with other herbal medicinal ingredients mixed in; ghee is often added as a preserving agent. The final product is rolled into small balls, which are taken orally.

4. UNICEF, "India: Age at Marriage," http://www.unicef.org/india/Media_AGE_AT_MAR RIAGE_in.pdf (accessed March 31, 2010). Interestingly, this same report indicates that, although the age at marriage for Tamil Nadu is slightly higher than the national average, the difference between the age of women and men at marriage is greater in Tamil Nadu than in most other states. In 2001 the average age at marriage in Tamil Nadu was 19.9 for women and 25.5 for men. This may be due to Dravidian kinship patterns in which women sometimes marry their maternal uncles.

5. Interview with Dr. S. Rajasekaran, deputy superintendent of the Government Hospital for Thoracic Medicine, May 31, 2004.

Bibliography

Abu-Lughod, Lila. 1993. *Women Writing Worlds: Bedouin Stories*. Berkeley: University of California Press.

Agarwal, Bina. 1994. *A Field of One's Own: Gender and Land Rights in South Asia*. Cambridge, UK: Cambridge University Press.

Ahearn, Laura. 2001. *Invitations to Love: Literacy, Love Letters, and Social Change in Nepal*. Ann Arbor: University of Michigan Press.

Alter, Joseph. 1992. *The Wrestler's Body: Identity and Ideology in North India*. Berkeley: University of California Press.

———. 1997. "Seminal Truth: A Modern Science of Male Celibacy in North India." *Medical Anthropology Quarterly* 11(3): 275–79.

Anandhi, S. 2005. "Women, Work, and Abortion Practices in Kancheepuram District, Tamil Nadu." Draft report. Chennai: Madras Institute of Development Studies.

Ananth, Prasanna, and Cheryl Koopman. 2003. "HIV/AIDS Knowledge, Beliefs, and Behavior Among Women of Childbearing Age in India." *AIDS Education and Prevention* 15(6): 529–46.

Arnold, David. 1993. *Colonizing the Body: State Medicine and Epidemic Disease in Nineteenth-Century India*. Berkeley: University of California Press.

Ashraf, Shahid, and Peter Godwin. 1998. "Gender Differentials and the Special Vulnerability of Women." In Peter Godwin, ed., *The Looming Epidemic: The Impact of HIV/AIDS in India*, 171–84. New Delhi: Mosaic Books.

Asthana, Sheena, and Robert Oostvogels. 1996. "Community Participation in HIV Prevention Problems and Prospects for Community-Based Strategies Among Female Sex Workers in Madras." *Social Science and Medicine* 43(2): 133–48.

Avert.org. 2010 (May 24). "AIDS, Drug Prices, and Generic Drugs." *http://www.avert.org.generic.htm*. Accessed June 9, 2010.

Banerjee, D. 2004. "The People and Health Service Development in India: A Brief Overview." *International Journal of Health Services* 34(1): 123–42.

Becker, Gay. 2000. *The Elusive Embryo: How Men and Women Approach New Reproductive Technologies*. Berkeley: University of California Press.

Berer, Marge. 1999. "HIV/AIDS, Pregnancy, and Maternal Mortality and Morbidity: Implications for Care." In Marge Berer and T. K. Sundari Ravindran, eds., *Safe Motherhood Initiative: Critical Issues*, 30–42. Oxford, UK: Blackwell Science.

Bhan, Nirojini, P. Mahajan, and M. Sondhi. 2004. "Awareness Regarding Sex Knowledge Among Adolescent Girls." *Anthropologist* 6(2): 101–103.

Bharadwaj, Aditya. 2002. "Why Adoption Is Not an Option in India: The Visibility of Infertility, the Secrecy of Donor Insemination, and Other Cultural Complexities." *Social Science and Medicine* 56: 1867–80.

———. 2011. "Reproductive Viability and the State: Embryonic Stem Cell Research in India." In Carole Browner and Carolyn Sargent, eds., *Reproduction, Globalization, and the State: New Theoretical and Ethnographic Perspectives*, 113–25. Durham, NC: Duke University Press.

———. 2013. *Conceptions: Infertility and Procreative Modernity in India*. New York: Berghahn Books (in press).

Bhaskaran, Suparna. 2004. *Made in India: Decolonizations, Queer Sexualities, Trans/national Projects*. New York: Palgrave Macmillan.

Biehl, João. 2005. *Vita: Life in a Zone of Social Abandonment*. Berkeley: University of California Press.

———. 2007. *Will to Live: AIDS Therapies and the Politics of Survival*. Princeton, NJ: Princeton University Press.

Biehl, João, Denise Coutinho, and Ana Luzia Outeiro. 2001. "Technology and Affect: HIV/AIDS Testing in Brazil." *Culture, Medicine, and Psychiatry* 25:87–129.

Bilheimer, Robert, dir. 2003. *A Closer Walk: A Film About AIDS in the World*. Worldwide Documentaries.

Biradavolu, Monica Rao, S. Burris, A. George, A. Jena, and K. M. Blankenship. 2009. "Can Sex Workers Regulate Police? Learning from an HIV Prevention Project for Sex Workers in Southern India." *Social Science and Medicine* 68: 1541–47.

Bloom, Shelah S., and Paula L. Griffiths. 2007. "Female Autonomy as a Contributing Factor to Women's HIV-Related Knowledge and Behavior in Three Culturally Contrasting States in India." *Journal of Biosocial Science* 39(4): 557–73.

Blystad, Astrid, and Karen Moland. 2009. "Technologies of Hope? Motherhood, HIV, and Infant Feeding in Eastern Africa." *Anthropology and Medicine* 16(2): 105–18.

Bond, Virginia, Levy Chilikwela, Sue Clay, Titus Kafuma, Laura Nyblade, and Nadia Bettega. 2003. *Kanayaka: "The Light Is On"—Understanding HIV and AIDS Related Stigma in Urban and Rural Zambia*. Lusaka, Zambia: Zambart Project.

Bourdier, Frédéric. 1997. "Women and AIDS in Southern India: Accusation and Reconstruction of Immorality." *Journal des Anthropologies* 68(9): 156–64.

———. 1998. "AIDS Epidemic in Southern India and Its Social Consequences in Gender Relations." *Eastern Anthropologist* 51(1): 63–72.

———. 2004. "Management of HIV/AIDS Epidemic in India." In Patrice Cohen and Suniti Solomon, eds., *AIDS and Maternity in India: From Public Health to Social Science Perspectives—Emerging Themes and Debates*, 83–102. Pondicherry, India: Institut Français de Pondichéry.

Browner, Carole, and Nancy Ann Press. 1995. "The Normalization of Prenatal Diagnostic Screening." In Faye Ginsburg and Rayna Rapp, eds., *Conceiving the New World Order: The Global Politics of Reproduction*, 307–22. Berkeley: University of California Press.

Bumiller, Elisabeth. 1990. *May You Be the Mother of a Hundred Sons: A Journey Among the Women of India*. New Delhi: Penguin Books.

Campbell, Catherine. 2004. "Migrancy, Masculine Identities, and AIDS: The Psychosocial Context of HIV Transmission on the South African Gold Mines." In E. S. Craddock, J. R. Oppong, and J. Gosh, eds., *HIV and AIDS in Africa: Beyond Epidemiology*, 144–54. Cambridge, MA: Blackwell.

Carpenter, Joel A. 1998. "Review of 'On the Boundaries of American Evangelicalism: The Postwar Evangelical Coalition.'" *Church History* 67(4): 822–24.

Carsten, Janet, ed. 2000. *Cultures of Relatedness: New Approaches to the Study of Kinship.* Cambridge, UK: Cambridge University Press.

——. 2004. *After Kinship.* Cambridge, UK: Cambridge University Press.

CDC (Centers for Disease Control and Prevention). 2006 (September 22). "Revised Recommendations for HIV Testing of Adults, Adolescents, and Pregnant Women in Health-Care Settings." MMWR Recommendations and Reports 55(RR14). *http://www.cdc.gov/mmwr/preview/mmwrhtml/rr5514a1.htm.* Accessed September 1, 2009.

Center for Reproductive Rights. 2005. "Pregnant Women Living with HIV/AIDS: Protecting Human Rights in Programs to Prevent Mother-to-Child Transmission of HIV." Briefing Paper. New York: Center for Reproductive Rights.

CFAR (Center for Advocacy and Research) and PWN+ (Positive Women's Network). 2003. *Positive Speaking: Voices of Women Living with HIV/AIDS.* New Delhi: United Nations Development Fund for Women (UNIFEM).

Chandra, Prabha S., V. Ravi, A. Desai, and D. K. Subbakrishna. 1998. "Anxiety and Depression Among HIV-Infected Heterosexuals: A Report from India." *Journal of Psychosomatic Research* 45(5): 401–409.

Chandrasekaran, Padma, G. Dallabetta, V. Loo, S. Rao, H. Gayle, and A. Alexander. 2006. "Containing HIV/AIDS in India: The Unfinished Agenda." *Lancet* 6: 508–21.

Chatterjee, Partha. 1989. "The Nationalist Resolution of the Women's Question." In Kumkum Sangari and Sudesh Vaid, eds., *Recasting Women: Essays in Indian Colonial History*, 233–53. New Brunswick, NJ: Rutgers University Press.

Cohen, Lawrence. 1997. "Semen, Irony, and the Atom Bomb." *Medical Anthropology Quarterly* 11(3): 301–303.

——. 2004. "Operability: Surgery at the Margin of the State." In Veena Das and Deborah Poole, eds., *Anthropology in the Margins of the State*, 165–90. Oxford, UK: Oxford University Press.

——. 2005. "Operability, Bioavailability, and Exception." In Aihwa Ong and Stephen Collier, eds., *Global Assemblages: Technology, Politics, and Ethics as Anthropological Problems*, 79–90. Malden, MA: Blackwell.

Cohen, Patrice, and Suniti Solomon, eds. 2004. *AIDS and Maternity in India: From Public Health to Social Science Perspectives—Emerging Themes and Debates.* Pondicherry, India: Institut Français de Pondichéry.

Cook, R. J., and B. M. Dickens. 2002. "Human Rights and HIV-Positive Women." *International Journal of Gynecology and Obstetrics* 77: 55–63.

Coutsoudis, Anna, Hoosen M. Coovadia, and Catherine M. Wilfert. 2008. "HIV, Infant Feeding, and More Perils for Poor People: New WHO Guidelines Encourage Review of Formula Milk Policies." *Bulletin of the World Health Organization* 86(3): 210–14.

Cruz, Marcelo. 1999. "Competing Strategies for Modernization in the Ecuadorean Andes." *Current Anthropology* 40: 377–83.

Daniel, Valentine. 1984. *Fluid Signs: Being a Person the Tamil Way.* Berkeley: University of California Press.

Das, Veena. 1995. "National Honor and Practical Kinship: Unwanted Women and Children." In Faye Ginsburg and Rayna Rapp, eds., *Conceiving the New World Order: The Global Politics of Reproduction*, 212–33. Berkeley: University of California Press.

Davis-Floyd, Robbie E. 1992. *Birth as an American Rite of Passage.* Berkeley: University of California Press.

Davis-Floyd, Robbie, and Carolyn F. Sargent, eds. 1997. *Childbirth and Authoritative Knowledge: Cross-Cultural Perspectives.* Berkeley: University of California Press.

Dawson, Jill, Ray Fitzpatrick, J. McLean, G. Hart, and M. Boulton. 1991. "The HIV Test and Sexual Behavior in a Sample of Homosexually Active Men." *Social Science and Medicine* 32(6): 683–88.

de Bruyn, Maria. 2002. *Reproductive Choice and Women Living with HIV/AIDS.* Chapel Hill, NC: Ipas.

————. 2005. *HIV/AIDS and Reproductive Health: Sensitive and Neglected Issues—A Review of the Literature; Recommendations for Action.* Chapel Hill, NC: Ipas.

de Paoli, Marina Manuela, Rachel Manongi, and Knut-Inge Klepp. 2002. "Counselors' Perspectives on Antenatal HIV Testing and Infant Feeding Dilemmas Facing Women with HIV in Northern Tanzania." *Reproductive Health Matters* 10(20): 144–56.

Desclaux, Alice. 2004. "Socio-Cultural Obstacles to the Prevention of HIV: Transmission Through Breastfeeding in West Africa." In Patrice Cohen and Suniti Solomon, eds., *AIDS and Maternity in India: From Public Health to Social Science Perspectives—Emerging Themes and Debates*, 185–94. Pondicherry, India: Institut Français de Pondichéry.

Desclaux, Alice, and Chiara Alfieri. 2009. "Counseling and Choosing Between Infant-Feeding Options: Overall Limits and Local Interpretations by Health Care Providers and Women Living with HIV in Resource-Poor Countries (Burkina Faso, Cambodia, Cameroon)." *Social Science and Medicine* 69: 821–29.

Dictionary of Contemporary Tamil (Tamil-Tamil-English), Pavoorchatram Rajagopal Subramanian, ed. 1992. Madras: Cre-A.

Doherty, Tanya, M. Chopra, D. Jackson, A. Goga, M. Colvin, and L. A. Persson. 2007. "Effectiveness of the WHO/UNICEF Guidelines on Infant Feeding for HIV-Positive Women: Results from a Prospective Cohort Study in South Africa." *AIDS* 21(13): 1791–97.

Doyal, Lesley, and Jane Anderson. 2005. "My Fear Is to Fall in Love Again: How HIV-Positive African Women Survive in London." *Social Science and Medicine* 60: 1729–38.

Dube, Siddharth. 2000. *Sex, Lies, and AIDS.* New Delhi: Harper Collins.

Dumont, Louis. 1970. *Homo Hierarchicus: The Caste System and Its Implications.* Chicago: University of Chicago Press.

Dyson, T., and M. Moore. 1983. "On Kinship Structure, Female Autonomy, and Demographic Behavior in India." *Population and Development Review* 9(1): 35–60.

Epele, Maria Esther. 2002. "Gender, Violence, and HIV: Women's Survival in the Streets." *Culture, Medicine, and Psychiatry* 26: 33–54.

Estroff, Susan. 1993. "Identity, Disability, and Schizophrenia: The Problem with Chronicity." In Shirley Lindenbaum and Margaret Lock, eds., *Knowledge, Power, and Practice: The Anthropology of Medicine and Everyday Life*, 247–86. Berkeley: University of California Press.

Farmer, Paul. 1992. *AIDS and Accusation: Haiti and the Geography of Blame.* Berkeley: University of California Press.

————. 1999. *Infections and Inequalities: The Modern Plagues.* Berkeley: University of California Press.

Farmer, Paul, and Arthur Kleinman. 2001 [1989]. "AIDS as Human Suffering" In Aaron Podolefsky and Peter Brown, eds., *Applying Anthropology: An Introductory Reader*, 6th ed., 352–60. Mountain View, CA: Mayfield.

Fassin, Didier. 2007. *When Bodies Remember: Experiences and Politics of AIDS in South Africa.* Berkeley: University of California Press.

Ferro-Luzzi, Gabriella Eichinger. 1974. "Women's Pollution Periods in Tamilnad (India)." *Anthropos* 69: 113–61.

Finn, Mark, and Srikant Sarangi. 2008. "Quality of Life as a Mode of Governance: NGO Talk of HIV 'Positive' Health in India." *Social Science and Medicine* 66: 1568–78.

Foucault, Michel. 1978. *The History of Sexuality.* New York: Pantheon.

Franklin, Sarah, and Helena Ragoné, eds. 1998. *Reproducing Reproduction: Kinship, Power, and Technological Innovation.* Philadelphia: University of Pennsylvania Press.

Freidson, Eliot. 1970. *Professional Dominance: The Social Structure of Medical Care.* New York: Atherton Press.

Ganatra, Bela. 2000. "Abortion Research in India: What We Know and What We Need to Know." In Radhika Ramasubban and Shireen J. Jejeebhoy, eds., *Women's Reproductive Health in India*, 186–235. New Delhi: Rawat Publications.

Geetha, K. 2004. "HIV/AIDS Infection: A Perceptual Study on Urban Working Women." In Patrice Cohen and Suniti Solomon, eds., *AIDS and Maternity in India: From Public Health to Social Science Perspectives—Emerging Themes and Debates*, 169–82. Pondicherry, India: Institut Français de Pondichéry.

Ghose, Toorjo, Dallas Swendeman, Sheba George, and Debasish Chowdhury. 2008. "Mobilizing Collective Identity to Reduce HIV Risk Among Sex Workers in Sonagachi, India: The Boundaries, Consciousness, Negotiation Framework." *Social Science and Medicine* 67: 311–20.

Ghosh, Jayati, V. Wadhwa, and E. Kalipeni. 2009. "Vulnerability to HIV/AIDS Among Women of Reproductive Age in the Slums of Delhi and Hyderabad, India." *Social Science and Medicine* 68: 638–42.

Giddens, Anthony. 1979. *Central Problems in Social Theory: Action, Structure and Contradiction in Social Analysis.* Berkeley: University of California Press.

Ginsburg, Faye D., and Rayna Rapp. 1995. "Introduction." In Faye Ginsburg and Rayna Rapp, eds., *Conceiving the New World Order: The Global Politics of Reproduction*, 1–17. Berkeley: University of California Press.

Godwin, Peter, ed. 1998. *The Looming Epidemic: The Impact of HIV/AIDS in India.* New Delhi: Mosaic Books.

Goffman, Erving. 1963. *Stigma: Notes on the Management of Spoiled Identity.* New York: Simon & Schuster.

Goldin, Carol S. 1994. "Stigmatization and AIDS: Critical Issues in Public Health." *Social Science and Medicine* 39: 1359–66.

Good, Mary-Jo DelVecchio. 1995. "Cultural Studies of Biomedicine: An Agenda for Research." *Social Science and Medicine* 41(4): 461–73.

———. 2001. "Biotechnical Embrace." *Culture, Medicine, and Psychiatry* 25(4): 395–410.

Goparaju, Lakshmi. 1998. *Ignorance and Inequality: Youth Sexuality in India and Its Implications to HIV Spread.* Ph.D. dissertation, Department of Anthropology, Syracuse University.

Gosh, Shohini. 2005. "The Troubled Existence of Sex and Sexuality: Feminists Engage with Censorship." In Mala Khuller, ed., *Writing the Women's Movement: A Reader*, 482–514. Delhi: Zubaan.

Greene, Margaret E., and Ann E. Biddlecom. 2000. "Absent and Problematic Men: Demographic Accounts of Male Reproductive Roles." *Population and Development Review* 26(1): 81–115.

Guntupalli, Aravinda Meera. 2008. "Qualitative Research on Reproductive Health and HIV/AIDS with Mumbai Sex Workers." In Devi Sridhar, ed., *Anthropologists Inside Organizations: South Asian Case Studies*, 36–54. New Delhi: Sage.

Gupta, Akhil, and James Ferguson, eds. 1997. *Anthropological Locations: Boundaries and Grounds of Field Science.* Berkeley: University of California Press.

Gupta, R. N. 2004. "An Overview of HIV/AIDS Epidemic and Its Prevention in India." In Patrice Cohen and Suniti Solomon, eds., *AIDS and Maternity in India: From Public Health to Social Science Perspectives—Emerging Themes and Debates*, 39–64. Pondicherry, India: Institut Français de Pondichéry.

Hancart Petitet, P. 2004. "Anthropological Perspectives on HIV/AIDS Transmission During Delivery." In Patrice Cohen and Suniti Solomon, eds., *AIDS and Maternity in India: From*

Public Health to Social Science Perspectives—Emerging Themes and Debates, 211–24. Pondicherry, India: Institut Français de Pondichéry.

Hankins, Catherine. 2000. "Preventing Mother-to-Child Transmission of HIV in Developing
Countries: Recent Developments and Ethical Implications." *Reproductive Health Matters* 8(15):
57–62.

Hart, George. 1973. "Woman and the Sacred in Ancient Tamilnad." *Journal of Asian Studies* 32(2):
233–50.

Herdt, Gilbert, ed. 1997. *Sexual Cultures and Migration in the Era of AIDS: Anthropological and
Demographic Perspectives*. New York: Clarendon.

Higgins, Donna, Christine Galavoti, Kevin R. O'Reilly, Daniel J. Schnell, Melinda Moore, Deborah L. Rugg, and Robert Johnson. 1991. "Evidence of the Effects of HIV Antibody Counseling
and Testing on Risk Behaviors." *Journal of the American Medical Association* 266(17): 2419–29.

Hofmann, Jennifer, Manuela De Allegri, Malabika Sarkar, Mamadou Sanon, and Thomas Böhler.
2009. "Breast Milk as the 'Water That Supports and Preserves Life': Socio-Cultural Constructions of Breastfeeding and Their Implications for the Prevention of Mother to Child Transmission of HIV in Sub-Saharan Africa." *Health Policy* 89: 322–28.

Hopkins, Kristine, R. Maria Barbosa, D. Riva Knauth, and J. E. Potter. 2005. "The Impact of Health
Care Providers on Female Sterilization Among HIV-Positive Women in Brazil." *Social Science
and Medicine* 61: 541–54.

Humsafar Trust. 1995. *Emerging Gay Identities in South Asia: Implications for HIV/AIDS and Sexual
Health*. Bombay: Humsafar Trust, Naz Project.

Hyde, Sandra. 2007. *Eating Spring Rice: The Cultural Politics of AIDS in Southwest China*. Berkeley:
University of California Press.

Ickovics, Jeannette R., Allison C. Morill, S. E. Beren, U. Walsh, and J. Rodin. 1994. "Limited Effects of HIV Counseling and Testing for Women." *Journal of the American Medical Association* 272(6): 443–48.

Inhorn, Marcia, and Frank van Balen, eds. 2002. *Infertility Around the Globe: New Thinking on Childlessness, Gender, and New Reproductive Technologies*. Berkeley: University of California Press.

Irschick, Eugene. 1969. *Politics and Social Conflict in South India: The Non-Brahmin Movement and
Tamil Separatism, 1916–1929*. Berkeley: University of California Press.

Jain, Kalpana. 2002. *Positive Lives: The Story of Ashok Pillai and Others with HIV*. New Delhi: Penguin.

Jain, Sandhya. 2003. "The Right to Family Planning, Contraception, and Abortion: The Hindu
View." In Daniel C. Maguire, ed., *Sacred Rights: The Case for Contraception and Abortion in
World Religions*, 129–43. Oxford, UK: Oxford University Press.

Jana, Smarajit, Suparna Ghosh, Debashis Bose, Sanchita Choudhury, and Kamala Mukherjee. 2002.
"Female Commercial Sex Workers: An Innovative Intervention from West Bengal." In Samiran
Panda, Anindya Chatterjee, and Abu S. Abdul-Quader, eds., *Living With the AIDS Virus: The
Epidemic and the Response in India*, 150–65. New Delhi: Sage.

Jeffery, Patricia, and Roger Jeffery. 1997. *Population, Gender, and Politics: Demographic Change in
Rural North India*. Cambridge, UK: Cambridge University Press.

Jeffery, Patricia, Roger Jeffery, and Andrew Lyon. 1989. *Labour Pains and Labour Power: Women and
Childbearing in India*. London: Zed Books.

Jeffery, Roger. 1988. *The Politics of Health in India*. Berkeley: University of California Press.

Jejeebhoy, Shireen J. 2000. "Adolescent Sexual and Reproductive Behaviour: A Review of the Evidence from India." In Radhika Ramasubban and Shireen J. Jejeebhoy, eds., *Women's Reproductive Health in India*, 40–101. New Delhi: Rawat Publications.

Jordan, Brigitte. 1993. *Birth in Four Cultures: A Crosscultural Investigation of Childbirth in Yucatan,
Holland, Sweden, and the United States*, 4th ed. Prospect Heights, IL: Waveland Press.

Joseph, Sherry. 2005. *Social Work Practice and Men Who Have Sex with Men*. New Delhi: Sage Publications India.

Joshi, Poornima. 2003 (June 9). "Condom, Condemned: Health Experts Are Flummoxed by Sushma Swaraj's Moral Turn on AIDS Awareness." http://www.outlookindia.com/article.aspx?220387. Accessed October 6, 2010.

Kavi, Ashok Row. 2007. "Kothis Versus Other MSM: Identity Versus Behavior in the Chicken and Egg Paradox." In Brinda Bose and Subhabrata Bhattacharyya, eds., *The Phobic and the Erotic: The Politics of Sexualities in Contemporary India*, 391–98. Calcutta: Seagull Books.

Kerr, Rachel Bezner, Laifolo Dakishoni, Lizzie Shumba, Rodgers Msachi, and Marko Chirwa. 2008. "'We Grandmothers Know Plenty': Breastfeeding, Complementary Feeding, and the Multifaceted Role of Grandmothers in Malawi." *Social Science and Medicine* 66:1095–1105.

Kielmann, Karina, Deepali Deshmukh, Sucheta Deshpande, Vinita Datye, John Porter, and Sheela Rangan. 2005. "Managing Uncertainty Around HIV/AIDS in an Urban Setting: Private Medical Providers and Their Patients in Pune, India." *Social Science and Medicine* 61: 1540–50.

Kirshenbaum, Sheri, A. Elizabeth Hirky, Jacqueline Correale, Rise B. Goldstein, Mallory O. Johnson, Mary Jane Rotheram-Borus, and Anke A. Ehrhardt. 2004. "'Throwing the Dice': Pregnancy Decision-Making Among HIV-Positive Women in Four U.S. Cities." *Perspectives on Sexual and Reproductive Health* 36(3): 106–13.

Klaits, Frederick. 2010. *Death in a Church of Life: Moral Passion During Botswana's Time of AIDS*. Berkeley: University of California Press.

Kleinman, Arthur. 1995. *Writing at the Margins*. Berkeley: University of California Press.

Kuganantham, P. 2004. "UNICEF Programme for the Prevention of Parent-to-Child HIV/AIDS Transmission, Tamil Nadu." In Patrice Cohen and Suniti Solomon, eds., *AIDS and Maternity in India: From Public Health to Social Science Perspectives—Emerging Themes and Debates*, 117–28. Pondicherry, India: Institut Français de Pondichéry.

Lakhani, Aruna, K. Gandhi, and M. Collumbien. 2001. "Addressing Semen Loss Concerns: Towards Culturally Appropriate HIV/AIDS Interventions in Gujarat, India." *Reproductive Health Matters* 9(18): 49–59.

Lakshmi, C. S. 1990. "Mother, Mother-Community, and Mother-Politics in Tamil Nadu." *Economic and Political Weekly* 15(42–43): WS72–WS83.

Lamb, Sarah. 2000. *White Saris and Sweet Mangoes: Aging, Gender, and Body in North India*. Berkeley: University of California Press.

Lane, Sandra, R. A. Rubinstein, R. H. Keefe, N. Webster, D. A. Cibula, A. Rosenthal, and J. Dowdell. 2004. "Structural Violence and Racial Disparity in HIV Transmission." *Journal of Health Care for the Poor and Underserved* 15: 319–35.

Libman, Howard, and Michael Stein. 2003. "Primary Care and Prevention of HIV Disease: Part I." In Howard Libman and Harvey J. Makadon, eds., *HIV: First Indian Edition*, 39–64. Philadelphia: American College of Physicians.

Lingam, Lakshmi, and Siddhi Mankad. 2004. "Breastfeeding and Infant Feeding Practices in India: A Critical Review." In Patrice Cohen and Suniti Solomon, eds., *AIDS and Maternity in India: From Public Health to Social Science Perspectives—Emerging Themes and Debates*, 195–210. Pondicherry, India: Institut Français de Pondichéry.

Lipner, Julius J. 1989. "The Classical Hindu View on Abortion and the Moral Status of the Unborn." In Harold G. Coward, Julius J. Lipner, and Katherine K. Young, eds., *Hindu Ethics: Purity, Abortion, and Euthanasia*, 41–69. Albany: SUNY Press.

Lock, Margaret, and Patricia Kaufert. 1998. "Introduction." In Margaret Lock and Patricia Kaufert, eds., *Pragmatic Women and Body Politics*, 1–27. Cambridge, UK: Cambridge University Press.

Lupton, Deborah, Sophie McCarthy, and Simon Chapman. 1995. "'Doing the Right Thing': The

Symbolic Meanings and Experiences of Having an HIV Antibody Test." *Social Science and Medicine* 41(2): 173–80.

Lyttleton, Chris. 2004. "Fleeing the Fire: Transformation and Gendered Belonging in Thai HIV/AIDS Support Groups." *Medical Anthropology* 23: 1–40.

MacLeod, Arlene E. 1991. *Accommodating Protest: Working Women, the New Veiling, and Change in Cairo.* New York: Columbia University Press.

MacNaughton, Gillian. 2004. *Women's Human Rights Related to Health-Care Services in the Context of HIV/AIDS.* Health and Human Rights Working Paper Series No. 5. London: Interights.

Mahajan, Payal, and Neeru Sharma. 2005. "Awareness Level of Adolescent Girls Regarding HIV/AIDS: A Comparative Study of Rural and Urban Areas of Jammu." *Journal of Human Ecology* 17(4): 313–14.

Majumdar, Basanti. 2004. "An Exploration of Socioeconomic, Spiritual, and Family Support Among HIV-Positive Women in India." *Journal of the Association of Nurses in AIDS Care* 15(3): 37–46.

Mankekar, Purnima. 1999. *Screening Culture, Viewing Politics: An Ethnography of Television, Womanhood, and Nation in Postcolonial India.* Durham, NC: Duke University Press.

Marriott, McKim. 1976. "Hindu Transactions: Diversity Without Dualism." In Bruce Kapfrerer, ed., *Transaction and Meaning: Directions in the Anthropology of Exchange and Symbolic Behavior,* 109–42. Philadelphia: Institute for the Study of Human Issues.

Martin, Emily. 1987. *The Woman in the Body: A Cultural Analysis of Reproduction.* Boston: Beacon Press.

McGilvray, Dennis. 1994. "Sexual Power and Fertility in Sri Lanka: Batticaloa Tamils and Moors." In C. MacCormack, ed., *Ethnography of Fertility and Birth,* 15–63. Prospect Heights, IL: Waveland Press.

Mill, Judy E., and John K. Anarfi. 2002. "HIV Risk Environment for Ghanaian Women: Challenges to Prevention." *Social Science and Medicine* 54: 325–37.

Miller, Barbara. 1981. *The Endangered Sex.* Ithaca, NY: Cornell University Press.

Misra, Kavita. 2006. "Politico-Moral Transactions in Indian AIDS Service: Confidentiality, Rights, and New Modalities of Governance." *Anthropological Quarterly* 79(1): 33–74.

Mohanty, Chandra Talpade. 1991. "Under Western Eyes: Feminist Scholarship and Colonial Discourses." In Chandra T. Mohanty, Anna Russo, and Lourdes Torres, eds., *Third World Women and the Politics of Feminism,* 51–80. Bloomington: Indiana University Press.

NACO (National AIDS Control Organization). 2005. "HIV Estimates—2004." http://www.nacoon line.org/facts_hivestimates04.htm. Accessed July 7, 2005.

———. 2007a. "Integrated Counseling and Testing Centre (ICTC)." http://www.nacoonline.org/National_AIDS_Control_Program/Services_for_Prevention/Integrated_Counselling_and_Testing__ICT/. Accessed July 28, 2009.

———. 2007b. *Operational Guidelines for Integrated Counseling and Testing Centres.* Delhi: National AIDS Control Organization, Ministry of Health and Family Welfare.

———. 2008 (October). *HIV Sentinel Surveillance and HIV Estimation in India 2007: A Technical Brief.* Delhi: NACO, Ministry of Health and Family Welfare.

———. 2009. *Annual Report 2008–09.* Delhi: Department of AIDS Control, Ministry of Health and Family Welfare.

Nag, Moni. 1996. *Sexual Behaviour and AIDS in India.* New Delhi: Vikas.

Nanda, Serena. 1990. *Neither Man nor Woman: The Hijras of India.* Belmont, CA: Wadsworth.

Narain, Jai P., ed. 2004. *AIDS in Asia: The Challenge Ahead.* New Delhi: Sage.

Natarajan, Shyamala. 2004. "Bridging Counseling and Care in the HIV/AIDS Epidemic: General Perspectives and the Case of Women." In Patrice Cohen and Suniti Solomon, eds., *AIDS and*

Maternity in India: From Public Health to Social Science Perspectives—Emerging Themes and Debates, 129–46. Pondicherry, India: Institut Français de Pondichéry.

National Institute of Allergy and Infectious Diseases. n.d. *2007–2008 Biennial Report on Women's Health Research*. http://www.niaid.nih.gov/topics/womenshealth/Documents/biennialreport wh.pdf. Accessed December 18, 2009.

Nguyen, Vinh-Kim. 2010. *The Republic of Therapy: Triage and Sovereignty in West Africa's Time of AIDS*. Durham, NC: Duke University Press.

Nguyen, V. K., C. Y. Ako, P. Niamba, A. Sylla, and I. Tiendrebeogo. 2007. "Adherence as Therapeutic Citizenship: Impact of the History of Access to Antiretroviral Drugs on Adherence to Treatment." *AIDS* 21: 31–35.

Nichter, Mark, and Mimi Nichter. 1996. "Cultural Notions of Fertility in South Asia and Their Impact on Sri Lankan Family Planning Practices." In Mark Nichter and Mimi Nichter, eds., *Anthropology and International Health: Asian Case Studies*, 3–34. Amsterdam: Gordon & Breach.

Obbo, Christine. 1995. "Gender, Age, and Class: Discourses on HIV Transmission and Control in Uganda." In H. T. Brummelhuis and G. Herdt, eds., *Culture and Sexual Risk: Anthropological Perspectives on AIDS*, 79–95. Amsterdam: Gordon & Breach.

O'Flaherty, Wendy Doniger. 1976. *The Origins of Evil in Hindu Mythology*. Berkeley: University of California Press.

Ogden, Jessica, and Laura Nyblade. 2005. *Common at Its Core: HIV-Related Stigma Across Contexts*. Washington, DC: International Center for Research on Women (ICRW).

O'Neil, John, T. Orchard, R. C. Swarankar, J. F. Blanchard, K. Gurav, and S. Moses. 2004. "Dhanda, Dharma, and Disease: Traditional Sex Work and HIV/AIDS in Rural India." *Social Science and Medicine* 54(4): 851–60.

Ong, Aihwa, and Stephen Collier. 2005. *Global Assemblages: Technology, Politics, and Ethics as Anthropological Problems*. Malden, MA: Blackwell.

Orchard, Treena Rae. 2007. "Girl, Woman, Lover, Mother: Towards a New Understanding of Child Prostitution Among Young Devadasis in Rural Karnataka, India." *Social Science and Medicine* 64: 2379–90.

Panda, Samiran, Anindya Chatterjee, and Abu S. Abdul-Quader, eds. 2002. *Living with the AIDS Virus: The Epidemic and the Response in India*. New Delhi: Sage.

Parameswaran, Gowri. 2004. "Stemming the Tide: Successes and Lessons Learned in Tamil Nadu, India." *Dialectical Anthropology* 28: 397–414.

Pardasani, Manoj P. 2005. "HIV Prevention and Sex Workers: An International Lesson in Empowerment." *International Journal of Social Welfare* 14: 116–26.

Parker, Richard, and Peter Aggleton. 2003. "HIV and AIDS-Related Stigma and Discrimination: A Conceptual Framework for Action." *Social Science and Medicine* 57: 13–24.

Petryna, Adriana. 2009. *When Experiments Travel: Clinical Trials and the Global Search for Human Subjects*. Princeton, NJ: Princeton University Press.

Pigg, Stacy Leigh. 2001. "Languages of Sex and AIDS in Nepal: Notes on the Social Production of Commensurability." *Cultural Anthropology* 14(4): 481–541.

Puri, Jyoti. 1999. *Woman, Body, Desire in Post-Colonial India: Narratives of Gender and Sexuality*. New York: Routledge.

Quinn, Thomas C., and Julie Overbaugh. 2005. "HIV/AIDS in Women: An Expanding Epidemic." *Science* 308(5728): 1582–83.

Rabinow, Paul. 1999. "Artificiality and Enlightenment: From Sociobiology to Biosociality." In Mario Biagiolo, ed., *The Social Science Reader*, 407–16. New York: Routledge.

Raheja, Gloria, and Ann Gold. 1996. *Listen to the Heron's Words: Reimagining Gender and Kinship in North India*. Berkeley: University of California Press.

Raman, Anuradha. 2009 (June). "DMK: The Wives and Wherefores." http://www.outlookindia.com/ TheWives&Wherefores. Accessed November 6, 2009.

Ramasubban, Radhika, and Shireen Jejeebhoy, eds. 2000. *Women's Reproductive Health in India.* New Delhi: Rawat Publications.

Ramaswamy, Sumathi. 1997. *Passions of the Tongue: Language Devotion in Tamil India, 1891–1970.* Berkeley: University of California Press.

Raphael, Dana, ed. 1979. *Breastfeeding and Food Policy in a Hungry World.* San Francisco: Academic.

Rapp, Rayna. 2000. *Testing Women, Testing the Fetus: The Social Impact of Amniocentesis in America.* New York: Routledge.

Reddy, Gayathri. 2005. *With Respect to Sex: Negotiating Hijra Identity in South India.* Chicago: University of Chicago Press.

Richey, Lisa Ann. 2011. "Antiviral but Pronatal? ARVs and Reproductive Health: The View from a South African Township." In Carolyn Sargent and Carole Browner, eds., *Reproduction, Globalization, and the State: New Theoretical and Ethnographic Perspectives,* 68–82. Durham, NC: Duke University Press.

Robins, S. 2006. "From 'Rights' to 'Ritual': AIDS Activism in South Africa." *American Anthropologist* 108(2): 312–23.

Sargent, Carolyn, and Joan Rawlins. 1992. "Transformations in Maternity Services in Jamaica." *Social Science and Medicine* 35(10): 1225–32.

Schoepf, Brooke Grundfest. 1992. "Women at Risk: Case Studies from Zaire." In Gilbert Herdt and Shirley Lindenbaum, eds., *The Time of AIDS: Social Analysis, Theory, and Method,* 259–86. Newbury Park, CA: Sage.

Seizer, Susan. 2005. *Stigmas of the Tamil Stage: An Ethnography of Special Drama Artists in South India.* Durham, NC: Duke University Press.

Sethi, Geeta. 2002. "AIDS in India: The Government's Response." In Samiran Panda, Anindya Chatterjee, and Abu S. Abdul-Quader, eds., *Living with the AIDS Virus: The Epidemic and the Response in India,* 36–61. New Delhi: Sage.

Shanti, K. 2004. "Gender and Health in India: The Imperatives for Engendering Health Policy, Administration, and Research." In Patrice Cohen and Suniti Solomon, eds., *AIDS and Maternity in India: From Public Health to Social Science Perspectives—Emerging Themes and Debates,* 149–68. Pondicherry, India: Institut Français de Pondichéry.

Shiffman, Jeremy. 2006. "HIV/AIDS and the Rest of the Global Health Agenda." *Bulletin of the World Health Organization* 84(12): 923.

———. 2008. "Has Donor Prioritization of HIV/AIDS Displaced Aid for Other Health Issues?" *Health Policy and Planning* 23: 95–100.

Shilts, Randy. 1988. *And the Band Played On: Politics, People, and the AIDS Epidemic.* New York: Penguin.

Singer, Merrill. 1994a. "AIDS and the Health Crisis of the U.S. Urban Poor: The Perspective of Critical Medical Anthropology." *Social Science and Medicine* 39: 931–48.

———. 1994b. "The Politics of AIDS: Introduction." *Social Science and Medicine* 38: 1321–24.

Smith, Stephanie. 2009 (May). *Public Health and Maternal Mortality in India.* Ph.D. dissertation, Syracuse University.

Smith-Rosenberg, Carol. 1985. *Disorderly Conduct: Visions of Gender in Victorian America.* New York: Oxford University Press.

Sontag, Susan. 1989. *AIDS and Its Metaphors.* New York: Farrar, Strauss & Giroux.

Steward, Wayne T., Gregory M. Herek, Jayashree Ramakrishna, Shalini Bharat, and Sara Chandy. 2008. "HIV-Related Stigma: Adapting a Theoretical Framework for Use in India." *Social Science and Medicine* 67: 1225–35.

Strathern, Marilyn. 1995. "Displacing Knowledge: Technology and the Consequences for Kinship." In Faye Ginsburg and Rayna Rapp, eds., *Conceiving the New World Order: The Global Politics of Reproduction*, 346–64. Berkeley: University of California Press.

Swendenman, Dallas, I. Basu, S. Das, S. Jana, and M. J. Rotheram-Borus. 2009. "Empowering Sex Workers in India to Reduce Vulnerability to HIV and Sexually Transmitted Diseases." *Social Science and Medicine* 69: 1157–66.

SWEN (Six-Week Extended-Dose Nevirapine) Study Team. 2008. "Extended-Dose Nevirapine to 6 Weeks of Age for Infants to Prevent HIV Transmission via Breastfeeding in Ethiopia, India, and Uganda: An Analysis of Three Randomized Controlled Trials." *Lancet* 372: 300–13.

Taylor, Janelle S. 1998. "An Image of Contradiction: Obstetrical Ultrasound in American Culture." In Helena Ragoné and Sarah Franklin, eds., *Reproducing Reproduction: Kinship, Power, and Technological Innovation*, 15–45. Philadelphia: University of Pennsylvania Press.

Thandaveswara, Sri. 1972. "The Bearing of Traditional, Cultural, Social, and Moral Attitudes on the Ethical Issues in Abortion: A Hindu View." *Bulletin of the Christian Institute for the Study of Religion and Society* 19(2): 24–32.

TNSACS (Tamil Nadu State AIDS Control Society). 2004a. *PPTCT (Prevention of Parent to Child Transmission of HIV): A Report, 2003.* Chennai: TNSACS, Government of Tamil Nadu.

———. 2004b. *The Sentinel Surveillance for HIV in Tamil Nadu 2003.* Chennai: TNSACS, Government of Tamil Nadu.

Traoré, Annick Tijou, M. Querre, H. Brou, V. Leroy, A. Desclaux, and A. Desgrées-du-Loû. 2009. "Couples, PMTCT Programs, and Infant Feeding Decision-Making in Ivory Coast." *Social Science and Medicine* 69: 830–37.

Trawick, Margaret. 1992. *Notes on Love in a Tamil Family.* Berkeley: University of California Press.

UNAIDS (Joint United Nations Programme on HIV/AIDS). 2006. "UNAIDS: Uniting the World Against AIDS: India." http://www.unaids.org/en/Regions_Countries/Countries/india.asp. Accessed January 25, 2006.

———. 2008. "UNAIDS Report on Global AIDS Epidemic." Technical Report. *http://www.unaids .org/en/KnowledgeCentre/HIVData/GlobalReport/2008/2008_Global_report.asp.* Accessed August 9, 2009.

———. 2009. "India." http://www.unaids.org/en/CountryResponses/Countries/india.asp. Accessed August 31, 2009.

———. 2010. "Global Report: UNAIDS Report on the Global AIDS Epidemic." http://www.unaids .org/globalreport/documents/20101123_GlobalReport_full_en.pdf. Accessed May 18, 2012.

Van Esterik, Penny. 1989. *Beyond the Breast-Bottle Controversy.* New Brunswick, NJ: Rutgers University Press.

———. 2002. "Contemporary Trends in Infant Feeding Research." *Annual Review of Anthropology* 31: 257–78.

Van Hollen, Cecilia. 1998. "Moving Targets: Routine IUD Insertions in Maternity Wards in Tamil Nadu, India." *Reproductive Health Matters* 6(11): 98–106.

———. 2002. "'Baby Friendly' Hospitals and Bad Mothers: Maneuvering Development in the Postpartum Period in Tamil Nadu, South India." In Shanti Rozario and Geoffrey Samuel, eds., *The Daughters of Hariti: Birth and Female Healers in South and Southeast Asia*, 63–181. New York: Routledge.

———. 2003a. *Birth on the Threshold: Childbirth and Modernity in South India.* Berkeley: University of California Press.

———. 2003b. "Invoking *Vali*: Painful Technologies of Modern Birth in South India." *Medical Anthropology Quarterly* 7(1): 49–77.

———. 2005. "Nationalism, Transnationalism, and the Politics of 'Traditional' Indian Medicine for HIV/AIDS." In Joseph Alter, ed., *Asian Medicine and Globalization*, 88–106. Philadelphia: University of Pennsylvania Press.

———. 2007. "Navigating HIV, Pregnancy, and Childbearing in South India: Pragmatics and Constraints in Women's Decision-Making." *Medical Anthropology* 26(7): 7–52.

———. 2010. "HIV/AIDS and the Gendering of Stigma in Tamil Nadu, South India." *Culture, Medicine, and Psychiatry* 34(4): 633–57.

———. 2011a. "Birth in the Age of AIDS: Local Responses to Global Policies and Technologies in South India." In Carolyn Sargent and Carole Browner, eds., *Reproduction, Globalization, and the State: New Theoretical and Ethnographic Perspectives*, 83–95. Durham, NC: Duke University Press.

———. 2011b. "Breast or Bottle? HIV-Positive Women's Responses to Global Health Policy on Infant Feeding in India." *Medical Anthropology Quarterly* 25(4): 499–518.

———. 2011c. "HIV/AIDS: Global Policies, Local Realities." In Isabelle Clark-Decès, ed., *Companion to the Anthropology of India*, 464–81. Oxford, UK: Blackwell and Wiley.

Verma, Ravi K, Pertti Pelto, Stephen Schensul, and Archana Joshi, eds. 2004. *Sexuality in the Time of AIDS: Contemporary Perspectives from Communities in India*. New Delhi: Sage.

Wadley, Susan, ed. 1980. *The Powers of Tamil Women*. Foreign and Comparative Studies/South Asia Series, No. 6. Syracuse, NY: Syracuse University.

Whiteford, Linda, and Lenore Manderson, eds. 2000. *Global Health Policy, Local Realities: The Fallacy of the Level Playing Field*. London: Lynne Rienner.

WHO (World Health Organization). 2002. "Prevention of HIV in Infants and Young Children: Review of Evidence and WHO's Activities." http://www.who.int/hiv/mtct/ReviewofEvidence.pdf. Accessed January 7, 2010.

———. 2007. "HIV and Infant Feeding: Update." Paper based on the technical consultation held on behalf of the Inter-Agency Task Team (IATT) on Prevention of HIV Infection in Pregnant Women, Mothers, and Their Infants, Geneva, October 25–27, 2006. Geneva: WHO, UNAIDS, UNICEF, UNFPA.

Whyte, Susan R., Michael A. Whyte, and David Kyaddondo. 2010. "Health Workers Entangled: Confidentiality and Certification." In Hansjörg Dilger and Ute Luig, eds., *Morality, Hope, and Grief: Anthropologies of AIDS in Africa*, 80–101. New York: Berghahn.

Winslow, Miron. 1979 [1862]. *Winslow's: A Comprehensive Tamil and English Dictionary*. Madras: Asian Educational Services.

World Vision. 1998. "Population and Poverty: What's the Connection? Topic Sheet." Education Services Bureau, World Vision, Melbourne, Australia. http://www.worldvision.com.au/resources/files/populationpoverty_9811.pdf. Accessed March 15, 2006.

Yadav, Priya. 2001. "HIV Positive Women Prefer Abortions." *Times of India*, May 13 (cited in Maria de Bruyn, *HIV/AIDS Pregnancy and Abortion: A Review of the Literature* [Chapel Hill, NC: Ipas, 2003]).

Zurbrigg, Sheila. 1984. *Rakku's Story: Structures of Ill-Health and the Source of Change*. Bangalore, India: Center for Social Action.

Index

Page numbers in italic indicate illustrations.